W9-BBO-928

Pulmonary Disease in Non-Pulmonary Malignancy

Editors

GUANG-SHING CHENG
JENNIFER D. POSSICK

CLINICS IN CHEST MEDICINE

www.chestmed.theclinics.com

June 2017 • Volume 38 • Number 2

ELSEVIER

1600 John F. Kennedy Boulevard • Suite 1800 • Philadelphia, Pennsylvania, 19103-2899

http://www.theclinics.com

CLINICS IN CHEST MEDICINE Volume 38, Number 2
June 2017 ISSN 0272-5231, ISBN-13: 978-0-323-53001-9

Editor: Katie Pfaff
Developmental Editor: Casey Potter

© **2017 Elsevier Inc. All rights reserved.**

This periodical and the individual contributions contained in it are protected under copyright by Elsevier, and the following terms and conditions apply to their use:

Photocopying
Single photocopies of single articles may be made for personal use as allowed by national copyright laws. Permission of the Publisher and payment of a fee is required for all other photocopying, including multiple or systematic copying, copying for advertising or promotional purposes, resale, and all forms of document delivery. Special rates are available for educational institutions that wish to make photocopies for non-profit educational classroom use. For information on how to seek permission visit www.elsevier.com/permissions or call: (+44) 1865 843830 (UK)/(+1) 215 239 3804 (USA).

Derivative Works
Subscribers may reproduce tables of contents or prepare lists of articles including abstracts for internal circulation within their institutions. Permission of the Publisher is required for resale or distribution outside the institution. Permission of the Publisher is required for all other derivative works, including compilations and translations (please consult www.elsevier.com/permissions).

Electronic Storage or Usage
Permission of the Publisher is required to store or use electronically any material contained in this periodical, including any article or part of an article (please consult www.elsevier.com/permissions). Except as outlined above, no part of this publication may be reproduced, stored in a retrieval system or transmitted in any form or by any means, electronic, mechanical, photocopying, recording or otherwise, without prior written permission of the Publisher.

Notice
No responsibility is assumed by the Publisher for any injury and/or damage to persons or property as a matter of products liability, negligence or otherwise, or from any use or operation of any methods, products, instructions or ideas contained in the material herein. Because of rapid advances in the medical sciences, in particular, independent verification of diagnoses and drug dosages should be made.

Although all advertising material is expected to conform to ethical (medical) standards, inclusion in this publication does not constitute a guarantee or endorsement of the quality or value of such product or of the claims made of it by its manufacturer.

Clinics in Chest Medicine (ISSN 0272-5231) is published quarterly by Elsevier Inc., 360 Park Avenue South, New York, NY 10010-1710. Months of issue are March, June, September, and December. Periodicals postage paid at New York, NY and additional mailing offices. Subscription prices are $352.00 per year (domestic individuals), $652.00 per year (domestic institutions), $100.00 per year (domestic students/residents), $388.00 per year (Canadian individuals), $810.00 per year (Canadian institutions), $479.00 per year (international individuals), $810.00 per year (international institutions), and $230.00 per year (international and Canadian students/residents). International air speed delivery is included in all Clinics subscription prices. All prices are subject to change without notice. **POSTMASTER:** Send address changes to Clinics in Chest Medicine, Elsevier Health Sciences Division, Subscription Customer Service, 3251 Riverport Lane, Maryland Heights, MO 63043. **Customer Service: Telephone: 1-800-654-2452** (U.S. and Canada); **1-314-447-8871** (outside U.S. and Canada). **Fax: 1-314-447-8029. E-mail: journalscustomerservice-usa@elsevier.com (for print support); journalsonlinesupport-usa@elsevier.com (for online support).**

Reprints. For copies of 100 or more of articles in this publication, please contact the Commercial Reprints Department, Elsevier Inc., 360 Park Avenue South, New York, NY 10010-1710. Tel.: 212-633-3874; Fax: 212-633-3820; E-mail: reprints@elsevier.com.

Clinics in Chest Medicine is covered in *MEDLINE/PubMed (Index Medicus), Current Contents/Clinical Medicine, EMBASE/ Excerpta Medica, Science Citation Index,* and *ISI/BIOMED.*

Printed in the United States of America.

Contributors

EDITORS

GUANG-SHING CHENG, MD
Assistant Member, Clinical Research
Division, Fred Hutchinson Cancer Research
Center, Assistant Professor, Division of
Pulmonary, Critical Care and Sleep Medicine,
Department of Internal Medicine, University of
Washington School of Medicine, Seattle,
Washington

JENNIFER D. POSSICK, MD
Medical Director, Winchester Chest Clinic,
Yale-New Haven Hospital, Assistant Professor,
Section of Pulmonary, Critical Care, and Sleep
Medicine, Yale University School of Medicine,
New Haven, Connecticut

AUTHORS

KATHLEEN M. AKGÜN, MD, MS
Assistant Professor, Section of
Pulmonary, Critical Care and Sleep Medicine,
Department of Internal Medicine,
VA Connecticut Healthcare System, Yale
University School of Medicine, West Haven,
Connecticut

ELIE AZOULAY, MD, PhD
Professor, Medical Intensive Care Unit, Hôpital
Saint-Louis, Paris, France

LARA BASHOURA, MD
Department of Pulmonary Medicine,
The University of Texas MD Anderson Cancer
Center, Houston, Texas

ANNE BERGERON, MD, PhD
Respiratory Medicine Department,
AP-HP, Hôpital Saint-Louis, Sorbonne
Paris Cité, UMR 1153 CRESS, Biostatistics
and Clinical Epidemiology Research Team,
Univ Paris Diderot, Paris, France

TREVOR J. BLEDSOE, MD
Department of Therapeutic Radiology,
Smilow Cancer Hospital at Yale-New Haven,
New Haven, Connecticut

GUANG-SHING CHENG, MD
Assistant Member, Clinical Research
Division, Fred Hutchinson Cancer Research
Center, Assistant Professor, Division of
Pulmonary, Critical Care and Sleep Medicine,
Department of Internal Medicine, University of
Washington School of Medicine, Seattle,
Washington

ROY H. DECKER, MD, PhD
Department of Therapeutic Radiology,
Smilow Cancer Hospital at Yale-New Haven,
New Haven, Connecticut

GEORGE A. EAPEN, MD
Department of Pulmonary Medicine, The
University of Texas MD Anderson Cancer
Center, Houston, Texas

SCOTT E. EVANS, MD, FCCP
Associate Professor, Division of Internal
Medicine, Department of Pulmonary Medicine,
The University of Texas MD Anderson Cancer
Center, Houston, Texas

SAADIA A. FAIZ, MD
Department of Pulmonary Medicine,
The University of Texas MD Anderson Cancer
Center, Houston, Texas

LIBRARY
ALLEGANY COLLEGE OF MD LIBRARY
12401 WILLOWBROOK ROAD, SE
CUMBERLAND, MD 21502-2596

ALEXANDER I. GEYER, MD
Assistant Member, Pulmonary Service,
Department of Medicine, Memorial Sloan
Kettering Cancer Center, Weill Cornell Medical
College, New York, New York

MARGARET L. GREEN, MD, MPH
Clinical Assistant Professor, University of
Washington, Affiliate Investigator, Fred
Hutchinson Cancer Research Center, Seattle,
Washington

BIANCA HARRIS, MD, MSc
Instructor, Pulmonary Service, Department of
Medicine, Memorial Sloan Kettering Cancer
Center, New York, New York

PAUL LEGER, MD
Internal Medicine Resident, Division of Internal
Medicine, Vanderbilt University Medical
Center, Nashville, Tennessee

VIRGINIE LEMIALE, MD
Medical Intensive Care Unit, Hôpital
Saint-Louis, Paris, France

ANDREW H. LIMPER, MD
Walter and Leonore Annenberg Professor of
Pulmonary Medicine, Division of Pulmonary
and Critical Care Medicine, Mayo Clinic,
Rochester, Minnesota

DAVID K. MADTES, MD
Full Member, Fred Hutchinson Cancer
Research Center, Associate Professor,
University of Washington, Seattle, Washington

FABIEN MALDONADO, MD
Associate Professor of Medicine and Thoracic
Surgery, Division of Allergy, Pulmonary and
Critical Care Medicine, Vanderbilt University
Medical Center, Nashville, Tennessee

ANNE-SOPHIE MOREAU, MD
Centre de réanimation, Hôpital Salengro,
CHU-Lille, Lille, France

SAMEER K. NATH, MD
Department of Therapeutic Radiology, Smilow
Cancer Hospital at Yale-New Haven, New
Haven, Connecticut

STEVEN A. PERGAM, MD, MPH, FIDSA
Assistant Member, Fred Hutchinson Cancer
Research Center, Assistant Professor,
University of Washington, Director, Infection
Prevention, Seattle Cancer Care Alliance,
Seattle, Washington

OLIVIER PEYRONY, MD
Medical Intensive Care Unit, Hôpital
Saint-Louis, Paris, France

JENNIFER D. POSSICK, MD
Medical Director, Winchester Chest Clinic,
Yale-New Haven Hospital, Assistant Professor,
Section of Pulmonary, Critical Care, and Sleep
Medicine, Yale University School of Medicine,
New Haven, Connecticut

JONATHAN PUCHALSKI, MD, MEd
Associate Professor of Medicine, Yale
University School of Medicine, New Haven,
Connecticut

AYMAN O. SOUBANI, MD
Service Chief, Pulmonary and Critical Care,
Karmanos Cancer Center, Medical Director,
Medical ICU, Harper University Hospital,
Professor of Medicine, Wayne State University
School of Medicine, Detroit, Michigan

LISA K. VANDE VUSSE, MD, MSc
Assistant Member, Fred Hutchinson Cancer
Research Center, Assistant Professor,
University of Washington, Seattle, Washington

JUSTIN L. WONG, MD
Clinical Fellow, Division of Internal Medicine,
Department of Pulmonary, Critical Care and
Sleep Medicine, The University of Texas Health
Sciences Center, Houston, Texas

LARA ZAFRANI, MD, PhD
Medical Intensive Care Unit, Hôpital Saint-
Louis, Paris, France

Contents

Pulmonary Manifestations of Non-Pulmonary Malignancy

> The lungs are a common site of metastatic disease. Pulmonary metastases develop due to local blood flow and cellular or biochemical properties of tumor cells. Metastases develop from any type of malignancy and may occur via hematogenous, lymphatic, aerogenous, and/or direct spread. Metastatic disease may present with symptoms indistinguishable from primary lung cancer, including dyspnea, hemoptysis, and chest pain. Radiographically, these may present as parenchymal lung disease, mediastinal lymphadenopathy, airway obstruction, or pleural and vascular disease. No part of the thorax is spared from metastatic potential. This review highlights complications of non-pulmonary solid malignancies based on sites of anatomic metastases.

> Pulmonary manifestations of lymphoma and leukemia may involve multiple structures within the thoracic cavity. Malignant lymphoma typically originates in lymph nodes, but concomitant or primary presentations with parenchymal, pleural, or tracheobronchial disease may occur. Once infection is excluded, leukemic infiltrates may be related to malignancy, hemorrhage, or secondary pulmonary alveolar proteinosis. Confirmation with cytology or flow cytometry is recommended to diagnose malignant pleural effusions in hematologic malignancies. In chronic leukemia with progressive pulmonary findings, exclusion of a synchronous malignancy or Richter syndrome should be performed. Venous thromboembolism may present in patients with leukemia and lymphoma despite the presence of thrombocytopenia.

Complications of Cancer Treatment

> Radiation-induced lung injury is a well-known complication of thoracic radiation for patients with breast, lung, thymic, and esophageal malignancies, and mediastinal lymphomas. Improvements in radiation technique, as well as the understanding of the pathophysiology of radiation injury, have led to lower rates of pneumonitis and improved symptom control. Here, the authors provide an overview of the pathophysiology, diagnosis, and management of patients with radiation pneumonitis as a complication of treatment of chest malignancies.

Pulmonary Toxicities from Conventional Chemotherapy

Paul Leger, Andrew H. Limper, and Fabien Maldonado

Despite significant recent progress in precision medicine and immunotherapy, conventional chemotherapy remains the cornerstone of the treatment of most cancers. Chemotherapy-induced lung toxicity represents a serious diagnostic challenge for health care providers and requires careful consideration because it is a diagnosis of exclusion with significant impact on therapeutic decisions. This review aims to provide clinicians with a valuable guide in assessing their patients with possible chemotherapy-induced lung toxicity.

Pulmonary Toxicities from Checkpoint Immunotherapy for Malignancy

Jennifer D. Possick

Checkpoint immunotherapy with agents targeting PD-1 and CTLA-4 has transformed the landscape of oncologic therapy. Immune-related adverse events (IRAEs), including significant pulmonary toxicities, have been observed in patients treated with these agents. The incidence, timing, clinical features, and outcomes of pulmonary IRAEs are quite variable, emphasizing the importance for clinical vigilance as these therapies become more ubiquitous in the treatment of a spectrum of malignancies. Outcomes are generally favorable when toxicity is recognized early and treated promptly.

Early Onset Noninfectious Pulmonary Syndromes after Hematopoietic Cell Transplantation

Lisa K. Vande Vusse and David K. Madtes

This article reviews the noninfectious pulmonary syndromes that cause morbidity and mortality early after hematopoietic cell transplantation with an emphasis on risk factors, clinical manifestations, treatment, and outcomes. The first section covers idiopathic pneumonia syndrome and its subtypes: peri-engraftment respiratory distress syndrome, diffuse alveolar hemorrhage, delayed pulmonary toxicity syndrome, and cryptogenic organizing pneumonia. The second section covers pulmonary toxicities of chemotherapies and immunosuppressive agents used in this setting. The final section covers less common syndromes, including pulmonary alveolar proteinosis, venous thromboembolism, pulmonary cytolytic thrombi, pulmonary venoocclusive disease, and transfusion-related acute lung injury.

Late-Onset Noninfectious Pulmonary Complications After Allogeneic Hematopoietic Stem Cell Transplantation

Anne Bergeron

Late-onset noninfectious pulmonary complications (LONIPCs), most of which occur between 3 months and 2 years following allogeneic hematopoietic stem cell transplantation (HSCT), have a significant effect on patient outcomes and are highly associated with mortalities and morbidities. LONIPCs can involve all anatomic lung regions: bronchi, parenchyma, vessels, and pleura; this diversity can lead to various clinical entities. Bronchiolitis obliterans syndrome is the most frequent LONIPC. Most LONIPCs are associated with graft-versus-host disease. Evaluation of prophylactic strategies for LONIPCs is necessary to improve outcomes in high-risk allogeneic HSCT recipients.

Pulmonary Infections in Patients with Malignancy

Justin L. Wong and Scott E. Evans

Bacterial pneumonias exact unacceptable morbidity on patients with cancer. Although the risk is often most pronounced among patients with treatment-induced cytopenias, the numerous contributors to life-threatening pneumonias in cancer populations range from derangements of lung architecture and swallow function to complex immune defects associated with cytotoxic therapies and graft-versus-host disease. These structural and immunologic abnormalities often make the diagnosis of pneumonia challenging in patients with cancer and impact the composition and duration of therapy. This article addresses host factors that contribute to pneumonia susceptibility, summarizes diagnostic recommendations, and reviews current guidelines for management of bacterial pneumonia in patients with cancer.

Steven A. Pergam

Invasive fungal infections, which occur primarily as a consequence of prolonged neutropenia and immunosuppression, are a life-threatening complication seen among patients with hematologic malignancies. The routine use of triazole antifungal prophylaxis, enhanced diagnostics, and newer antifungal agents have led to improvements in the care of fungal pneumonias, but invasive fungal infections remain a major cause of morbidity and mortality. This article covers risk factors for major fungal infections, diagnostic approaches, and treatment options for specific fungal pathogens, including *Aspergillus* and Mucorales species, and discusses current approved strategies for prevention of common and uncommon fungal pneumonias.

Margaret L. Green

Viral pneumonia is a common complication for patients with hematologic malignancies and after hematopoietic cell transplantation causing significant morbidity, and often mortality. Infections are predominantly caused by herpes viruses, either by reactivation of latent infection, or less commonly primary infection, or community respiratory viruses. High-resolution CT scan is useful for diagnosis but is nonspecific; generally, bronchoalveolar lavage is required. Prevention strategies are not pathogen-specific but include vaccination, chemoprophylaxis, preemptive treatment, and effective infection-prevention strategies during community outbreaks. Directed antiviral treatment is available for some pathogens. Toxicities and viral resistance are perennial challenges.

Evaluation of Pulmonary Disease in Patients with Malignancy

Guang-Shing Cheng

Pretransplant pulmonary function tests provide baseline data by which to reference subsequent respiratory impairment, as well as important prognostic information, for the hematopoietic cell transplant (HCT) recipient. Abnormalities in forced expiratory volume in 1 second and diffusing capacity of carbon monoxide are associated with early respiratory failure and increased all-cause mortality after allogeneic HCT. These parameters have been incorporated into risk assessment calculators that may aid in clinical decision making. This article discusses the clinical implications of pulmonary function parameters and other risk factors for pulmonary complications in the context of evolving allogeneic HCT practice.

Pulmonary complications (PC) of hematologic malignancies and their treatments are common causes of morbidity and mortality. Early diagnosis is challenging due to host risk factors, clinical instability, and provider preference. Delayed diagnosis impairs targeted treatment and may contribute to poor outcomes. An integrated understanding of clinical risk and radiographic patterns informs a timely approach to diagnosis and treatment. There is little prospective evidence guiding optimal modality and timing of minimally invasive lung sampling; however, a low threshold for diagnostic bronchoscopy during the first 24 to 72 hours after presentation should be a guiding principle in high-risk patients.

Critical Care of the Patient with Malignancy

Advances in cancer treatment and patient survival are associated with increasing number of these patients requiring intensive care. Over the last 2 decades, there has been a steady improvement in the outcomes of critically ill patients with cancer. This review provides data on the use of the intensive care unit (ICU) and short and long-term outcomes of critically ill patients with cancer, the ICU system practices that influence patients outcomes, and the role of the different clinical variables in predicting the prognosis of these patients.

Acute respiratory failure occurs in up to 50% of patients treated for hematologic malignancies and is associated with a high case fatality rate. Because of residual organ dysfunction and time spent receiving respiratory care, underlying disease control is affected. Early admission to an intensive care unit for acute respiratory failure has proven benefit because it is the best place for rapid implementation of noninvasive diagnostic and therapeutic strategies. This article reviews the clinical approach and diagnostic strategies for acute respiratory failure in patients with hematologic malignancies.

Patients with cancer continue to have unmet palliative care needs. Concurrent palliative care is tailored to the needs of patients as well as their families to relieve suffering. Specialty palliative care referral is associated with improved symptom management, improved end-of-life quality, and higher family-rated satisfaction. Optimal timing for palliative care referral has not been determined. Barriers to palliative care referral include workforce limitations, provider attitudes and perceptions, and potential ethnic and racial disparities in access to palliative care. Future work should focus on novel, patient-centered approaches to identify and address unmet palliative care needs for patients living with cancer.

PROGRAM OBJECTIVE

The goal of the *Clinics in Chest Medicine* is to provide provide practitioners with state-of-the-art information that is clinically useful, concise, well referenced, and comprehensive.

TARGET AUDIENCE

All practicing physicians and health care professionals who provide patient care utilizing findings from *Chest Medicine Clinics of North America*.

LEARNING OBJECTIVES

Upon completion of this activity, participants will be able to:
1. Review pulmonary manifestations of non-pulmonary malignancies.
2. Discuss management and palliative care for patients with malignancies.
3. Recognize pulmonary complications of non-pulmonary malignancies and their treatments.

ACCREDITATION

The Elsevier Office of Continuing Medical Education (EOCME) is accredited by the Accreditation Council for Continuing Medical Education (ACCME) to provide continuing medical education for physicians.

The EOCME designates this enduring material for a maximum of 15 *AMA PRA Category 1 Credit*(s)™. Physicians should claim only the credit commensurate with the extent of their participation in the activity.

All other health care professionals requesting continuing education credit for this enduring material will be issued a certificate of participation.

DISCLOSURE OF CONFLICTS OF INTEREST

The EOCME assesses conflict of interest with its instructors, faculty, planners, and other individuals who are in a position to control the content of CME activities. All relevant conflicts of interest that are identified are thoroughly vetted by EOCME for fair balance, scientific objectivity, and patient care recommendations. EOCME is committed to providing its learners with CME activities that promote improvements or quality in health care and not a specific proprietary business or a commercial interest.

The planning committee, staff, authors and editors listed below have identified no financial relationships or relationships to products or devices they or their spouse/life partner have with commercial interest related to the content of this CME activity:

Kathleen M. Akgün, MD, MS; Elie Azoulay, MD, PhD; Lara Bashoura, MD; Anne Bergeron, MD, PhD; Trevor J. Bledsoe, MD; Guang-Shing Cheng, MD; Roy H. Decker, MD, PhD; George A. Eapen, MD; Saadia A. Faiz, MD; Anjali Fortna; Alexander I. Geyer, MD; Bianca Harris, MD, MSc; Paul Leger, MD; Virginie Lemiale, MD; Andrew H. Limper, MD; David K. Madtes, MD; Fabien Maldonado, MD; Anne-Sophie Moreau, MD; Sameer K. Nath, MD; Oliver Peyrony, MD; Katie Pfaff; Jennifer D. Possick, MD; Jonathon Puchalski, MD, Med; Ayman O. Soubani, MD; Subhalakshmi Vaidyanathan; Lisa K. Vande Vusse, MD, MSc; Justin L. Wong, MD; Amy Williams; Lara Zafrani, MD, PhD.

The planning committee, staff, authors and editors listed below have identified financial relationships or relationships to products or devices they or their spouse/life partner have with commercial interest related to the content of this CME activity:

Scott E. Evans, MD, FCCP has stock ownership in, and receives royalties/patents from, Pulmotect.
Margaret L. Green, MD, MPH has research support from Merck & Co., Inc. and Astellas Pharma US Inc.
Steven A. Pergam, MD, MPH, FIDSA is a consultant/advisor for Merck & Co., Inc. and Optimer Pharmaceuticals Inc.

UNAPPROVED/OFF-LABEL USE DISCLOSURE

The EOCME requires CME faculty to disclose to the participants:
1. When products or procedures being discussed are off-label, unlabelled, experimental, and/or investigational (not US Food and Drug Administration [FDA] approved); and
2. Any limitations on the information presented, such as data that are preliminary or that represent ongoing research, interim analyses, and/or unsupported opinions. Faculty may discuss information about pharmaceutical agents that is outside of FDA-approved labelling. This information is intended solely for CME and is not intended to promote off-label use of these medications. If you have any questions, contact the medical affairs department of the manufacturer for the most recent prescribing information.

TO ENROLL

To enroll in the *Chest Medicine Clinics* Continuing Medical Education program, call customer service at 1-800-654-2452 or sign up online at http://www.theclinics.com/home/cme. The CME program is available to subscribers for an additional annual fee of USD $225.

METHOD OF PARTICIPATION

In order to claim credit, participants must complete the following:

1. Complete enrolment as indicated above.
2. Read the activity.
3. Complete the CME Test and Evaluation. Participants must achieve a score of 70% on the test. All CME Tests and Evaluations must be completed online.

CME INQUIRIES/SPECIAL NEEDS

For all CME inquiries or special needs, please contact elsevierCME@elsevier.com.

CLINICS IN CHEST MEDICINE

THE CLINICS ARE AVAILABLE ONLINE!
Access your subscription at:
www.theclinics.com

Preface

Pulmonary Disease in Non-Pulmonary Malignancy

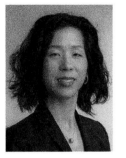 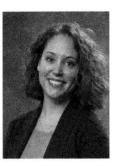

Guang-Shing Cheng, MD   Jennifer D. Possick, MD
Editors

The global burden of cancer is increasing yearly—in fact, the Centers for Disease Control and Prevention anticipates that the number of malignancies diagnosed annually will increase to 19 million by 2025, compared to 14 million cases diagnosed in 2012. Significant health care resources and biomedical research efforts are dedicated to prolonging the lives of patients with cancer. Improved treatment regimens, including the rational design of targeted immunological and cellular therapies, aggressive management of complications, and better supportive care, have turned many patients with cancer into cancer survivors.

Although lung cancer remains the most lethal malignancy worldwide, the overall cancer burden lies in other solid and liquid malignancies. Separate from the challenges of diagnosing and managing primary lung cancers, the lung's enormous alveolar and blood surface area make it particularly vulnerable to side effects from cytotoxic treatments for, and direct complications from, non-pulmonary malignancies. As a result, pulmonary/critical care practitioners and allied professionals are increasingly called upon to play an essential role in the care of these individuals.

As pulmonary/critical care physicians practicing in academic centers with sizable cancer populations, we encounter diagnostic and therapeutic challenges in our practices for which the scientific literature and evidence-based clinical guidance are diffuse and challenging to find, in part due to the multidisciplinary nature of cancer care. To address this gap, we assembled this issue of

Clinics in Chest Medicine to focus on pulmonary and critical care issues relevant to the care of patients with non-pulmonary malignancies, a first for this publication. We chose to cover a broad scope of clinical topics that cleave to recurrent themes, including the ways in which non-pulmonary malignancies and complications of cancer treatments manifest as lung disease. We also sought to highlight specific considerations for recipients of hematopoietic cell transplant, whose altered immunity and prolonged survivorship leave them vulnerable to specific pulmonary complications.

This issue opens with two comprehensive reviews of the pulmonary manifestations of non-pulmonary solid and hematologic malignancies, respectively. The varied presentations of metastatic malignancy throughout the bronchopulmonary anatomy—including parenchyma, airways, pleura, and vasculature—often pose challenges in diagnosis and management. Treatment depends on the site of involvement as well as the overall burden of disease. Primary presentations of lymphomas in the lung, as well extramedullary leukemia, often mimic infection and remain challenging to recognize and diagnose.

Complications of cancer treatment remain the primary reason that pulmonologists are consulted by oncologists. The second series of articles addresses pulmonary toxicities from radiation therapy and conventional chemotherapies as well as the spectrum of pulmonary complications observed with the checkpoint inhibitor immunotherapies now employed in the treatment of a growing number of malignancies. In addition, there

Clin Chest Med 38 (2017) xiii–xiv
http://dx.doi.org/10.1016/j.ccm.2017.03.001
0272-5231/17/© 2017 Published by Elsevier Inc.

chestmed.theclinics.com

is a discussion on the unique and devastating noninfectious pulmonary syndromes of idiopathic pneumonia syndrome and bronchiolitis obliterans syndrome in patients who receive hematopoietic cell transplant as curative therapy for malignancy and other hematologic diseases.

Infectious complications that arise from immune dysfunction due to the malignancies and corresponding treatments are discussed in the third group of articles. Impairment of mucosal integrity as a result of chemotherapy and aspiration risk make patients with cancer particularly vulnerable to bacterial infections. Invasive fungal infections cause considerable morbidity and mortality in profoundly neutropenic patients, and impaired cellular immunity predisposes these patients to serious opportunistic and community-acquired viral pneumonias.

The fourth section covers considerations in the diagnostic evaluation of pulmonary disease, focusing primarily on patients with hematologic malignancies and those patients receiving hematopoietic cell transplant. Best practices for evaluation of respiratory disease in this population remain an area of active clinical investigation, as efforts to reduce the morbidity and mortality from pulmonary complications are paramount to the overall success of hematopoietic cell transplantation.

This issue closes with considerations in the care of the critically ill patient with malignancy. As cancer treatments have advanced and survivorship has improved, an updated understanding of critical care outcomes in these populations must inform our discussions of goals of care, ICU utilization, and approach to acute respiratory failure. Recommendations for palliative and end-of-life care for patients with cancer, which are often neglected until patients are admitted to the ICU, are also addressed here.

We hope that this compendium of diverse articles will provide a state-of-the-art perspective on the pulmonary care of individuals with malignancy and may serve as a point of departure for future discussion, investigation, and collaboration as the field of cancer care continues to evolve.

We extend our sincere gratitude to all of the authors who contributed their time, passion, and expertise to this issue of *Clinics in Chest Medicine*. In addition, we thank Casey Potter for her steady guidance, and the entire Elsevier editorial staff for bringing this issue to fruition. Last, we are ever grateful to our families for their unflagging support in this endeavor.

Guang-Shing Cheng, MD
Fred Hutchinson Cancer Research Center
Mailstop D5-360
1100 Fairview Avenue N
Seattle, WA 98109, USA

Jennifer D. Possick, MD
Section of Pulmonary, Critical Care
and Sleep Medicine
Yale University School of Medicine
333 Cedar Street
PO Box 208057
New Haven, CT 06520-8057, USA

E-mail addresses:
gcheng2@fredhutch.org (G.-S. Cheng)
jennifer.possick@yale.edu (J.D. Possick)

Pulmonary Manifestations of Non-Pulmonary Malignancy

Pulmonary Manifestations of Solid Non-Pulmonary Malignancies

Jonathan Puchalski, MD, MEd

KEYWORDS

- Metastatic disease • Complications • Pulmonary metastases • Solid malignancies

KEY POINTS

- The lungs are a common site of metastatic disease and these include the lung parenchyma, airways, mediastinal lymph nodes, pleura, and vasculature.
- Metastatic disease may present without symptoms, with nonspecific symptoms, and with pulmonary symptoms, in addition to symptoms related to their anatomic origin.
- Treatment of pulmonary metastatic disease includes systemic therapy as well as local therapy based on the site of metastasis, including the airway and pleural space.

INTRODUCTION

The lungs are a common site of metastatic disease and these include the lung parenchyma, airways, mediastinal lymph nodes, pleura, and vasculature (**Table 1**). Metastatic disease may present without symptoms, with nonspecific symptoms such as anorexia or weight loss, and with pulmonary symptoms such as chronic cough, hemoptysis, dyspnea, and hoarseness, in addition to symptoms related to their anatomic origin.

Pulmonary metastases develop due to various mechanisms, including local blood flow and cellular or biochemical properties of tumor cells that thrive in an appropriate microenvironment for growth. These likely include growth factors and inhibitors, chemoattractants, and complex cellular interactions that may predispose tumor deposition based on distinct subtypes. Some diseases, such as melanoma, choriocarcinoma, and sarcoma, have thoracic metastatic invasion up to 80% to 100% of the time based on autopsy specimens. Other cancers with pulmonary metastatic lesions occurring more than 50% of the time include those of the breast, prostate, kidney, thyroid, and testes.[1]

PARENCHYMAL DISEASE

Metastatic disease is often identified as a solitary nodule, multiple pulmonary nodules, and infiltrates in a distribution consistent with lymphangitic spread. However, up to 50% of cases of lymphangitic spread may have normal chest radiograph, but are detected on computed tomography (CT).[1]

Nodules may appear small (miliary), large ("cannonball"), cavitary, calcified, and be either well-defined or poorly defined. Examples are demonstrated in **Fig. 1**, including metastatic disease from breast cancer, osteosarcoma, and thyroid cancer. Although calcification often represents benign disease, it occurs with metastatic osteogenic sarcoma and chondrosarcoma, among others. Cavitation is most commonly seen with metastatic squamous cell carcinoma, and in this scenario may occur up to 75% of the time.[1] A recent study suggested the presence of multiple nodules and cavitation most commonly represented metastatic disease but suggested biopsy to confirm malignancy because almost 10% had nonmetastatic deposits.[2]

Lymphangitic features are characterized by reticular or reticulonodular infiltrates and nodular

Financial Disclosures: None.
Conflicts of Interest: None.
Yale University School of Medicine, 15 York Street, LCI 100, New Haven, CT 06510, USA
E-mail address: jonathan.puchalski@yale.edu

Clin Chest Med 38 (2017) 177–186
http://dx.doi.org/10.1016/j.ccm.2016.12.002
0272-5231/17/© 2017 Elsevier Inc. All rights reserved.

Table 1
Pulmonary manifestations of extrathoracic malignancies and treatment considerations

Site of Disease	Evaluation	Treatment Possibilities
Lung parenchyma	Biopsy (bronchoscopy, CT-guided, surgical resection)	Systemic therapy Metastatectomy Palliative care
Endobronchial disease	Bronchoscopy	Systemic therapy Radiation therapy Bronchoscopic including electrocautery, APC, laser, cryotherapy, stenting Palliative care
Mediastinal lymph nodes	EBUS EUS Mediastinoscopy CT-guided biopsies	Systemic therapy Palliative care
Pleural effusion	Thoracentesis Thoracoscopy CT-guided biopsies	Systemic therapy Thoracentesis Tunneled pleural catheter Pleurodesis Palliative care
Pericardial Effusion	Echocardiography	Systemic therapy Catheter drainage Surgical window Palliative care
Pulmonary vascular disease	CT angiogram V/Q scan	Systemic therapy Anticoagulation Palliative care
Paraneoplastic syndrome	PET scan Brain MRI	Systemic therapy Palliative care

Abbreviations: APC, argon plasma coagulation; CT, computed tomography; EBUS, endobronchial ultrasound; EUS, endoscopic ultrasound.

septal thickening without architectural distortion. This pattern is associated most frequently with adenocarcinoma, namely breast, prostate, stomach, and pancreas carcinomas.[1] An example of metastatic adenocarcinoma of the lung is shown in **Fig. 1**. The differential diagnosis includes infection or pulmonary toxicity from chemotherapy, and thus further investigation may be required in the form of bronchoscopy, transthoracic biopsy, or, occasionally, surgical biopsy.

Treatment for metastatic parenchymal disease is often systemic cytotoxic chemotherapy and/or hormonal manipulation aimed at the underlying malignancy. Radiation may be used as part of a palliative approach, such as those tumors causing significant hemoptysis.

Although surgery is often the primary treatment modality for limited stage cancer, occasionally pulmonary metastatectomy may be considered for oligometastatic disease in the absence of extrathoracic sites of disease. In these cases of carefully defined oligometastatic disease, the number and site of metastatic tumors are limited and represent a distinct scenario from more extensive metastatic disease. As described by Weichselbaum and Hellman,[3] "successful results of curative resection of lung metastases have been described for almost all types of cancer." In the report from the International Registry of Lung Metastases, 4572 patients almost equally divided between epithelial tumors and sarcomas who underwent complete resection of metastatic tumors had a 5-year survival rate of 36% and a 10-year survival rate of 26%.[4] Multiple studies have since been performed to identify specific cohorts with the greatest chance of benefit. In an analysis of 19 papers, investigators determined that patients most likely to benefit from pulmonary metastatectomy in colorectal carcinoma included those with smaller size and number of metastatic deposits, lower carcinoembryonic antigen levels, absence of intrathoracic lymph node involvement, and response to induction chemotherapy.[5] In a more recent single-center retrospective study of 188 patients with solitary metastatic colorectal carcinoma, the 5-year overall survival was 53% (95% confidence interval, 44%–60%) and progression-free survival was 33% (95% confidence interval,

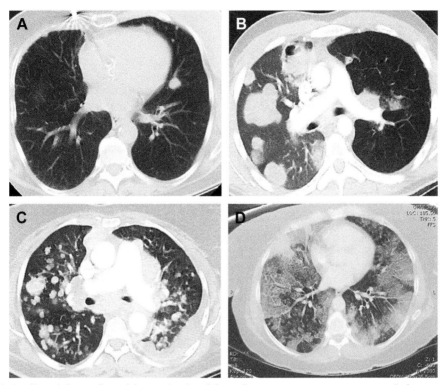

Fig. 1. (*A*) Small nodule confirmed by navigational bronchoscopy to represent metastatic breast cancer. (*B*) Metastatic disease with large and small nodules, one of which is cavitary, owing to metastatic osteosarcoma. (*C*) Significant small and large nodules, as well as mediastinal lymphadenopathy and a left pleural effusion owing to metastatic papillary thyroid carcinoma. (*D*) Diffuse lymphangitic spread owing to metastatic lung adenocarcinoma.

25%–42%). Multivariate adjusted analysis showed that TNM stages (*P* = .019), number of resected lung metastases of 5 or fewer (*P* = .009), and lymph node involvement (*P*<.0001) were independent factors of a poor prognosis.[6] A recent editorial citing a 5-year overall survival of 40% after pulmonary metastatectomy for various metastatic tumors criticized the available literature for a lack of randomized, controlled trials and concluded no evidence exists to justifiably guide metastatectomy when the purpose is to improve survival.[7] Thus, at present, some controversy exists as to which patients should be considered when evaluating patients for metastatectomy.

Assuming a defined benefit of aggressive management of pulmonary metastases, comorbidities may preclude an operative approach. Alternative treatment approaches include stereotactic body radiotherapy as well as ablative techniques, such as cryoablation[8] and percutaneous radiofrequency thermal ablation.[9] It is likely that many factors will ultimately determine not only who are candidates for metastatectomy, but also which modality should be used based on costs,[10] tumor type,[11] and expected benefit from mutation-based systemic treatment and immunotherapy for the underlying disease.

ENDOBRONCHIAL DISEASE AND AIRWAY OBSTRUCTION

Tumors may metastasize to the airways via hematogenous, lymphatic, or aerogenous spread, or invade the bronchus through adjacent lung parenchyma or lymph nodes. They may also compress the airways from extraluminal but adjacent growth. Metastatic airway tumors frequently manifest with dyspnea, wheezing, postobstructive pneumonia, or hemoptysis, or they may be asymptomatic.[12] The incidence is variable and depends in part on tumor type. In 1 study of 943 consecutive bronchoscopies, 18 (1.9%) had endobronchial metastases. Of these, the most common primary tumors included breast, kidney, bone, and soft tissue. Tumor deposits were identified in the trachea, mainstem bronchi, and lobar bronchi. The median survival in this population was 122 days.[13] In a review of the literature in 2000, the most common solid tumors with endobronchial metastases were breast, kidney, and colorectal carcinoma. In this review, survival was typically 1 to 2 years.[14] Finally, a retrospective analysis of 174 patients collected from 2 institutions over 18 years demonstrated endobronchial metastases from extrathoracic malignancies in 4% of total cases. Again, breast, colorectal, and kidney cancers were the most common primary tumors. The mean latency period between the appearance of primary and metastatic endobronchial tumor was 136 months (range, 1–300). In 5% of cases, endobronchial disease was the first manifestation of malignancy, particularly in patients with previously undiagnosed renal cell carcinoma.[15]

Short-term mortality in the presence of some endobronchial malignancies is high. In a recent retrospective study of 19 patients with melanoma, endobronchial metastases occurred at a median of 48 months after the primary tumor diagnosis. The median overall survival at diagnosis of endobronchial disease was 6 months and factors predicting poor survival included multiple sites of metastases, and pleural and soft tissue involvement. Different treatment modalities, including chemotherapy, surgery, radiotherapy, and bronchoscopic therapy, showed no effect on survival.[16]

Although the mainstay of management for metastatic disease is systemic therapy, airway obstruction from endoluminal and extrinsic disease may require therapies with a more immediate impact, particularly when respiratory distress is present. Radiation therapy (RT) may be used for both central and more distal (lobar) obstruction. In conjunction with the American Society for Radiation Oncology Guidelines for Palliative Lung Cancer Care and the Third International Cancer Workshop, surveys determined support for palliative thoracic RT depending on patient performance status, pulmonary function, anticipated RT volume, and other factors. The survey determined that RT is generally indicated for patients with advanced stage III and IV disease with "significant and troublesome current or impending symptoms."[17] Depending on tumor radiosensitivity, its effect may not be immediate and, in fact, inflammation and subsequent edema from RT may temporarily worsen the degree of airway impingement.

Several bronchoscopic techniques may be used for the palliative treatment of endobronchial disease, often as part of a multimodality approach (**Fig. 2**). Rigid bronchoscopy may core out endobronchial disease efficiently and be useful for stent placement, particularly silicone stents.[18] Larger forceps may debulk endoluminal tumor quicker than those used via flexible bronchoscopy. However, a variety of instruments may be placed through the working channel of the flexible

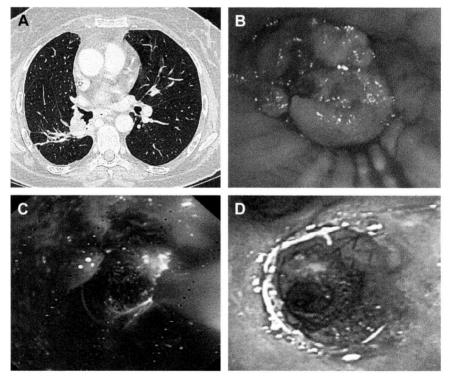

Fig. 2. (*A*) Computed tomography scan showing endobronchial disease (*B*) confirmed on bronchoscopy to be metastatic colorectal cancer. (*C*) Endobronchial therapy may include heat therapies such as argon plasma coagulation or (*D*) implantation of airway stents.

bronchoscope to debride the tumor and reestablish airway patency. These include balloons (such as controlled radial expansion balloons and Fogarty balloons), devices that deliver heat (electrocautery, argon plasma coagulation, laser, photodynamic therapy, and brachytherapy), as well as cryoablation probes. Balloon bronchoplasty involves the use of balloons, typically filled with saline, that expand in diameter under the operator's guidance. Available in 4- to 20-mm sizes, airway dilation is performed with resultant improvement in airway diameter, at least temporarily.[19] Heat modalities are also used to ablate endobronchial tumor. Endobronchial electrosurgery, carried out with probes or "knives" advanced through the working channel of the bronchoscope, became mainstream in 1985. Heat generated by high-frequency alternating electrical current can cut, vaporize, or coagulate tissue in the airways. Argon plasma coagulation uses ionized argon gas to conduct an electrical current between the tissue and the delivery probe, creating evaporation of water in tissue and subsequent coagulation and tissue destruction. Laser, usually used with a power of 40 W or less, allows for immediate tissue destruction with both photocoagulation ad vaporization of tissue.[19,20]

Additional bronchoscopic techniques using heat ablation include photodynamic therapy and brachytherapy. Photodynamic therapy combines a photosensitizer with light at a wavelength matching the drug absorption (laser plus a photosensitizer) to generate tissue destruction.[19] It has been shown to decrease the level of obstruction and improve dyspnea, cough, hemoptysis, and quality of life in patients with endobronchial obstruction from non-pulmonary metastatic disease.[21] Brachytherapy is accomplished by placing a radiation source, most commonly iridium-192, within or alongside a tumor via bronchoscopic guidance. Radiation dose depends on the diameter and length of the treatment field, and it may be administered with high-dose rates (12 Gy/h).[22] It is not recommended typically in patients who have not first received external beam radiation and evidence of its effectiveness for metastatic endobronchial lesions is limited.[23]

Cryotherapy uses extremes of cold to cause cell death. Ice crystal formation damages organelles and causes transcellular fluid shifts to result in immediate, direct cell injury. Delayed cell death is also caused by local vasoconstriction and potentially by immune-mediated phenomena. The standard technique involves repeated freeze–thaw cycles and subsequent sloughing of the devitalized tissue. Another technique, called cryorecanalization, stabilizes the cryoprobe onto the lesion while freezing it and removing pieces while still frozen (cryoadhesion). Evidence of efficacy is mostly case series based, but seems to be promising for malignant central airway obstruction.[24]

Airway stents may be placed in the trachea, mainstem bronchi, or bronchus intermedius in conjunction with the aforementioned techniques as 1 component of a multimodality approach to reestablish airway patency. Whereas the prior techniques are for endobronchial disease, stents may be used for both endoluminal disease and obstruction from extrinsic compression. Typically 10 to 18 mm in diameter and of various lengths, relief of airflow obstruction is often immediate.[25] These therapeutic bronchoscopic techniques are typically part of a palliative approach to symptoms, especially dyspnea, and may be used concurrent with systemic therapies. They have been shown to improve dyspnea, quality of life, and pulmonary function, among other outcomes.[26–30] In light of mucus plugging, granulation tissue development, dislodgement, and other complications, their potential risks should be evaluated against their benefits.[31]

METASTATIC LYMPHADENOPATHY

Metastases to intrathoracic lymph nodes portend a poor prognosis. In 1 study evaluating the role of endobronchial ultrasound (EBUS) imaging and PET/CT scanning, the most common metastases were from colorectal, breast, stomach, head and neck, and urogenital carcinomas.[32] Another study found 17 of 103 patients being evaluated for metastatectomy in the setting of presumed oligometastatic disease had metastatic nodal involvement from colorectal, kidney, melanoma, breast, and other cancers.[33] Given the impact of metastatic nodal involvement, screening for mediastinal/hilar lymph node involvement is recommended when pulmonary metastatectomy is being considered.[5]

Although CT scanning may detect nodal involvement and PET-CT may suggest malignant disease, neither adequately confirms the presence of metastatic disease. In these cases, tissue confirmation is essential to determine the most appropriate treatment. Techniques to biopsy the mediastinum and hilum include CT-guided biopsies (limited by number of nodes sampled and location), mediastinoscopy (relatively invasive and expensive), video-assisted thoracoscopic biopsies (relatively invasive and expensive), endoscopic ultrasound (does not reach right paratracheal, pretracheal or hilar nodes) and convex probe EBUS.

Although EBUS, endoscopic ultrasound imaging, and mediastinosocopy may be combined in a maximal effort to increase diagnostic yield, EBUS has shown promising results as an independent nonsurgical diagnostic modality. Using real-time ultrasound examination, a needle may be passed into mediastinal and hilar lymph nodes, as well as centralized lung masses, to attain tissue. A metaanalysis of 533 patients showed a 0.85 sensitivity (0.80–0.89), 0.99 specificity (0.95–1.00), and diagnostic accuracy of 0.8588.[34] Serious complications are rare (0.16%).[35] This and other needle techniques represent a less invasive and less expensive approach to mediastinal lymph node sampling than mediastinoscopy.[36]

Treatment for mediastinal and hilar lymph node involvement from extrathoracic metastases is typically systemic therapy. There may be a limited role for surgical resection (mediastinal lymphadenectomy) in very well-defined scenarios.[37]

MALIGNANT PLEURAL EFFUSION

Metastatic disease accounts for the majority of malignant pleural disease. There are approximately 150,000 annual cases of malignant pleural effusion (MPE) in the United States and 40,000 cases in the United Kingdom. Lung cancer is the most common cause of a MPE and approximately 25% of patients with breast and 10% of those with lymphoma develop MPEs.[1] Ovarian and gastric cancers round out the top 5 causes and together these account for 80% of all MPE.[38,39] **Fig. 3** provides examples of malignant pleural disease.

Pleural effusions may be associated with breathlessness, pain, and significant quality of life limitations in addition to shortened life expectancy.[40,41] Management of MPE may include repeated thoracentesis, placement of a tunneled pleural catheter (TPC), or instillation of agents for pleurodesis. Regardless of the modality, improvements in dyspnea and quality of life seem to be similar between the techniques. Repeated

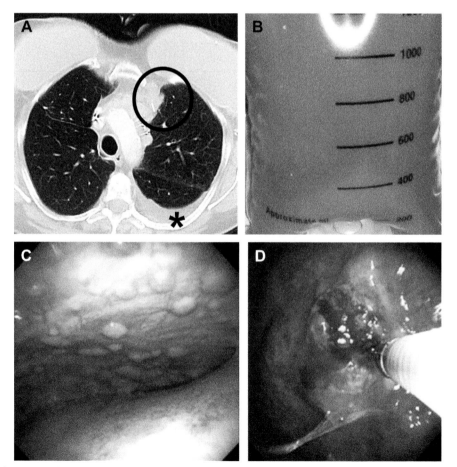

Fig. 3. (A) Computed tomography scan shows metastatic mediastinal deposit (*circle*) and a pleural effusion (*) (B) confirmed to represent metastatic breast cancer. (C) Pleural metastases are visualized and (D) biopsied in different patients confirming metastatic involvement.

thoracentesis is generally preferred when life expectancy is extremely short (days to weeks). TPC placement is often performed because it can be accomplished without the need for hospitalization and owing to its technical ease. Pleurodesis occurs at 29 to 59 days in 45% to 70% of patients depending in part on extent of lung reexpansion and likely the underlying pathology.[42] Although not significant at 42 days, dyspnea improved more in patients undergoing TPC placement at 6 months compared with pleurodesis in the TIME2 trial (Therapeutic Intervention in Malignant Effusion-2).[43] There also seems to be less of a need for repeat ipsilateral intervention in patients undergoing TPC placement compared with pleurodesis. However, pleurodesis offers the benefit of eliminating effusions in a short time period without the sustained burden of an indwelling catheter and its associated management needs such as drainage by visiting nurses or family members. This can be accomplished by video-assisted thoracoscopic surgery, thoracoscopy (pleuroscopy), or by chest tube insertion with instillation of different pleurodesing agents. Success of pleurodesis is 60% to 100%, depending on which agent is used, among which options include talc, doxycycline, povidone-iodine, and others.[42] Talc poudrage seems to offer the greatest pleurodesis efficacy, although more data are required as noted in a recent Cochrane database metaanalysis.[44] Although the initial costs of the procedure and associated hospitalization are higher, ongoing drainage via TPC can surpass these expenses in patients with longer life expectancies, such as those with breast cancer. Ultimately, the modality of managing MPE is based on the patient's preferences, comorbidities, functional status prognosis, and local procedural expertise.

Although pleural effusions are encountered much more commonly, pneumothorax may be associated with malignancy and pleural fistula development. In some cases, the tumor erodes into the adjacent pleura. In others, a cavitary lesion may result in pneumothorax. Cancer-related therapies may also be related to pneumothorax. One study highlighted the associated morbidity and mortality associated with sarcoma. Investigators found that spontaneous pneumothorax was associated with virtually every cell type of sarcoma. It frequently recurred and was associated with a poor prognosis. Mechanisms felt to be responsible for development of the pneumothorax included direct involvement of the pleura with tumor or extension of cavitary lesions. Necrosis of tumors owing to chemotherapy was also felt to be associated.[45] Pneumothoraces have also been described in patients with metastatic breast cancer,[46] pancreatic, adrenal, and renal, among others, although those associated with sarcomas seem to be the most prevalant.[47]

MALIGNANT PERICARDIAL EFFUSION

The symptoms of malignant pericardial effusion may include dyspnea, chest discomfort, and tachycardia. Other manifestations such as hypotension, tamponade, and cardiogenic shock can be life threatening. Pericardial effusions may be due to direct tumor extension from breast and esophageal cancer, obstruction of lymphatic drainage owing to mediastinal lymphadenopathy, or via hematogenous or lymphatic spread of tumor (melanoma, thymic cancer, and others). Finally, many patients with pericardial effusions also have concurrent pleural effusions. In addition to treatment of the malignancy, procedures to relieve symptoms of pericardial effusions include pericardiocentesis, placement of pericardial catheters for long-term drainage, pericardial sclerosis, and percutaneous balloon pericardiotomy. Surgical approaches include pericardial fenestration (pericardial "window"), pericardiectomy, and creation of a pericardial–peritoneal shunt.[48,49]

PULMONARY VASCULAR DISEASE IN MALIGNANCY

Cancer increases the risk of venous thromboembolism by 7-fold, especially in patients with metastases and during chemotherapy.[50] The pathogenesis involves the tumor's capacity to interact with and activate the host hemostatic system. Advanced stages of malignancy and sites of cancer, including the lung, stomach, kidney, pancreas, bladder and brain, are cancer-specific factors related to thrombotic risk.[51]

Pulmonary vascular disease in the setting of malignancy may be life threatening. In addition to the hypercoagulable state in cancer, pulmonary thromboembolism occurs when aggregates of tumor cells lodge in the pulmonary vasculature either as emboli from distal vascular sites or by direct extension of tumor. Cancers that frequently cause tumor embolism include breast, liver, gastric, kidney, prostate, and choriocarcinoma. In renal cell carcinoma, local tumor extension from the involved renal vein or inferior vena cava may metastasize or even extend proximally the distance to the pulmonary artery. Symptoms and physical examination findings are similar to those of venous thromboembolism, which include chest pain, dyspnea, and hemoptysis. Evaluation may include a V/Q scan or CT pulmonary angiogram to assess for emboli and echocardiogram to assess for right heart strain. Whereas these radiographic results are indistinguishable from nontumor emboli, certain tests may help to separate the etiologies. Pulmonary microvascular cytology can be obtained by placing a pulmonary artery catheter into the wedged position and subsequently aspirating samples for cytologic analysis.[52] Convex probe EBUS has also been used to biopsy abnormalities within the pulmonary arteries to confirm tumor emboli.[53]

Pulmonary tumor thrombotic microangiopathy is a distinct pulmonary vascular manifestation of malignancy characterized by microembolic nests of tumor and associated with the activation of coagulation and obliterative intimal proliferation. The proliferating intimal cells in the pulmonary arteries and veins are both endothelial and nonendothelial (myofibroblastic) in origin. This phenomenon is most often associated with gastric carcinoma, but also carcinoma of the breast, bladder, ovaries (clear cell), liver, and gallbladder. This phenomenon may lead to pulmonary hypertension. Treatment of these disorders includes anticoagulation for thrombosis and systemic therapy for the underlying cancer. For pulmonary tumor thrombotic microangiopathy, antiinflammatory or antiproliferative therapy (glucocorticoids, imatinib) in addition to pulmonary vasodilators may be useful, but studies are lacking.[54] There are questions as to whether pulmonary tumor thrombotic microangiopathy represents a paraneoplastic syndrome.[55]

Superior and inferior vena cava syndromes represent another vascular spectrum of malignancy. Up to 10% of cases of superior vena cava syndrome are related to metastatic disease. Manifestations may include cough, dyspnea, stridor and hoarseness among others. An in-depth overview is referenced.[56]

PARANEOPLASTIC SYNDROME

Although lung cancers are the most common cause, other malignancies with or without pulmonary metastases may be associated with paraneoplastic syndromes. Symptoms are not due to the tumor itself, but due to functional peptides or hormones secreted by the tumor or an immune cross-reaction between tumor and normal tissue. In the latter case, the central or peripheral nervous system are typically affected. Gynecologic and breast cancers produce anti-Yo and anti-Ri antibodies that are associated with paraneoplastic cerebellar degeneration and resultant ataxia. Germ cell tumors of the testis and breast cancer are associated with antiamphiphysin that causes stiff-man syndrome and encephalomyelitis. Thymoma is

associated with antiacetylcholine receptor and anti–variable-gated potassium channel antibodies that leads to myasthenia gravis and limbic encephalitis, respectively.[57] Cough has been reported as a paraneoplastic-presenting symptom of renal cell carcinoma. Breast cancer has been associated with bilateral diaphragm paralysis.[52] The full scope of paraneoplastic syndromes include multiple organ systems.[58]

SUMMARY

Pulmonary metastases from extrathoracic malignancies may affect all components of the respiratory system. The spectrum extends from the pulmonary vasculature to the parenchyma and includes patients without symptoms and those with life-threatening emergencies. This review highlights the wide potential of metastatic involvement, including both diagnostic and therapeutic strategies for this highly morbid and potentially lethal condition.

REFERENCES

1. Whitesell PL, Peters SG. Pulmonary manifestations of extrathoracic malignant lesions. Mayo Clin Proc 1993;68:483–91.
2. Caparica RM, Milena PM, Rocha CH, et al. Pulmonary nodules in patients with nonpulmonary cancer: not always metastases. J Glob Oncol 2016;2(3):138–44.
3. Weichselbaum RR, Hellman S. Oligometastases revisited. Nat Rev Clin Oncol 2011;8:378–82.
4. Pastorino U, Buyse M, Friedel G, et al. Long-term results of lung metastasectomy: prognostic analyses based on 5206 cases. J Thorac Cardiovasc Surg 1997;113:37–49.
5. Tsitsias T, Toufektzian L, Routledge T, et al. Are there recognized prognostic factors for patients undergoing pulmonary metastasectomy for colorectal carcinoma? Interact Cardiovasc Thorac Surg 2016; 23(6):962–9.
6. Guerrera F, Mossetti C, Ceccarelli M, et al. Surgery of colorectal cancer lung metastases: analysis of survival, recurrence and re-surgery. J Thorac Dis 2016;8:1764–71.
7. Aberg T, Treasure T. Analysis of pulmonary metastasis as an indication for operation: an evidence-based approach. Eur J Cardiothorac Surg 2016; 50(5):792–8.
8. de Baere T, Tselikas L, Woodrum D, et al. Evaluating cryoablation of metastatic lung tumors in patients–safety and efficacy: the ECLIPSE trial–interim analysis at 1 year. J Thorac Oncol 2015;10:1468–74.
9. Thanos L, Mylona S, Pomoni M, et al. Percutaneous radiofrequency thermal ablation of primary and

metastatic lung tumors. Eur J Cardiothorac Surg 2006;30:797–800.

10. Lester-Coll NH, Rutter CE, Bledsoe TJ, et al. Cost-effectiveness of surgery, stereotactic body radiation therapy, and systemic therapy for pulmonary oligometastases. Int J Radiat Oncol Biol Phys 2016;95:663–72.

11. Ricardi U, Badellino S, Filippi AR. Clinical applications of stereotactic radiation therapy for oligometastatic cancer patients: a disease-oriented approach. J Radiat Res 2016;57(S1):i58–68.

12. Lee SH, Jung JY, Kim DH, et al. Endobronchial metastases from extrathoracic malignancy. Yonsei Med J 2013;54:403–9.

13. Dalar L, Ozdemir C, Sokucu SN, et al. Bronchoscopic palliation to treat endobronchial metastasis of the tracheobronchial tree. Respir Investig 2016;54:116–20.

14. Katsimbri PP, Bamias AT, Froudarakis ME, et al. Endobronchial metastases secondary to solid tumors: report of eight cases and review of the literature. Lung Cancer 2000;28:163–70.

15. Marchioni A, Lasagni A, Busca A, et al. Endobronchial metastasis: an epidemiologic and clinicopathologic study of 174 consecutive cases. Lung Cancer 2014;84:222–8.

16. Chaussende A, Hermant C, Tazi-Mezalek R, et al. Endobronchial metastases from melanoma: a survival analysis. Clin Respir J 2016. [Epub ahead of print].

17. Rodrigues G, Macbeth F, Burmeister B, et al. Consensus statement on palliative lung radiotherapy: Third International Consensus Workshop on Palliative Radiotherapy and Symptom Control. Clin Lung Cancer 2012;13:1–5.

18. Cavaliere S, Venuta F, Foccoli P, et al. Endoscopic treatment of malignant airway obstructions in 2,008 patients. Chest 1996;110:1536–42.

19. Folch E, Mehta AC. Airway interventions in the tracheobronchial tree. Semin Respir Crit Care Med 2008;29:441–52.

20. Puchalski J, Feller-Kopman D. The pulmonologist's diagnostic and therapeutic interventions in lung cancer. Clin Chest Med 2011;32:763–71.

21. McCaughan JS Jr. Survival after photodynamic therapy to non-pulmonary metastatic endobronchial tumors. Lasers Surg Med 1999;24:194–201.

22. Mahmood K, Wahidi MM. Ablative therapies for central airway obstruction. Semin Respir Crit Care Med 2014;35:681–92.

23. Donovan E, Timotin E, Farrell T, et al. Brachytherapy for endobronchial metastasis: an effective method of achieving palliative relief of symptoms. Int J Radiat Oncol Biol Phys 2016;96:E439–40.

24. DiBardino DM, Lanfranco AR, Haas AR. Bronchoscopic cryotherapy. clinical applications of the cryoprobe, cryospray, and cryoadhesion. Ann Am Thorac Soc 2016;13:1405–15.

25. Puchalski J, Musani AI. Tracheobronchial stenosis: causes and advances in management. Clin Chest Med 2013;34:557–67.

26. Stratakos G, Gerovasili V, Dimitropoulos C, et al. Survival and quality of life benefit after endoscopic management of malignant central airway obstruction. J Cancer 2016;7:794–802.

27. Oviatt PL, Stather DR, Michaud G, et al. Exercise capacity, lung function, and quality of life after interventional bronchoscopy. J Thorac Oncol 2011;6:38–42.

28. Amjadi K, Voduc N, Cruysberghs Y, et al. Impact of interventional bronchoscopy on quality of life in malignant airway obstruction. Respiration 2008;76:421–8.

29. Neumann K, Sundset A, Espinoza A, et al. Changes in quality of life, dyspnea scores, and lung function in lung cancer patients with airway obstruction after a therapeutic bronchoscopy. J Bronchology Interv Pulmonol 2013;20:134–9.

30. Ost DE, Ernst A, Grosu HB, et al. Therapeutic bronchoscopy for malignant central airway obstruction: success rates and impact on dyspnea and quality of life. Chest 2015;147:1282–98.

31. Herth FJ, Eberhardt R. Airway stent: what is new and what should be discarded. Curr Opin Pulm Med 2016;22:252–6.

32. Song JU, Park HY, Jeon K, et al. The role of endobronchial ultrasound-guided transbronchial needle aspiration in the diagnosis of mediastinal and hilar lymph node metastases in patients with extrapulmonary malignancy. Intern Med 2011;50:2525–32.

33. Eckardt J, Licht PB. Endobronchial ultrasound-guided transbronchial needle aspiration is a sensitive method to evaluate patients who should not undergo pulmonary metastasectomy dagger. Interact Cardiovasc Thorac Surg 2015;20:482–5 [discussion: 5].

34. Yang B, Li F, Shi W, et al. Endobronchial ultrasound-guided transbronchial needle biopsy for the diagnosis of intrathoracic lymph node metastases from extrathoracic malignancies: a meta-analysis and systematic review. Respirology 2014;19:834–41.

35. Caglayan B, Yilmaz A, Bilaceroglu S, et al. Complications of convex-probe endobronchial ultrasound-guided transbronchial needle aspiration: a multi-center retrospective study. Respir Care 2016;61:243–8.

36. Hegde PV, Liberman M. Mediastinal staging: endosonographic ultrasound lymph node biopsy or mediastinoscopy. Thorac Surg Clin 2016;26:243–9.

37. Riquet M, Berna P, Brian E, et al. Intrathoracic lymph node metastases from extrathoracic carcinoma: the place for surgery. Ann Thorac Surg 2009;88:200–5.

38. Egan AM, McPhillips D, Sarkar S, et al. Malignant pleural effusion. QJM 2014;107:179–84.

39. Karpathiou G, Stefanou D, Froudarakis ME. Pleural neoplastic pathology. Respir Med 2015;109:931–43.

40. DeBiasi EM, Pisani MA, Murphy TE, et al. Mortality among patients with pleural effusion undergoing thoracentesis. Eur Respir J 2015;46:495–502.

41. Argento AC, Murphy TE, Pisani MA, et al. Patient-centered outcomes following thoracentesis. Pleura (Thousand Oaks) 2015;2:1–12.

42. Fortin M, Tremblay A. Pleural controversies: indwelling pleural catheter vs. pleurodesis for malignant pleural effusions. J Thorac Dis 2015;7:1052–7.

43. Davies HE, Mishra EK, Kahan BC, et al. Effect of an indwelling pleural catheter vs chest tube and talc pleurodesis for relieving dyspnea in patients with malignant pleural effusion: the TIME2 randomized controlled trial. JAMA 2012;307:2383–9.

44. Clive AO, Jones HE, Bhatnagar R, et al. Interventions for the management of malignant pleural effusions: a network meta-analysis. Cochrane Database Syst Rev 2016;(5):CD010529.

45. Hoag JB, Sherman M, Fasihuddin Q, et al. A comprehensive review of spontaneous pneumothorax complicating sarcoma. Chest 2010;138:510–8.

46. Brufman G, Krasnokuki D, Schwartz A, et al. Spontaneous pneumothorax complicating lung metastases from carcinoma of the breast. Radiol Clin (Basel) 1977;46:38–41.

47. Wright FW. Spontaneous pneumothorax and pulmonary malignant disease–a syndrome sometimes associated with cavitating tumours. Report of nine new cases, four with metastases and five with primary bronchial tumours. Clin Radiol 1976;27:211–22.

48. Jama GM, Scarci M, Bowden J, et al. Palliative treatment for symptomatic malignant pericardial effusion dagger. Interact Cardiovasc Thorac Surg 2014;19:1019–26.

49. Burazor I, Imazio M, Markel G, et al. Malignant pericardial effusion. Cardiology 2013;124:224–32.

50. Donadini MP, Squizzato A, Ageno W. Treating patients with cancer and acute venous thromboembolism. Expert Opin Pharmacother 2016;17:535–43.

51. Falanga A, Marchetti M, Russo L. The mechanisms of cancer-associated thrombosis. Thromb Res 2015;135(Suppl 1):S8–11.

52. Agrawal A, Sahni S, Iftikhar A, et al. Pulmonary manifestations of renal cell carcinoma. Respir Med 2015;109:1505–8.

53. Desai NR, Greenhill SR, Vance M, et al. Pulmonary tumor embolism diagnosed by endobronchial ultrasound. J Bronchology Interv Pulmonol 2015;22:e16–9.

54. Price LC, Wells AU, Wort SJ. Pulmonary tumour thrombotic microangiopathy. Curr Opin Pulm Med 2016;22:421–8.

55. Carter CA, Scicinski JJ, Lybeck HE, et al. Pulmonary tumor thrombotic microangiopathy: a new paraneoplastic syndrome? Case Rep Oncol 2016;9:246–8.

56. Wilson LD, Detterbeck FC, Yahalom J. Clinical practice. Superior vena cava syndrome with malignant causes. N Engl J Med 2007;356:1862–9.

57. Braik T, Evans AT, Telfer M, et al. Paraneoplastic neurological syndromes: unusual presentations of cancer. A practical review. Am J Med Sci 2010;340:301–8.

58. Kanaji N, Watanabe N, Kita N, et al. Paraneoplastic syndromes associated with lung cancer. World J Clin Oncol 2014;5:197–223.

Pulmonary Manifestations of Lymphoma and Leukemia

Lara Bashoura, MD, George A. Eapen, MD, Saadia A. Faiz, MD*

KEYWORDS

- Hematologic malignancies • Cancer • Pleural disease • Lymphoma • Leukemia
- Pulmonary hypertension • Lymphadenopathy

KEY POINTS

- Malignant lymphoma typically originates in the lymph nodes, but concomitant or primary presentations may also include parenchymal, endobronchial, or pleural disease.
- Myeloid sarcoma is an extramedullary manifestation of myeloid leukemia, which may occur before, during, or after cancer diagnosis. It may rarely present in the form of a pulmonary mass, endobronchial disease, pleural disease, or intrathoracic lymphadenopathy.
- Confirmation with cytology and/or flow cytometry is recommended to diagnose malignant pleural effusions in lymphoma and leukemia.
- After infection is excluded, pleural effusions in acute leukemia and myelodysplastic syndrome are often related to malignancy.
- Venous thromboembolism may present in patients with leukemia and lymphoma despite the presence of thrombocytopenia.

INTRODUCTION

Pulmonary disease can occur across the entire disease spectrum of hematologic malignancies. Although infectious processes are common in these immunosuppressed individuals, noninfectious causes account for up to half of the pulmonary manifestations found in hematologic malignancies and should be kept in mind when evaluating enigmatic pulmonary findings in this population.

Significant overlap exists among variants of lymphoma and leukemia. Lymphoid neoplasms may evolve into a leukemic picture, and leukemia may present with a mass lesion, more classically suggestive of a lymphoma. Intrathoracic disease is common in lymphoid disorders. In fact, 85% of individuals with Hodgkin lymphoma (HL) and 66% of those with non-Hodgkin lymphoma (NHL) may have pulmonary findings.[1] Although the most common abnormality affecting the respiratory system in myeloid disease includes infection, myelogenous leukemia and its precursors have distinct pulmonary presentations as well. This review highlights prominent noninfectious pulmonary complications of lymphoma, leukemia, and their precursors.

Mediastinal Lymphadenopathy

Malignant lymphomas are neoplasms of the lymphatic system that include HL and a heterogeneous group of tumors referred to as NHL. These malignancies initially affect lymph node groups with subsequent spread to other organs. Lymphoma typically affects the anterior mediastinum

Department of Pulmonary Medicine, The University of Texas MD Anderson Cancer Center, 1400 Pressler Unit 1462, Houston, TX 77030-1402, USA
* Corresponding author.
E-mail address: safaiz@mdanderson.org

Clin Chest Med 38 (2017) 187–200
http://dx.doi.org/10.1016/j.ccm.2016.12.003
0272-5231/17/© 2016 Elsevier Inc. All rights reserved.

and may be part of more diffuse disease. The distribution of mediastinal lymphoma includes about 50% to 70% HL and 15% to 25% NHL.[2] Primary mediastinal lymphoma is rare and comprises 10% of lymphomas in the mediastinum. The 3 most common subtypes of mediastinal lymphoma include nodular sclerosing HL, lymphoblastic lymphoma, and large B-cell lymphoma.

HL and NHL are markedly different in tumor biology, clinical presentation, and therapeutic approach. HL has a bimodal incidence with a peak in young adulthood and again after the age of 50 years.[2] Reed-Sternberg cells are pathognomonic, and the nodular sclerosing subtype commonly affects the mediastinum.

Lymphoblastic lymphoma is a high-grade aggressive subtype of NHL that commonly affects the mediastinum at a mean age of 28 years.[2] Although blastic involvement of the bone marrow is common, if there is nodal predominant disease with less than 25% involvement in the bone marrow, it is categorized as a lymphoblastic lymphoma. Alternatively, if the disease burden is predominantly noted in the marrow and circulation with little nodal involvement, then it is categorized as T-cell acute lymphoblastic leukemia (ALL).[3]

Primary mediastinal B-cell lymphoma is a diffuse large B-cell lymphoma derived from the thymus, and it is the most common type of NHL involving the mediastinum in adults, with distinct clinical and biologic characteristics when compared with other lymphomas. It mainly affects young adults with a mean age of presentation of 30 years and a slight female predilection.[2,4] It accounts for 5% of aggressive lymphomas and

typically presents with a rapidly growing anterior or superior mediastinal mass often resulting in tracheal compression.[5,6] HL and primary mediastinal B-cell lymphoma share several similarities, including similar genetic mutations and prominent fibrosis, but the presence of Reed-Sternberg cells and tumor markers enables histologic differentiation.[6] Patients may present with superior vena cava (SVC) syndrome, phrenic nerve palsy, dysphagia, hoarseness, bilateral breast swelling or chest pain, and productive cough.[4] Although initial involvement of the bone marrow or extrathoracic structures is not common, primary mediastinal B-cell lymphoma often invades within the thoracic cavity to the lungs, pleura, or pericardium.

The pattern of mediastinal involvement in HL is distinct compared with NHL (**Table 1**). Approximately 85% of patients with HL will have intrathoracic lymphadenopathy at the time of initial diagnosis, compared with 50% of individuals with NHL.[7,8] Intrathoracic disease may be incidentally detected on imaging studies due to a lack of respiratory symptoms, while occasionally symptoms related to compression of mediastinal structures ranging from mild cough to SVC syndrome may prompt the workup.

Other lymphoid neoplasms including ALL and chronic lymphocytic leukemia (CLL) may affect the mediastinum similar to lymphoma. Hilar and mediastinal involvement by CLL has been reported in autopsy and radiographic series.[9] Although it is classically an indolent disease, CLL may also evolve into malignant lymphoma. Richter syndrome is described in up to 10% of patients and is characterized by transformation into

Table 1 Radiographic patterns of lymphoma		
Characteristics of	Hodgkin Lymphoma	Non-Hodgkin Lymphoma
Mediastinal disease	Nodular sclerosis most common abnormality Progressive and contiguous Asymmetric pattern Unilateral disease and single lymph node involvement less common	Large B-cell and lymphoblastic lymphoma most common abnormality Less predictable progression Less bulky Frequently not contiguous Single lymph node involvement may occur
Mediastinal predilection	Anterior mediastinum Superior mediastinum (prevascular, paratracheal), hilar, subcarinal, cardiophrenic, posterior mediastinum, internal mammary	Anterior mediastinum Posterior mediastinum Paracardiac node
Parenchymal disease	Often associated with mediastinal or hilar adenopathy	Frequently occurs in the absence of mediastinal disease

Data from Refs.[1,20,22,24,101,102]

an aggressive lymphoma. Manifestations may include systemic symptoms, extranodal involvement, or rapid increase in lymphadenopathy.[10] The associated prognosis is poor with an estimated survival of 10 months.[11] Patients with CLL are also at a higher risk for developing other secondary malignancies, including melanoma, sarcoma, and lung cancer.[12,13] Tissue sampling to differentiate between Richter syndrome versus a synchronous malignancy is therefore important.

Acute myelogenous leukemia (AML) has been demonstrated in autopsy series to affect the mediastinum, but this is typically not clinically significant unless it occurs in the form of a myeloid sarcoma (MS).[14] MS is a rare extramedullary tumor consisting of immature cells, and the mediastinum is the most common site for pulmonary involvement.[15,16] In most of these cases, the intrathoracic MS presented before or at the time of initial diagnosis of myelogenous leukemia.

Sampling of mediastinal tissue is required to confirm the diagnosis in patients with new or increased mediastinal lympadenopathy. Several studies have described the utility of endobronchial ultrasound-guided transbronchial needle aspiration in the diagnosis of de novo mediastinal lymphomas, identification of lymphoma subtypes, and differentiation from other alternate diagnoses.[17–19]

Parenchymal Disease

Infiltrates

Parenchymal disease is more common in HL, for as a group it affects the thorax more frequently, whereas up to 60% of NHL will present with intra-abdominal disease.[20,21] Distinct clinical and radiographic patterns have been described with the pattern of involvement closely correlating with lymphatic anatomy.[8,22] Sites of disease tend to occur at bifurcation points of the bronchi and pulmonary vasculature. Clinical symptoms vary, and if present, may include cough, chest discomfort, pleurisy, or respiratory insufficiency. Similar presentations may be noted on imaging (**Table 2**).

Primary HL arising in the lung without lymph node involvement is not common, but can occur.[20,22–24] Radiographic changes seen with pulmonary involvement include direct invasion from involved lymph nodes or via the bronchopulmonary lymphatics with peribronchial infiltrates, patchy pneumonic infiltrates, or parenchymal nodules (see **Table 2**).[21] Bronchial obstruction and associated atelectasis have also been described, but atelectasis is usually suggestive of concomitant endobronchial disease.

Table 2 Specific radiographic lymphomatous patterns of parenchymal disease	
Radiographic Pattern	Characteristics
Bronchovascular or lymphangitic	Most common in HL due to direct invasion from lymph nodes or via bronchopulmonary lymphatics Subsegmental or segmental distribution Air bronchograms
Nodular	Most common in NHL Single or multiple nodules, which may be round, oval, or ill defined. Nodules may vary in size May be located subpleural, parenchymal, or perihilar. Subpleural disease may appear to be plaquelike or as a mass May traverse lobar fissures Multiple, unilateral, or bilateral More common in lower lobes Cavitation may occur
Pneumonic (alveolar)	Segmental or lobar Unilateral or bilateral Often patchy Radiographically indistinguishable from bacterial pneumonia Typically does not cause volume loss
Miliary	Mostly noted with NHL due to hematogenous spread

Data from Refs.[1,20–22,24]

The radiographic patterns of NHL involvement in the lung may include nodular, pneumonic-alveolar, bronchovascular-lymphangitic, and miliary-hematogenous forms (see **Table 2**).[8] There is tendency for these patterns to overlap, and patients may present with several simultaneously.[1] Lymphomatous pulmonary nodules are the most frequent manifestation (**Fig. 1**). Initially, there is very little destruction of the alveolar wall by NHL, but eventually the lymphomatous infiltration tends to coalesce. Rarely, cavitation may be present. Lymphomatous infiltrates may spread in a perivascular and peribronchial distribution and result in coarse linear and reticulonodular infiltrates radiating outwards from the hilum. With more

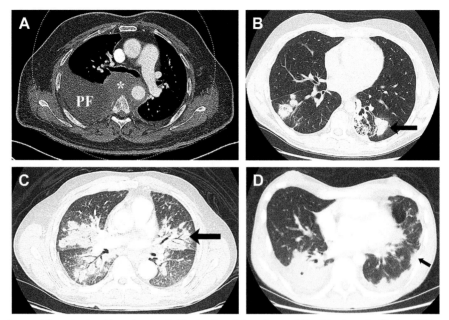

Fig. 1. Radiographic variants of lymphoma. Follicular B-cell lymphoma (*A*) with pleural effusion (PF) and mediastinal lymphadenopathy (*asterisk*). Peripheral T-cell lymphoma (*B*) with bilateral peripheral nodular opacities (*arrow*). Lymphomatoid granulomatosis (*C*) with widespread bilateral nodular consolidation (*arrow*) with air bronchograms. HL (*D*) with pleural-based nodularity (*arrow*) and parenchymal consolidation (*asterisk*).

extensive disease, a patchy infiltrate resembling bronchopneumonia may be present.

Radiographic patterns similar to lymphoma may be seen in patients with lymphoid leukemia such as ALL and CLL.[25] In those with CLL, infiltrates have also been reported to follow a peribronchial and perivascular pattern, with interstitial, centrilobular, and nodular patterns described.[9,26] In a series of 110 hospitalized patients with CLL, 9% had leukemic involvement affecting the lungs.[27] Tissue diagnosis may be obtained via transbronchial biopsies.[9]

Earlier autopsy series in leukemia patients documented pulmonary involvement, but clinical symptoms and/or radiographic findings were not present.[28,29] Patients with high levels of circulating malignant cells incidentally had more severe leukemic involvement at autopsy of the lungs, but infection, edema, and hemorrhage were the main sources of clinical symptoms.[14,29] Infection is still the predominant cause of pulmonary infiltrates in this immunosuppressed population, and bronchoalveolar lavage (BAL) is the preferred diagnostic modality.[30]

Pulmonary hemorrhage is more pronounced in those with severe thrombocytopenia, and clinically, this may manifest as diffuse alveolar hemorrhage.[29,31] Symptoms of dyspnea, cough, and hemoptysis along with radiographic imaging revealing diffuse bilateral ground glass opacities should raise clinical suspicion for this condition. Although BAL may provide additional diagnostic support, clinical correlation is essential, for localized bleeding may also occur in areas of infection and inflammation. These patients are often empirically treated with antimicrobial therapy along with correction of abnormal hematologic parameters.

Myeloid sarcoma

MS is an unusual extramedullary tumor of immature myeloid cells that is variably referred to as chloroma, granulocytic sarcoma, extramedullary leukemia, or myeloblastoma.[15,16,32] It may precede, accompany, or follow the diagnosis of acute or chronic leukemia. Approximately 2% to 5% of AML may develop MS, but it may also be seen in myelodysplastic syndrome (MDS) and myeloproliferative neoplasms.[32] The bone, periosteum, soft tissue, lymph nodes, and skin are most commonly involved, but reports have included descriptions of lung masses, intrathoracic lymphadenopathy, pleural-based nodules, and tracheobronchial disease.[16,33–37] In the series of intrathoracic MS by Takasugi and colleagues,[16] lung involvement was present in 18% of patients. Infiltrates have been described as either nodular, interstitial, or air space disease.[16] Biopsy of tissue may yield diagnosis based on morphology and special stains, including myeloperoxidase and immunohistochemical analysis.[38] The presence of MS has generally been associated with poor outcome and shorter overall survival, but the lack of concurrent AML may be favorable.[32,39]

Extramedullary hematopoiesis

Extramedullary hematopoiesis is the production of blood cells outside of the bone marrow, and this typically occurs when there is inadequate production of blood cells. It is a rare disorder, but has been described in myelofibrosis, chronic myeloid leukemia (CML), polycythemia vera, and MDS.[40] This phenomenon typically occurs in the spleen, liver, and lymph nodes but has been reported in all organs. The locations for extramedullary hematopoiesis usually correlate with sites of hematopoietic production during fetal life and early stages of life, so the marrow of vertebral bodies, sternum, ribs, femora, and tibiae are often involved.[41] Frequently, these are incidental findings on imaging studies, but they may present with symptomatic disease in the form of pleural effusions or pleural-based tumors, pulmonary hypertension (PH), subglottic stenosis, or acute respiratory failure.[40] Most cases of pulmonary extramedullary hematopoiesis have been reported concurrently with a known hematologic malignancy, but rarely, some cases present de novo. For example, a patient with a right lower lobe stenotic bronchus with no discrete endobronchial lesion was found to have extramedullary hematopoiesis following surgical resection and subsequently developed CML within a year.[42]

The most common intrathoracic manifestations are paraspinal masses, which are usually discovered incidentally. The paraspinal masses are typically bilateral, smooth-surfaced, soft tissue masses with areas of fat attenuation and no calcifications.[41] Diagnosis may be confirmed with surgical biopsy, fine needle aspiration, or technetium (Tc99m) radionuclide scanning. A single case report described a patient with acute respiratory failure due to pulmonary interstitial extramedullary hematopoiesis associated with myelofibrosis diagnosed via transbronchial biopsy.[43] Ectopic hematopoietic tissue is extremely sensitive to low doses of radiation, so in addition to treatment of underlying disorder, radiation may be therapeutic.[40] Two cases of PH and lung infiltrates attributed to extramedullary hematopoeisis have been reported to regress with radiation therapy, but the durability of this response has not been established.[44–46]

Pulmonary alveolar proteinosis

Pulmonary alveolar proteinosis (PAP) is a rare disorder characterized by deposition of intra-alveolar periodic acid-Schiff-positive protein and lipid-rich material. It is considered an autoimmune disease and is associated with a high titer of antibodies to granulocyte-macrophage colony stimulating factor (GM-CSF). Secondary PAP has been described in patients with hematologic malignancies, and although the GM-CSF pathway does not appear to be involved, macrophage dysfunction is postulated to contribute mechanistically.[47] Most cases have been described with myeloid neoplasms and their precursors, but lymphoid disorders have also been implicated. These patients may present with cough, dyspnea, or respiratory failure. Radiographic findings may vary from geographic ground-glass opacities, septal thickening, and consolidation to diffuse ground glass opacities.[48]

Diagnosis may be confirmed with BAL with retrieval of periodic acid-Schiff-positive proteinaceous material.[49] The combination of underlying immunosuppression, concomitant cytopenias, and loss of local pulmonary immunity places patients at risk for infection before, during, or after diagnosis of PAP. In particular, they are susceptible to a wide range of both common and unusual opportunistic pathogens, including aspergillosis, nocardiosis, and mycobacteria. Resolution of hematologic malignancy–associated PAP requires effective treatment of the underlying malignancy with chemotherapy or hematopoietic stem cell transplantation.[47]

Primary pulmonary lymphoma

Primary pulmonary lymphoma is a distinct entity that arises from lung tissue de novo.[50] Most likely originating from bronchus-associated lymphoid tissue, it represents a monoclonal proliferation of lymphoid tissue in the lungs with no detectable extrathoracic lymphoma for at least 3 months after initial diagnosis.[6] The most common type is low-grade marginal zone B-cell lymphoma or mucosa-associated lymphoid tissue (MALT) lymphoma. Other forms may include diffuse large B-cell lymphoma, follicular lymphoma, Burkitt lymphoma, T-cell lymphoma, and lymphomatoid granulomatosis. These variants may present with systemic symptoms or with localized respiratory complaints. This group has pulmonary manifestations similar to lymphoma.

Endobronchial Disease

Endobronchial disease has been described mostly in lymphoma, but can also occur in acute and chronic leukemia. Symptom severity varies widely and may include cough, dyspnea, wheezing, or stridor. Atelectasis, tracheal deviation, or an endobronchial mass seen on imaging may suggest airway disease. Lesions may present as a solitary mass or may be due to contiguous disease from the adjacent mediastinum or lung parenchyma.

Endobronchial lymphoma has been reported in both types of lymphoma, but more commonly with HL.[1] Rose and associates[51] described 2 distinct patterns of lymphomatous involvement (**Table 3**). Type 1 is the most common and occurs in patients with clinically apparent systemic lymphoma (**Fig. 2**). The presence of systemic disease suggests either hematogenous or lymphatic spread to bronchi. Some authors have suggested a preferential distribution at airway bifurcations.[52] Type 2 consists of a solitary mass involving the central airways without evidence of systemic lymphoma.[51] In those with regional adenopathy, endobronchial lymphoma may result from tumor extension from regional lymph nodes. Variants of B-cell (CLL) and T-cell (ALL) neoplasms may present similarly.[53–55]

AML affects the tracheobronchial tree in the form of bronchial chloroma (**Fig. 3**).[37,56,57] Diagnostic evaluation in the airway with endobronchial biopsy or fine needle aspiration may yield the diagnosis.

Pleural Disease

Pleural effusion

In patients with hematologic malignancies, pleural effusions may herald the diagnosis or indicate relapse. In those with symptoms, cough, dyspnea, chest pain, and pleurisy are prevalent. Given the inherent immune dysfunction, the possibility of infection is particularly concerning. In fact, in both autopsy and clinical series, parapneumonic effusions were the most common cause of pleural effusions in acute leukemia.[29,58] Certain therapeutic agents such as dasatinib are known to cause pleural effusions, and these may require initiation of steroids or dose interruption in addition to fluid drainage.[59] Other potential systemic causes, including thrombosis, liver dysfunction, cardiomyopathy, or renal insufficiency, should be excluded.

Diagnostic evaluation of a pleural effusion provides valuable information for clinical management. Cytology may not always reveal malignant cells or may contain circulating blood cells from the procedure itself (**Fig. 4**). Ascribing a pleural effusion to the underlying malignancy requires a process of eliminating other diagnoses. Confirmatory testing with cytology and flow cytometry is recommended even in those with transudative effusions.[58,60] The diagnostic yield of cytology in lymphoma and leukemia has been estimated to range from 61% to 75%.[58,60,61] In those with recurrent exudative pleural effusions without a clear diagnosis, pleural biopsies and/or bone marrow biopsy may be helpful.[62]

Lymphomas are the most common hematologic malignancies associated with pleural disease. Effusions occur in 30% of individuals with HL and in up to 20% of those with NHL, but are rarely the sole manifestation.[1] Concomitant mediastinal lymphadenopathy is present in 90% of HL and in 20% to 70% of NHL, but 90% of NHL will have extrathoracic disease.[1] The effusions are typically serous or serosanguinous and exudative by Light's criteria. Chylous effusions may be found in 19% of NHL and 3% of HL.[23,63,64] Pleural effusions are postulated to develop by either lymphomatous pleural infiltration, blockage of pleural lymphatic drainage by tumor, or adenopathy and obstruction of thoracic duct by tumor with resultant chylous effusion.

The prognostic impact of pleural effusions in lymphoma remains controversial. The presence of a pleural effusion in intermediate grade NHL at initial presentation does not seem to have an adverse effect on survival, but in a retrospective study of 91 patients with follicular low-grade

Table 3
Endobronchial patterns of lymphoma

	Type 1	Type 2
Lymphoma	Systemic Common with NHL	No systemic involvement Common with HL De novo[a] within BALT
Signs and symptoms	Pneumonitis	Airway obstruction, wheezing, cough
Airway involvement	Diffuse submucosal nodules in airway	Solitary mass
Other radiographic findings	Parenchymal infiltrates, mediastinal lymphadenopathy	Atelectasis, lymph node enlargement in proximity

Abbreviation: BALT, bronchial-associated lymphoid tissue.
[a] In cases with no regional involvement, lesions may arise de novo within bronchial-associated lymphoid tissue.
Data from Refs.[1,51,52]

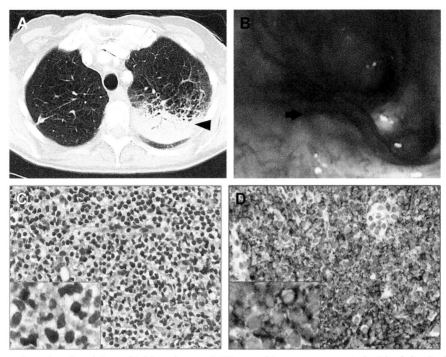

Fig. 2. Parenchymal and endobronchial lymphoma. A 75-year-old woman presented with abdominal mass and pulmonary infiltrate. Computed tomographic (CT) scan (*A*) showed left upper lobe consolidative opacities (*arrowhead*). (*B*) Bronchoscopy revealed smooth raised lesions (*arrow*) found overlying the left mainstem carina near the left upper lobe. Biopsies of the endobronchial abnormality and left upper lobe were obtained and revealed MALT lymphoma. Similar histologic features of both areas were noted with a dense lymphoid infiltrates composed of predominantly small lymphocytes with irregular nuclei, condensed chromatin, and small to moderate amounts of pale cytoplasm (*C*, H&E stain, original magnification ×20, Inset ×50). Occasionally, large cells and plasma cells are present. Anti-CD20 immunohistochemistry demonstrates lymphocytes are B-cells in endobronchial biopsy (*D*, H&E stain, original magnification ×20, Inset ×50). (Bronchoscopic images *Courtesy of* Roberto F. Casal, MD; and pathologic images *Courtesy of* Wei Wang, MD, Houston, TX.)

lymphoma, pleural effusions did adversely affect survival.[65,66] Another smaller study of 57 patients with high-grade NHL revealed an overall 50% disease-free survival after initial treatment, but pleural effusions were noted in 17 patients at presentation and associated with an extremely poor outcome.[67]

Pleural effusions in CLL are less commonly described, but autopsy studies revealed pleural involvement in 3% to 16% of CLL.[9] Pleural fluid analysis typically reveals a lymphocytic exudate, but chylous and hemorrhagic effusions have also been reported.[62] Malignant pleural effusions (MPEs) have primarily been described in patients with advanced disease, and in the largest series following 110 patients hospitalized over 9 years, the incidence was 7%.[27] Interestingly, although 7 had CLL, 2 were found to have Richter's syndrome and 1 had adenocarcinoma. A new exudative effusion in a patient with CLL should therefore heighten clinical suspicion for either disease progression or synchronous malignancy.

Pleural effusions in acute leukemia, MDS, and myeloproliferative neoplasms are rare. The effusion may be the manifestation of systemic disease or rarely a form of extramedullary hematopoiesis (most notably in myeloproliferative disease). A recent large series described 111 such patients over a 10-year period, and the most frequent cause for the effusions was infection (47%), followed by malignancy (36%).[58] MPEs were typically exudates, serosanguinous or sanguineous, and larger in volume (greater than 1.5 L). The study found that overall survival correlated with the underlying malignancy rather than the presence of a pleural effusion, but a pleural effusion did portend more aggressive disease if the malignancy was diagnosed within 6 months.[58]

In solid organ malignancies, the presence of an MPE is a hallmark of advanced disease and poor prognosis, but the prognostic impact of MPEs in hematologic malignancies is less clear. With the exception of lymphoma, the data regarding MPEs in hematologic malignancies are sparse. A retrospective review in hospitalized patients

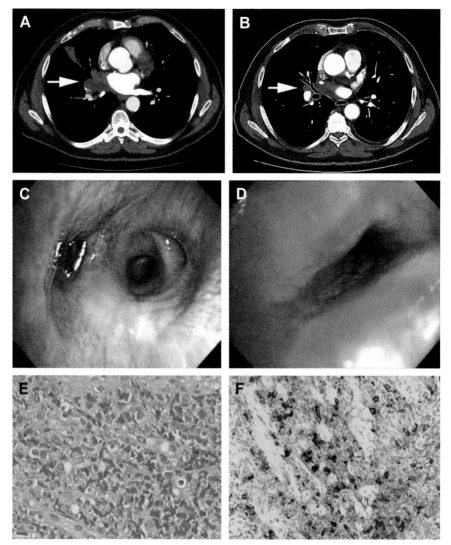

Fig. 3. Bronchial chloroma. A 64-year-old man with AML in remission undergoing consolidation chemotherapy presented with right middle lobe infiltrate with a hilar mass (*arrow*) occluding the right middle lobe bronchus (*A*). Imaging after treatment revealed reduction in right hilar mass (*arrow*) and resolution of narrowing of right middle lobe aperture (*B*). Bronchoscopy revealed narrowed right middle lobe aperture (*C, D*) and endobronchial biopsy demonstrated AML in the bronchial mucosa (*E*, H&E, original magnification ×20). Immunohistochemical studies demonstrated positive for myeloperoxidase in neoplastic cells (*F*, original magnification ×20). (*Reprinted from* Faiz SA, Ordonez NG, Morice RC, et al. Bronchial chloroma. Am J Respir Crit Care Med 2014;190(2):e5–6; with permission of the American Thoracic Society.)

with lymphoproliferative disorders and MPEs identified a high pleural fluid to serum lactate dehydrogenase level as a predictor of malignant pleural involvement and hospital mortality.[68] Interestingly, in a recently validated prognostic score, the presence of a hematologic malignancy was found to be favorable, but the proportion of hematologic malignancies in their cohorts was less than 7% overall.[69] It appears the significance of MPEs in these patients varies based on the characteristics of the underlying malignancy, but further study is needed.

Vascular Complications

Leukostasis

Leukostasis is characterized by diffuse accumulations of leukemic cells in minor vessels. It tends to occur in brain, lungs, heart, and testes in myeloid leukemia.[70] In autopsy studies, patients typically had hyperleukocytosis, and pulmonary leukostasis was characterized by leukemic cells occupying significant portions of the vascular lumen, with or without the presence of fibrin.[29] Involvement of small arteries, arterioles, capillaries, and venules

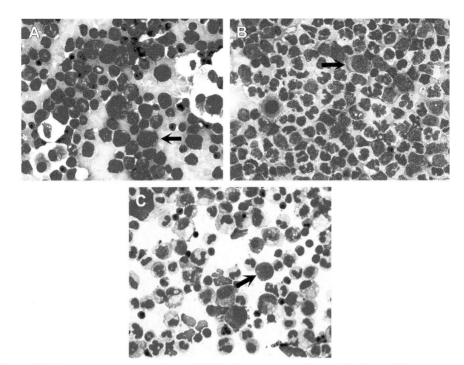

Fig. 4. Pleural fluid cytology in acute leukemia (Diff-Quik stain, original magnification ×400). Acute lymphocytic leukemia noted to have exudative pleural effusion with numerous lymphoblasts (A). A lymphoblast (*arrow*) is a naive lymphocyte that further differentiates and is characterized as round large cells with less distinct nucleoli, condensed chromatin, and scant cytoplasm. AML with progressive disease noted to have exudative pleural effusion with numerous blasts (B). Myeloblasts (*arrow*) are immature granulocytic cells with large nuclei, prominent nucleoli, less condensed nuclear chromatin, and variable amounts of cytoplasmic granules. (C) A patient with AML and an underlying exudative effusion, but in contrast to others, there are immature granulocytes and rare blasts (*arrow*) noted on the slide. Clinical correlation was needed to discern if these findings represented peripheral blood contamination due to circulating blasts in the blood or are more consistent with MPE. The latter was decided clinically. (Pathologic images *Courtesy of* John Stewart, MD, Houston, TX.)

was noted. Radiographically, leukostasis is unlikely to be detected on chest radiographs, but it should be suspected in those developing pulmonary edema with hyperleukocytosis.[70] Cytoreductive therapy may reduce pulmonary leukostasis.

Pseudohypoxemia

Arterial blood gas sampling is commonly used to determine adequate gas exchange in patients; however, in those with significant hyperleukocytosis or thrombocytosis, pseudohypoxemia may be observed. Initially described by Hess and colleagues,[71] the Pao_2 of blood at room temperature decreases at a faster rate in patients with increased numbers of circulating leukocytes or platelets and may thus result in a factitious diagnosis of hypoxemia. In vitro studies demonstrated a decline in Pao_2 due to oxygen consumption by both normal and abnormal leukocytes, but the leukocyte oxygen consumption in those with extreme and immature leukocytosis was extremely rapid.[72] Also referred to as "leukocyte larceny," this phenomenon should be suspected in those with hypoxemia out of proportion to pulmonary symptoms and/or a paucity of pulmonary abnormality on imaging.[73,74] Cooling of arterial blood samples and rapid analysis may improve the reliability of such Pao_2 readings. Pulse oximetry will typically be normal in these patients.

Superior vena cava syndrome

SVC syndrome refers to a constellation of symptoms resulting from either extrinsic compression or intrinsic obstruction of the SVC. The severity of symptoms varies depending on the degree of SVC compromise and acuity of onset. Common symptoms may include facial and neck swelling, cough, dyspnea, and orthopnea. Symptoms typically worsen with bending over or lying down. Hoarseness, stridor, syncope, headache, dizziness, and facial plethora are rare.[75,76] Physical examination may reveal facial and periorbital edema, jugular venous distention, venous collaterals on the chest and abdomen, and edema of the neck and upper chest, and rarely, papilledema (**Fig. 5**).

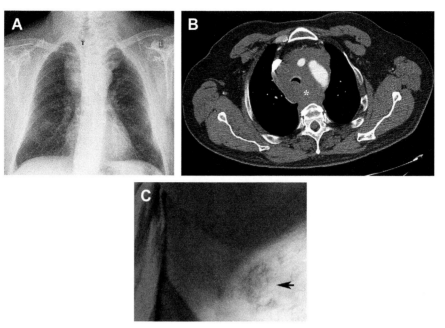

Fig. 5. SVC syndrome. A 65-year-old man with follicular B-cell lymphoma who presented with periorbital and facial edema with neck swelling. Chest radiograph (*A*) revealed mediastinal widening with tracheal (T) deviation from left to right. CT chest scan (*B*) reveals soft tissue abnormality extending from the left supraclavicular region encasing the vessels, and extending down into the mediastinum to surround the aorta (*asterisk*). Differential includes thymoma, metastatic lung malignancy, and lymphoma. Venous collaterals (*arrow*) in a 65-year-old woman with SVC obstruction due to small cell lung cancer (*C*).

Clinical history and radiographic imaging can usually distinguish extrinsic versus intrinsic causes. Extrinsic compression typically involves a superior mediastinal mass located on the right side, and a histologic diagnosis is typically needed to direct further therapies.[77] Lung cancer accounts for most of the malignant causes of SVC syndrome, but lymphoma may be the culprit in up to 12%.[75] A large case series reported a 3.9% incidence of SVC syndrome among all patients with lymphoma, mainly large cell and lymphoblastic NHL.[78] There have only been a few isolated reports of HL resulting in SVC syndrome.[78] Rarely, MS may also present with SVC syndrome, and it typically has complex cytogenetics with poor prognosis.[79] The cause of the SVC syndrome dictates further management. Chemotherapy is the initial treatment for lymphoma, because it provides both local and systemic therapeutic effect. Radiotherapy after completion of chemotherapy may be beneficial in those with large cell lymphoma that have masses greater than 10 cm.[78]

Thromboembolic disease

The association between malignancy and venous thrombosis is well established, but the risk of thrombosis and hematologic malignancies has recently become more evident. In a large population-based, case-controlled study to identify risk factors for venous thrombosis, a 7-fold increase in overall risk of venous thrombosis in patients with malignancy and a 28-fold increase in those with hematologic malignancies compared with those without cancer were discovered.[80] The highest risk for venous thrombosis was in hematologic malignancies, followed by lung and gastrointestinal cancer. The risk was particularly elevated during the first few months after diagnosis and in the presence of distant metastases. Conversely, the risk for a new diagnosis of cancer appears elevated for at least 2 years after a first episode of venous thrombosis, and this was particularly significant in those with ovarian cancer, HL, and NHL.[81]

Thrombocytopenia and a diagnosis within 12 months were identified in most acute leukemia patients as a risk factor for venous thromboembolism, and in a large single-center 6-year study, 15% of ALL patients and 8% of AML patients developed pulmonary embolism.[82] Further studies specifically in patients with leukemia and lymphoma have demonstrated additional contributing factors for thrombosis, including central venous catheters, hematopoietic growth factors, high-dose corticosteroids, L-asparaginase, and new immunomodulatory agents.[83–86] Unfortunately, evidence-based trials for the treatment of venous thomboembolism in those with thrombocytopenia are lacking. Currently, guidelines recommend a reduction of therapeutic low-molecular-weight heparin by 50% with a platelet count of 25 to 50 K/uL and discontinuation of anticoagulation less than 25 K/uL.[87] Thromboprophylaxis is recommended in patients with cancer that are considered high risk for thrombosis due to their cancer or current therapy, those hospitalized with an acute medical illness, and those in the postoperative period following major surgery and/or abdominal or pelvic surgery for cancer.[88] Further study for both treatment and thromboprophylaxis in those with thrombocytopenia is needed.

Thrombotic disease is a significant cause of morbidity and mortality in Philadelphia-chromosome-negative myeloproliferative neoplasms, particularly polycythemia vera and essential thrombocythemia.[89] Their acquired thrombophilic states are attributed to a combination of abnormalities of blood cells resulting in a prothrombotic phenotype and the host inflammatory response. The spectrum of thrombotic manifestations varies from microcirculatory disturbances to venous and arterial thrombosis. Chronic thromboembolic pulmonary hypertension (CTEPH) was the presenting symptom in some patients diagnosed with myeloproliferative disease, and subsequent treatment with thromboendarterectomy and pulmonary vasodilators has been described.[90] Myelosuppressive drugs (eg, hydroxyurea) may reduce the patient's thrombotic risk, but it may also accelerate the rate of leukemic transformation.

Pulmonary hypertension

The role of malignancy in PH has not been well described, and patients with cancer may develop PH after cancer diagnosis or as a result of cancer-related treatments. In general, the diagnostic workup for PH should follow established guidelines, and treatment for those with pulmonary arterial hypertension (PAH) should be administered in conjunction with a PAH-specialized center.[91] Patients with myeloproliferative neoplasms and CML have been described to develop PH.[46,92] The literature to date has mostly been in the form of case reports and small series, so the true prevalence of PH in this population remains unclear.[90,93–97] Although the exact pathogenesis of PH in these patients may be variable, potential pathophysiologic mechanisms related to the underlying hematologic malignancies include CTEPH, portal hypertension, extramedullary hematopoiesis, toxicity due to chemotherapy, or occlusion of pulmonary capillary bed due to aberrant, excessive, or immature cells.[46] Therapies described for PH secondary to malignancy described include cytoreductive therapy, antithrombotic agents, hematologic control of the malignancy, and pulmonary-specific vasodilators, but randomized trials are lacking.[46] The authors' group has described the resolution of PAH and myelofibrosis after allogeneic hematopoietic transplantation in one patient.[98]

The most notable chemotherapeutic agent associated with PAH is dasatinib, which is a tyrosine kinase inhibitor used to treat CML and Philadelphia-positive ALL. It has rarely been reported to cause moderate to severe precapillary PAH with functional and hemodynamic impairment with an estimated incidence of 0.45%.[92,99] Duration of dasatinib treatment before PAH onset ranged from 1 week to 75 months.[99,100] Although cessation of drug and initiation of PAH-specific therapy is often needed, most patients will have improvement or resolution of PAH.[99,100] The cause of dasatinib-induced PAH remains unclear, but immune mechanisms are suspected. Screening of patients for cardiopulmonary disease before initiation of therapy and/or during therapy if symptoms develop has been recommended.[100]

SUMMARY

Intrathoracic lymph nodes, lung parenchyma, the pleura, and pulmonary vasculature may all be affected by lymphoma, leukemia, or their precursors. Patients may present with one or multiple pulmonary manifestations. Recognition of clinical and radiographic patterns will facilitate prompt diagnosis, and appropriate diagnostic interventions should be obtained in those with unclear causes. After possible infection and drug toxicity are addressed, treatment of the underlying malignancy is often the key to successful management.

REFERENCES

1. Berkman N, Breuer R, Kramer MR, et al. Pulmonary involvement in lymphoma. Leuk Lymphoma 1996; 20(3–4):229–37.
2. Duwe BV, Sterman DH, Musani AI. Tumors of the mediastinum. Chest 2005;128(4):2893–909.
3. Portell CA, Sweetenham JW. Adult lymphoblastic lymphoma. Cancer J 2012;18(5):432–8.
4. van Besien K, Kelta M, Bahaguna P. Primary mediastinal B-cell lymphoma: a review of pathology and management. J Clin Oncol 2001;19(6):1855–64.
5. Shaffer K, Smith D, Kirn D, et al. Primary mediastinal large-B-cell lymphoma: radiologic findings at

presentation. AJR Am J Roentgenol 1996;167(2):425–30.

6. Kligerman SJ, Franks TJ, Galvin JR. Primary extranodal lymphoma of the thorax. Radiol Clin North Am 2016;54(4):673–87.

7. Castellino RA. Diagnostic imaging evaluation of Hodgkin's disease and non-Hodgkin's lymphoma. Cancer 1991;67(4 Suppl):1177–80.

8. Balikian JP, Herman PG. Non-Hodgkin lymphoma of the lungs. Radiology 1979;132(3):569–76.

9. Berkman N, Polliack A, Breuer R, et al. Pulmonary involvement as the major manifestation of chronic lymphocytic leukemia. Leuk Lymphoma 1992;8(6):495–9.

10. Robertson LE, Pugh W, O'Brien S, et al. Richter's syndrome: a report on 39 patients. J Clin Oncol 1993;11(10):1985–9.

11. Jain P, O'Brien S. Richter's transformation in chronic lymphocytic leukemia. Oncology (Williston Park) 2012;26(12):1146–52.

12. Greene MH, Hoover RN, Fraumeni JF Jr. Subsequent cancer in patients with chronic lymphocytic leukemia–a possible immunologic mechanism. J Natl Cancer Inst 1978;61(2):337–40.

13. Tsimberidou AM, Wen S, McLaughlin P, et al. Other malignancies in chronic lymphocytic leukemia/small lymphocytic lymphoma. J Clin Oncol 2009;27(6):904–10.

14. Ross JS, Ellman L. Leukemic infiltration of the lungs in the chemotherapeutic era. Am J Clin Pathol 1974;61(2):235–41.

15. Wang HQ, Li J. Clinicopathological features of myeloid sarcoma: report of 39 cases and literature review. Pathol Res Pract 2016;212(9):817–24.

16. Takasugi JE, Godwin JD, Marglin SI, et al. Intrathoracic granulocytic sarcomas. J Thorac Imaging 1996;11(3):223–30.

17. Moonim MT, Breen R, Fields PA, et al. Diagnosis and subtyping of de novo and relapsed mediastinal lymphomas by endobronchial ultrasound needle aspiration. Am J Respir Crit Care Med 2013;188(10):1216–23.

18. Ko HM, da Cunha Santos G, Darling G, et al. Diagnosis and subclassification of lymphomas and non-neoplastic lesions involving mediastinal lymph nodes using endobronchial ultrasound-guided transbronchial needle aspiration. Diagn Cytopathol 2013;41(12):1023–30.

19. Grosu HB, Iliesiu M, Caraway NP, et al. Endobronchial ultrasound-guided transbronchial needle aspiration for the diagnosis and subtyping of lymphoma. Ann Am Thorac Soc 2015;12(9):1336–44.

20. Filly R, Bland N, Castellino RA. Radiographic distribution of intrathoracic disease in previously untreated patients with Hodgkin's disease and non-Hodgkin's lymphoma. Radiology 1976;120(2):277–81.

21. Bragg DG. The clinical, pathologic and radiographic spectrum of the intrathoracic lymphomas. Invest Radiol 1978;13(1):2–11.

22. MacDonald JB. Lung involvement in Hodgkin's disease. Thorax 1977;32(6):664–7.

23. Johnson DW, Hoppe RT, Cox RS, et al. Hodgkin's disease limited to intrathoracic sites. Cancer 1983;52(1):8–13.

24. Fishman EK, Kuhlman JE, Jones RJ. CT of lymphoma: spectrum of disease. Radiographics 1991;11(4):647–69.

25. Okada F, Ando Y, Kondo Y, et al. Thoracic CT findings of adult T-cell leukemia or lymphoma. AJR Am J Roentgenol 2004;182(3):761–7.

26. Moore W, Baram D, Hu Y. Pulmonary infiltration from chronic lymphocytic leukemia. J Thorac Imaging 2006;21(2):172–5.

27. Ahmed S, Siddiqui AK, Rossoff L, et al. Pulmonary complications in chronic lymphocytic leukemia. Cancer 2003;98(9):1912–7.

28. Green RANN. Pulmonary involvement in leukemia. Am Rev Respir Dis 1959;80:833–44.

29. Bodey GP, Powell RD Jr, Hersh EM, et al. Pulmonary complications of acute leukemia. Cancer 1966;19(6):781–93.

30. Chellapandian D, Lehrnbecher T, Phillips B, et al. Bronchoalveolar lavage and lung biopsy in patients with cancer and hematopoietic stem-cell transplantation recipients: a systematic review and meta-analysis. J Clin Oncol 2015;33(5):501–9.

31. Nanjappa S, Jeong DK, Muddaraju M, et al. Diffuse alveolar hemorrhage in acute myeloid leukemia. Cancer Control 2016;23(3):272–7.

32. Paydas S, Zorludemir S, Ergin M. Granulocytic sarcoma: 32 cases and review of the literature. Leuk Lymphoma 2006;47(12):2527–41.

33. Sathyanarayanan V, Sirsath NT, Das U, et al. An unusual case of pulmonary granulocytic sarcoma treated with combined chemotherapy and radiation. Ecancermedicalscience 2013;7:368.

34. Yam LT. Granulocytic sarcoma with pleural involvement. Identification of neoplastic cells with cytochemistry. Acta Cytol 1985;29(1):63–6.

35. Guimaraes MD, Marchiori E, Marom EM, et al. Pulmonary granulocytic sarcoma (chloroma) mimicking an opportunistic infection in a patient with acute myeloid leukemia. Ann Hematol 2014;93(2):327–8.

36. Thawani R, Chichra A, Mahajan A, et al. Granulocytic sarcoma of the lung in acute myeloid leukemia. Indian Pediatr 2014;51(2):145–6.

37. Genet P, Pulik M, Lionnet F, et al. Leukemic relapse presenting with bronchial obstruction caused by granulocytic sarcoma. Am J Hematol 1994;47(2):142–3.

38. Klco JM, Welch JS, Nguyen TT, et al. State of the art in myeloid sarcoma. Int J Lab Hematol 2011;33(6):555–65.

39. Tsimberidou AM, Kantarjian HM, Wen S, et al. Myeloid sarcoma is associated with superior event-free survival and overall survival compared with acute myeloid leukemia. Cancer 2008;113(6): 1370–8.

40. Koch CA, Li CY, Mesa RA, et al. Nonhepatosplenic extramedullary hematopoiesis: associated diseases, pathology, clinical course, and treatment. Mayo Clin Proc 2003;78(10):1223–33.

41. Roberts AS, Shetty AS, Mellnick VM, et al. Extramedullary haematopoiesis: radiological imaging features. Clin Radiol 2016;71(9):807–14.

42. Gowitt GT, Zaatari GS. Bronchial extramedullary hematopoiesis preceding chronic myelogenous leukemia. Hum Pathol 1985;16(10):1069–71.

43. Yusen RD, Kollef MH. Acute respiratory failure due to extramedullary hematopoiesis. Chest 1995; 108(4):1170–2.

44. Rumi E, Passamonti F, Boveri E, et al. Dyspnea secondary to pulmonary hematopoiesis as presenting symptom of myelofibrosis with myeloid metaplasia. Am J Hematol 2006;81(2):124–7.

45. Steensma DP, Hook CC, Stafford SL, et al. Low-dose, single-fraction, whole-lung radiotherapy for pulmonary hypertension associated with myelofibrosis with myeloid metaplasia. Br J Haematol 2002;118(3):813–6.

46. Machado RF, Farber HW. Pulmonary hypertension associated with chronic hemolytic anemia and other blood disorders. Clin Chest Med 2013; 34(4):739–52.

47. Chaulagain CP, Pilichowska M, Brinckerhoff L, et al. Secondary pulmonary alveolar proteinosis in hematologic malignancies. Hematol Oncol Stem Cell Ther 2014;7(4):127–35.

48. Chung JH, Pipavath SJ, Myerson DH, et al. Secondary pulmonary alveolar proteinosis: a confusing and potentially serious complication of hematologic malignancy. J Thorac Imaging 2009;24(2):115–8.

49. Cordonnier C, Fleury-Feith J, Escudier E, et al. Secondary alveolar proteinosis is a reversible cause of respiratory failure in leukemic patients. Am J Respir Crit Care Med 1994;149(3 Pt 1):788–94.

50. Solomonov A, Zuckerman T, Goralnik L, et al. Non-Hodgkin's lymphoma presenting as an endobronchial tumor: report of eight cases and literature review. Am J Hematol 2008;83(5):416–9.

51. Rose RM, Grigas D, Strattemeir E, et al. Endobronchial involvement with non-Hodgkin's lymphoma. A clinical-radiologic analysis. Cancer 1986;57(9): 1750–5.

52. Gallagher CJ, Knowles GK, Habeshaw JA, et al. Early involvement of the bronchi in patients with malignant lymphoma. Br J Cancer 1983;48(6): 777–81.

53. Chernoff A, Rymuza J, Lippmann ML. Endobronchial lymphocytic infiltration. Unusual manifestation of chronic lymphocytic leukemia. Am J Med 1984; 77(4):755–9.

54. Otsuka K, Kuronuma K, Otsuka M, et al. A case of adult T cell leukemia/lymphoma presenting as severe tracheal stenosis. Intern Med 2011;50(21):2637–41.

55. Milkowski DA, Worley BD, Morris MJ. Richter's transformation presenting as an obstructing endobronchial lesion. Chest 1999;116(3):832–5.

56. Faiz SA, Ordonez NG, Morice RC, et al. Bronchial chloroma. Am J Respir Crit Care Med 2014; 190(2):e5–6.

57. Stafford CM, Herndier B, Yi ES, et al. Granulocytic sarcoma of the tracheobronchial tree: bronchoscopic and pathologic correlation. Respiration 2004;71(5):529–32.

58. Faiz SA, Bashoura L, Lei X, et al. Pleural effusions in patients with acute leukemia and myelodysplastic syndrome. Leuk Lymphoma 2013;54(2):329–35.

59. Brixey AG, Light RW. Pleural effusions due to dasatinib. Curr Opin Pulm Med 2010;16(4):351–6.

60. Porcel JM, Esquerda A, Vives M, et al. Etiology of pleural effusions: analysis of more than 3,000 consecutive thoracenteses. Arch Bronconeumol 2014;50(5):161–5.

61. Johnston WW. The malignant pleural effusion. A review of cytopathologic diagnoses of 584 specimens from 472 consecutive patients. Cancer 1985;56(4):905–9.

62. Faiz SA, Sahay S, Jimenez CA. Pleural effusions in acute and chronic leukemia and myelodysplastic syndrome. Curr Opin Pulm Med 2014;20(4):340–6.

63. Xaubet A, Diumenjo MC, Marin A, et al. Characteristics and prognostic value of pleural effusions in non-Hodgkin's lymphomas. Eur J Respir Dis 1985;66(2):135–40.

64. Das DK, Gupta SK, Ayyagari S, et al. Pleural effusions in non-Hodgkin's lymphoma. A cytomorphologic, cytochemical and immunologic study. Acta Cytol 1987;31(2):119–24.

65. Elis A, Blickstein D, Mulchanov I, et al. Pleural effusion in patients with non-Hodgkin's lymphoma: a case-controlled study. Cancer 1998;83(8):1607–11.

66. Morel P, Dupriez B, Plantier-Colcher I, et al. Long-term outcome of follicular low-grade lymphoma. A report of 91 patients. Ann Hematol 1993;66(6): 303–8.

67. Kirn D, Mauch P, Shaffer K, et al. Large-cell and immunoblastic lymphoma of the mediastinum: prognostic features and treatment outcome in 57 patients. J Clin Oncol 1993;11(7):1336–43.

68. Ahmed S, Shahid RK, Rimawi R, et al. Malignant pleural effusions in lymphoproliferative disorders. Leuk Lymphoma 2005;46(7):1039–44.

69. Clive AO, Kahan BC, Hooper CE, et al. Predicting survival in malignant pleural effusion: development and validation of the LENT prognostic score. Thorax 2014;69(12):1098–104.

70. van Buchem MA, Wondergem JH, Kool LJ, et al. Pulmonary leukostasis: radiologic-pathologic study. Radiology 1987;165(3):739–41.

71. Hess CE, Nichols AB, Hunt WB, et al. Pseudohypoxemia secondary to leukemia and thrombocytosis. N Engl J Med 1979;301(7):361–3.

72. Chillar RK, Belman MJ, Farbstein M. Explanation for apparent hypoxemia associated with extreme leukocytosis: leukocytic oxygen consumption. Blood 1980;55(6):922–4.

73. Fox MJ, Brody JS, Weintraub LR. Leukocyte larceny: a cause of spurious hypoxemia. Am J Med 1979;67(5):742–6.

74. Horr S, Roberson R, Hollingsworth JW. Pseudohypoxemia in a patient with chronic lymphocytic leukemia. Respir Care 2013;58(3):e31–3.

75. Wilson LD, Detterbeck FC, Yahalom J. Clinical practice. Superior vena cava syndrome with malignant causes. N Engl J Med 2007;356(18):1862–9.

76. Cheng S. Superior vena cava syndrome: a contemporary review of a historic disease. Cardiol Rev 2009;17(1):16–23.

77. Armstrong BA, Perez CA, Simpson JR, et al. Role of irradiation in the management of superior vena cava syndrome. Int J Radiat Oncol Biol Phys 1987;13(4):531–9.

78. Perez-Soler R, McLaughlin P, Velasquez WS, et al. Clinical features and results of management of superior vena cava syndrome secondary to lymphoma. J Clin Oncol 1984;2(4):260–6.

79. Ramasamy K, Lim Z, Pagliuca A, et al. Acute myeloid leukaemia presenting with mediastinal myeloid sarcoma: report of three cases and review of literature. Leuk Lymphoma 2007;48(2):290–4.

80. Blom JW, Doggen CJ, Osanto S, et al. Malignancies, prothrombotic mutations, and the risk of venous thrombosis. JAMA 2005;293(6):715–22.

81. Murchison JT, Wylie L, Stockton DL. Excess risk of cancer in patients with primary venous thromboembolism: a national, population-based cohort study. Br J Cancer 2004;91(1):92–5.

82. Vu K, Luong NV, Hubbard J, et al. A retrospective study of venous thromboembolism in acute leukemia patients treated at the University of Texas MD Anderson Cancer Center. Cancer Med 2015;4(1):27–35.

83. Huybers P, Wunsch C. Paleophysical oceanography with an emphasis on transport rates. Annu Rev Mar Sci 2010;2:1–34.

84. Falanga A, Marchetti M, Russo L. Venous thromboembolism in the hematologic malignancies. Curr Opin Oncol 2012;24(6):702–10.

85. Elice F, Rodeghiero F. Hematologic malignancies and thrombosis. Thromb Res 2012;129(3):360–6.

86. Simkovic M, Vodarek P, Motyckova M, et al. Venous thromboembolism in patients with chronic lymphocytic leukemia. Thromb Res 2015;136(6):1082–6.

87. Carrier M, Khorana AA, Zwicker J, et al. Management of challenging cases of patients with cancer-associated thrombosis including recurrent thrombosis and bleeding: guidance from the SSC of the ISTH. J Thromb Haemost 2013;11(9):1760–5.

88. Lyman GH, Khorana AA, Kuderer NM, et al. Venous thromboembolism prophylaxis and treatment in patients with cancer: American Society of Clinical Oncology clinical practice guideline update. J Clin Oncol 2013;31(17):2189–204.

89. Falanga A, Marchetti M. Thrombotic disease in the myeloproliferative neoplasms. Hematology Am Soc Hematol Educ Program 2012;2012:571–81.

90. Guilpain P, Montani D, Damaj G, et al. Pulmonary hypertension associated with myeloproliferative disorders: a retrospective study of ten cases. Respiration 2008;76(3):295–302.

91. McLaughlin VV, Shah SJ, Souza R, et al. Management of pulmonary arterial hypertension. J Am Coll Cardiol 2015;65(18):1976–97.

92. Simonneau G, Gatzoulis MA, Adatia I, et al. Updated clinical classification of pulmonary hypertension. J Am Coll Cardiol 2013;62(25 Suppl):D34–41.

93. Garcia-Manero G, Schuster SJ, Patrick H, et al. Pulmonary hypertension in patients with myelofibrosis secondary to myeloproliferative diseases. Am J Hematol 1999;60(2):130–5.

94. Garypidou V, Vakalopoulou S, Dimitriadis D, et al. Incidence of pulmonary hypertension in patients with chronic myeloproliferative disorders. Haematologica 2004;89(2):245–6.

95. Marvin KS, Spellberg RD. Pulmonary hypertension secondary to thrombocytosis in a patient with myeloid metaplasia. Chest 1993;103(2):642–4.

96. Nand S, Orfei E. Pulmonary hypertension in polycythemia vera. Am J Hematol 1994;47(3):242–4.

97. Reisner SA, Rinkevich D, Markiewicz W, et al. Cardiac involvement in patients with myeloproliferative disorders. Am J Med 1992;93(5):498–504.

98. Faiz SA, Iliescu C, Lopez-Mattei J, et al. Resolution of myelofibrosis-associated pulmonary arterial hypertension following allogeneic hematopoietic stem cell transplantation. Pulm Circ 2016;6(4):611–3.

99. Montani D, Bergot E, Gunther S, et al. Pulmonary arterial hypertension in patients treated by dasatinib. Circulation 2012;125(17):2128–37.

100. Shah NP, Wallis N, Farber HW, et al. Clinical features of pulmonary arterial hypertension in patients receiving dasatinib. Am J Hematol 2015;90(11):1060–4.

101. Castellino RA, Blank N, Hoppe RT, et al. Hodgkin disease: contributions of chest CT in the initial staging evaluation. Radiology 1986;160(3):603–5.

102. North LB, Fuller LM, Hagemeister FB, et al. Importance of initial mediastinal adenopathy in Hodgkin disease. AJR Am J Roentgenol 1982;138(2):229–35.

Complications of Cancer Treatment

Radiation Pneumonitis

Trevor J. Bledsoe, MD, Sameer K. Nath, MD*, Roy H. Decker, MD, PhD

KEYWORDS

- Radiation pneumonitis • Radiation complications • Radiation fibrosis

KEY POINTS

- Patients undergoing thoracic radiotherapy are at risk for radiation pneumonitis.
- Symptoms include shortness of breath, low-grade fever, and cough.
- Diagnosis includes correlation between symptoms, imaging findings, and radiation history.
- Imaging studies often demonstrate patchy consolidation within the area of the high-dose radiation field and do not conform to normal lobar anatomy. Imaging findings may not correlate with symptoms.
- High-dose glucocorticoid therapy is the backbone of therapy and results in symptom improvement in most patients.

INTRODUCTION

Although radiation therapy provides the backbone of primary and adjuvant therapy for several thoracic malignancies, the lungs have long been known to be exquisitely sensitive to the deleterious effects of ionizing radiation. In fact, within three years of the discovery of x-rays, the first incidence of radiation pneumonitis was described in 1898 during the treatment of a patient with tuberculosis.[1] Radiation-induced lung injury is now a well-known complication of patients undergoing thoracic radiation for lung, esophageal, breast, thymic, and hematologic malignancies. This sensitivity of normal lung parenchyma typically remains the dose-limiting factor for radiotherapy of chest malignancies. However, with the advent of modern treatment planning and the adherence to well-established dosimetric predictors of pneumonitis, the risk of radiation pneumonitis has been significantly mitigated. Patients treated with thoracic radiation for non-lung cancers are typically treated using similar radiation techniques as patients with primary lung cancer. However, patients receiving radiotherapy for non-lung cancer malignancies are generally treated to a lower total radiation dose and volume of lung and therefore have a lower risk of developing radiation pneumonitis. As such, most of the data regarding radiation pneumonitis is derived from the treatment of lung cancer; however, this clinical syndrome is similar regardless of the primary tumor type, and therefore, extrapolation to non-pulmonary tumors is appropriate. In this article, the authors review the modern understanding of radiation-induced lung injury, including the pathophysiology, diagnosis, management options, and complications.

RADIOBIOLOGY OF RADIATION THERAPY

As radiation passes through soft tissue, energy is locally deposited in packets that have sufficient strength to break strong chemical bonds and generate free radicals, primarily in water molecules. These secondary free radicals may lead to interactions with DNA, and to a lesser degree, lipids and proteins, resulting in alterations to their biochemical structure. Because DNA is essential to the reproductive viability of the cell, injury to DNA leads to a complex series of downstream molecular effects that result in the death of cancer cells as well as the normal lung parenchymal cells

The authors have no conflicts of interest to disclose.
Department of Therapeutic Radiology, Smilow Cancer Hospital at Yale-New Haven, 35 Park Street, Ste LL 513, New Haven, CT 06511, USA
* Corresponding author.
E-mail address: Sameer.nath@yale.edu

Clin Chest Med 38 (2017) 201–208
http://dx.doi.org/10.1016/j.ccm.2016.12.004
0272-5231/17/© 2017 Elsevier Inc. All rights reserved.

via mitotic death, and, to a smaller degree, apoptosis. Although the primary radiochemical interaction occurs over a period of milliseconds, cellular effects and cell death occur over a much longer period of time as cells attempt to divide. Fractionating, or dividing the total radiation dose into small daily doses, allows normal epithelial cells time to recover from radiation injury to a greater extent than malignant cells, likely due to differences in DNA repair ability and intrinsic radiosensitivity, thereby increasing the therapeutic ratio and minimizing toxicity.[2] In addition to these direct cytotoxic effects on target cells, radiation can also induce a robust inflammatory response that contributes to the development of lung fibrosis and resultant late morbidity from lung radiation.[3]

PATHOPHYSIOLOGY

Although type I pneumocytes comprise the majority of epithelial lung cells, they are thought to be terminally differentiated and typically do not divide. Owing to the lack of cellular division, type I pneumocytes are thought to be relatively radioresistant. Therefore, the primary insult that drives radiation pneumonitis is likely due to cytotoxic damage to the type II pneumocytes and vascular endothelial cells, both of which can be induced to undergo mitosis after cellular injury and therefore are more susceptible to radiation-induced cellular death.[4,5] Within hours of the delivery of high-dose radiation, changes within irradiated lung tissue can be observed despite a latency period of several weeks to months before the onset of a clinical syndrome. These tissue changes include abnormalities of surfactant-containing lamellar bodies within type II pneumocytes seen on electron microscopy specimens within one hour of radiation and increases in surfactant production detected in bronchoalveolar lavage samples within hours of radiation.[6,7] The subsequent pathogenesis of radiation injury to the lung has been well studied in animal models and is classically divided into distinct sequential phases depending on the time from radiation exposure[8]:

- Immediate phase (hours to days) is characterized by an inflammatory response that causes a leukocytic infiltration, which results in intraalveolar edema and vascular congestion. This phase is clinically silent.
- Latent phase (days to weeks) is characterized by the accumulation of thick secretions due to an increase in goblet cells and ciliary malfunction.
- Acute exudative phase (weeks to months) consists of hyaline membrane formation, type II pneumocyte proliferation, epithelial and endothelial sloughing, and clinical symptoms of radiation pneumonitis.
- Intermediate phase (months) follows with progression of the aforementioned changes with variable repair, dissolution of hyaline membranes, migration of fibroblasts, and capillary regeneration.
- Fibrotic phase (months to years) represents the final phase of injury and consists of progressive fibrosis wherein fibroblasts deposit collagen that eventually distorts alveolar spaces and diminishes lung volumes.

Following cytoxic injury to the target lung cells, dysregulation of a cytokine signal transduction cascade is also thought to occur. This effect may begin early following exposure to radiation and leads to a perpetual cascade involving several cytokines (notably transforming growth factor-beta [TGF-β], proangiogenic hypoxia-inducible factor-1 alpha, and vascular endothelial growth factor), which mediate the aforementioned pathologic changes and resultant fibrosis.[3] Of these, TGF-β is the most well established, and serum levels may be predictive of the risk of pneumonitis.[9]

INCIDENCE

The exact incidence of radiation pneumonitis is not known because it varies by primary tumor site and whether one is describing radiographic changes only or clinically symptomatic disease.[10] Radiation pneumonitis may be graded in several ways; the following is the Common Toxicity Criteria for Adverse Events (Version 4.0)[11]:

- Grade 1: Asymptomatic, radiographic findings only
- Grade 2: Symptomatic, but not interfering with activities of daily living
- Grade 3: Symptomatic and interfering with activities of daily living, oxygen indicated
- Grade 4: Life threatening, ventilator support is indicated
- Grade 5: Death

In patients undergoing breast radiation, the risk of pneumonitis depends on the radiation dose, patient anatomy, amount of lung tissue in the treatment field, use of chemotherapy, and extent of regional nodal irradiation. The incidence of grade 1 pneumonitis among patients treated for breast cancer is not known, because patients with early-stage breast cancer do not typically undergo routine chest computed tomography (CT) in follow-up. Estimates of symptomatic pneumonitis from patients treated with modern approaches are typically around 1% or less.[12] In a recent large multi-institutional trial randomizing patients with early-stage breast cancer to standard whole breast radiation therapy with or without regional nodal radiation, the rate of grade 2 or higher pneumonitis was found to be 1.2% with regional nodal radiation versus 0.2% without regional nodal radiation.[13] Certain chemotherapeutic agents can also enhance the effects of radiation and increase the rates of symptomatic pneumonitis, confounding estimates.[14–17] A list of agents known to increase rates of radiation pneumonitis is presented in **Box 1**. Risks of radiation pneumonitis appear to be highest when these agents are delivered concurrently with radiotherapy. As an example, a retrospective review of 1624 patients treated with radiotherapy after conservative surgery found higher rates of radiation pneumonitis among patients treated with a 3-field radiation technique and concurrent chemotherapy (8.8%) compared with those who received sequential chemotherapy and radiotherapy (1.3%).[18] The incidence of radiation pneumonitis among all patients was 1%. A second study demonstrated that the use of paclitaxel concurrently with radiation during a course of breast radiotherapy was associated with a 14% rate of pneumonitis in comparison to 1.1% without paclitaxel.[15] Induction chemotherapy can also increase the risk of developing radiation pneumonitis.[19,20] A retrospective review of patients with esophageal cancer treated with chemoradiation found that patients treated with induction chemotherapy before chemoradiation were more likely to develop grade $\geq$2 radiation pneumonitis (49%) compared with patients who did not receive induction chemotherapy (14%).[21]

Box 1
Chemotherapeutic agents associated with increased rates of radiation pneumonitis

Taxanes (eg, paclitaxel and docetaxel)

Cyclophosphamide

Gemcitabine

Irinotecan

Bleomycin

Dactinomycin

Doxorubicin

Mitomycin C

Vincristine

Recombinant interferon-alpha

Bevacizumab

Radiotherapy techniques used for the treatment of lymphoma have undergone significant changes since the 1960s that have led to reduced toxicity from radiation therapy. Before the mid-1990s, an extended-field technique was used that targeted significant amounts of normal tissue and was associated with increased rates of second cancer and cardiac sequelae.[22] Today, patients are commonly treated with intensity-modulated radiation therapy (IMRT) using an involved-site technique that spares significant amounts of normal tissue.[23] A recent study of patients with Hodgkin and non-Hodgkin lymphoma treated with IMRT found that 14% of patients developed radiation pneumonitis (grades 1–3).[24] Several dosimetric parameters were found to be predictive of radiation pneumonitis, including mean lung dose greater than 13.5 Gy, V20 greater than 30%, and V5 greater than 55%. Patients who developed relapsed or refractory lymphoma who were treated with salvage chemotherapy or hematopoietic stem cell transplantation had the highest rates of radiation pneumonitis (25%).

In patients with lung cancer, estimates of radiation pneumonitis similarly depend on numerous factors. The most well-established parameter that is closely monitored by radiation oncologists is V20, which is the volume of normal lung receiving 20 Gy or more. In a classic study of patients receiving conventionally fractionated radiotherapy published by Graham and colleagues,[25] the V20 was found to significantly predict for the development of grade 2 or higher pneumonitis, as follows:

- V20 less than 22%: 0% risk by 24 months
- V20 22% to 31%: 7% risk by 24 months
- V20 32% to 40%: 13% risk by 24 months
- V20 greater than 40%: 36% risk by 24 months

In addition, metrics measuring the volume of lung receiving a low dose of radiation, such as the V5 or mean lung dose, have also been found to be important predictors of radiation pneumonitis in thoracic radiation, particularly with the advent of newer radiotherapy treatment technologies. In a study by Allen and colleagues,[26] 13 patients undergoing adjuvant radiation for mesothelioma following extrapleural pneumonectomy were treated with IMRT. Six of the 13 patients developed fatal pneumonitis, despite having a V20 within the acceptable range. The median V5 for patients who developed fatal pneumonitis was 98%, compared with 90% for those who did not, suggesting metrics such as the V5 should also be considered in addition to the V20, especially when using treatment modalities like IMRT.

Interestingly, the rates of pneumonitis appear much lower for patients undergoing treatment with stereotactic body radiation therapy (SBRT) for the definitive management of lung cancer.[27] Although surgery remains the mainstay of treatment of early-stage non–small cell lung cancer, SBRT is commonly used for the definitive management of patients with early-stage lung cancer who are unable or unwilling to undergo surgery. Lung SBRT consists of the delivery of high doses of radiation, typically in the range of 10 to 18 Gy per fraction, for a total of 3 to 5 fractions (although dose fractionation schemes vary). The primary reason for the lower rates of pneumonitis may be related to the reduced treatment volumes as well as potential underlying differences in radiobiologic interactions with high dose-per-fraction radiation. Dosimetric predictors of radiation pneumonitis are less well established for treatment with SBRT and may include measures of mean lung dose, V10 and V20.[28]

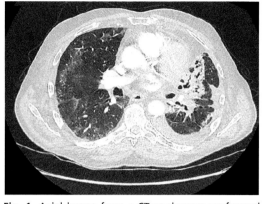

Fig. 1. Axial image from a CT angiogram performed 5 months after radiotherapy demonstrating consolidation and atelectasis consistent with radiation pneumonitis and fibrosis in a 64-year-old man with cT3N2M0, stage IIIA, squamous cell carcinoma of lung who completed a course of chemoradiotherapy to a total dose of 66 Gy in 33 fractions with concurrent cisplatin and etoposide.

DIAGNOSIS

The syndrome of radiation pneumonitis is diagnosed clinically based on the presence of classic symptoms, timing and history of radiation therapy, appropriate imaging findings, and exclusion of alternative causes, such as infection, cardiogenic edema, pulmonary embolus, drug-related toxicity, and other causes. Ruling out alternative diagnoses can be difficult; one study found that assigning a diagnosis of radiation-induced lung injury was challenging in 28% of patients due to confounding medical conditions.[29] Classic findings of radiation pneumonitis include the following:

- Onset of symptoms typically within 3 to 12 weeks of completion of radiotherapy; however, symptoms may arise later within the first year after radiation.
- Symptoms of low-grade fever, shortness of breath, nonproductive cough, and/or malaise.
- Nonspecific physical examination findings may include crackles on auscultation or skin erythema/hyperpigmentation in the treatment field.
- Laboratory studies suggestive of acute inflammation may be present with modest increases in white blood cell count, C-reactive protein, or erythrocyte sedimentation rate.
- Imaging findings suggestive of pneumonitis within the treatment field. Examples of the radiographic changes seen in patients who developed radiation pneumonitis are presented in **Figs. 1–4**. All patients undergoing radiotherapy directed at the lungs are

expected to develop some degree of radiographic change. However, radiographic changes may not correlate with clinical symptoms.[30] The classic portal-line effect that does not conform to normal lung anatomy is no longer seen as often due to modern radiation therapy techniques that often use multiple beam angles. Chest CT usually shows evidence of patchy consolidation roughly within the area of the high-dose radiation field and similarly does not conform to normal lobar anatomy.[31] Occasionally, progression outside of the field may be seen for unclear reasons, possibly due to a progressive immunologic response.[32,33]

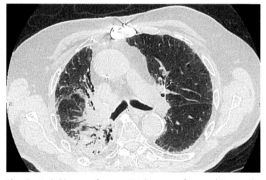

Fig. 2. Axial image from a CT chest performed 8 months after SBRT in an 82-year-old man with pT2bN0M0, stage IIA non–small cell lung cancer, who underwent SBRT to 50 Gy in 5 fractions. The image demonstrates airspace consolidation in the medial right middle lobe and superior right lower lobe with traction bronchiectasis and reticulation within the radiation field, consistent with evolution of radiation fibrosis.

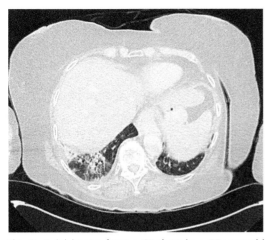

Fig. 3. Axial image from a CT chest in a 75 year old woman with stage I, T1N0 hepatocellular carcinoma in segment 7 of the liver who underwent definitive treatment with SBRT, receiving 48 Gy in 3 fractions. She developed mild shortness of breath and a slight cough approximately 3 months after completing treatment. Chest CT scan performed 3 months after treatment demonstrated patchy, peribronchovascular consolidation and ground glass opacities with associated dilated airways in the right lower lobe at the area of her recently completed radiotherapy. She was treated with a 4-week prednisone taper and experienced resolution of her symptoms.

Organizing pneumonia is rarely seen after high-dose lung radiation. It is characterized by lung infiltrations seen outside the area of treatment and does not result in pulmonary fibrosis.[32,34]

No single test confirms the diagnosis of radiation pneumonitis. Transbronchial biopsy can be performed to rule out alternative causes such as tumor spread and infection; however, tissue samples may be inadequate for diagnosis of radiation pneumonitis. Often patients are treated with a trial of antibiotics and steroids and monitored for a clinical response. If performed, pulmonary function testing usually demonstrates reductions in lung volumes and diffusing capacity of the lungs for carbon monoxide that may persist after therapy.[35]

RISK FACTORS FOR RADIATION PNEUMONITIS

Certain factors have been found to be protective of pneumonitis. Concurrent angiotensin converting enzyme inhibitor (ACE-I) use during radiotherapy has been correlated with a greater freedom from symptomatic pneumonitis in retrospective series of patients treated with both conventionally fractionated and SBRT.[36,37] The mechanism by which ACE-Is decrease risk of pneumonitis is not known, but may include mitigation of radiation-induced endothelial cell injury[38] or suppression of proinflammatory mediators.[39] Surprisingly, smoking during radiotherapy has also been shown in several studies to be associated with a decreased rate of radiation pneumonitis.[40,41]

TREATMENT AND PROGNOSIS

Treatment is typically instituted only for patients who become symptomatic. The backbone of therapy includes a long course of high-dose oral glucocorticoids. Prednisone is commonly prescribed at a starting dose of at least 40 to 60 mg daily (or 1 mg/kg daily) and is slowly tapered over 8 to 12 weeks while monitoring patient symptoms. Prophylaxis for *Pneumocystis pneumonia* should

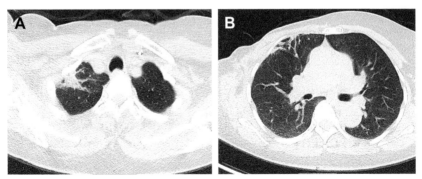

Fig. 4. (*A*, *B*) Axial images from a CT chest in a 79-year-old woman with a history of right breast invasive ductal carcinoma who underwent right modified radical mastectomy demonstrating a pT3N2aM0, stage III, breast cancer, estrogen receptor (ER)-positive, progesterone receptor (PR)-positive, and HER2-negative. She subsequently completed 12 cycles of adjuvant paclitaxel. She then underwent a course of radiotherapy: the right chest wall and internal mammary nodes were treated to a total dose of 50 Gy; the right supraclavicular fossa and axilla were treated to a total dose of 46 Gy. Chest CT scan performed 6 months after treatment demonstrated patchy opacification at the sites her previously completed radiotherapy. Despite radiographic changes, the patient never developed symptoms of radiation pneumonitis.

be considered due to the generally prolonged course. Symptoms typically improve shortly after initiation; however, relapse of symptoms following reduction in steroid dosing is common, requiring reinitiation of higher doses and a slower taper. For patients who have milder symptoms, a trial of nonsteroidal anti-inflammatory drugs or inhaled steroids could be considered.[42] In patients who cannot tolerate steroids or have significant refractory disease, other immunosuppressive agents such azathioprine and cyclosporine can be considered; however, evidence for their use is limited to case reports.[43,44] Other experimental agents include amifostine and pentoxifylline. Amifostine was found to reduce rates of radiation pneumonitis when given daily before radiotherapy in a randomized control trial of patients with advanced lung cancer.[45] Subsequent studies did not confirm this finding, and guidelines have not recommended its use.[46] In a small, randomized, placebo-controlled trial of 40 patients, pentoxifylline given 3 times daily during radiotherapy was shown to significantly decrease the rates of late pulmonary injury.[47] These results however require independent validation. Finally, although glucocorticoids are effective in the acute exudative phase of injury, they have minimal benefit after fibrosis has developed.[48] The benefit of antifibrotic agents, such as colchicine, is not known.

Patients who are properly diagnosed and appropriately treated with high-dose steroids have a good overall prognosis and can expect their symptoms to resolve. Pulmonary function recovers slowly and can occur up to 18 months following treatment. After 18 months, additional recovery is uncommon.[35] Although clinical symptoms typically resolve with treatment, most patients will develop progressive pulmonary fibrosis.[17] The development of pulmonary fibrosis appears to be related to the development of moderate (grade 2–3) radiation pneumonitis.[49] In cases of severe injury from a large field of radiation, chronic pulmonary insufficiency may develop and can progress to chronic cor pulmonale as a result of pulmonary hypertension, although this is uncommon.[50]

SUMMARY

The risk of radiation pneumonitis is often a significant concern when treating patients with thoracic malignancies and should be considered in the differential diagnosis of any patient who presents with pulmonary symptoms following radiation therapy. As radiation pneumonitis is diagnosed clinically, ruling out other causes of dyspnea is critical. Prompt treatment with high-dose steroids usually results in rapid improvement in most

patients, and a slow steroid taper should ensue. It is hoped that future studies will lead to better risk stratification, reduced lung injury, and more therapeutic options for affected patients.

FUTURE DIRECTIONS

Future studies may elucidate which patients are at highest risk for the development of pneumonitis and identify novel strategies to mitigate lung injury. Genomic analyses have identified single nucleotide polymorphisms in various genes, including those involved in the DNA repair pathway, that are associated with higher rates of radiation pneumonitis.[51,52] Whether these genetic markers can be used to select patients who require additional lung sparing during planning or utilization of a radioprotective agent during treatment is uncertain and requires further investigation. In a large meta-analysis, TGF-β1 polymorphisms were found to be associated with an increased risk of radiation pneumonitis, but differed in importance based on ethnicity.[53] Other methods of risk reduction, including the use of novel radiotherapy platforms, are being investigated. One approach uses proton therapy, which has been shown to reduce the amount of normal lung exposed to radiation during the treatment of early and advanced stage lung cancers.[54] Current trials exploring the use of proton therapy during lung radiation are ongoing and should provide additional insight regarding treatment tolerance and toxicity.

REFERENCES

1. Bergonie J, Teissier J. Rapport sur l'action des rayons X sur la tuberculose. Arch Electr Med 1898; 6:334.
2. Hall EJ, Giaccia AJ, Ovid Technologies Inc. Radiobiology for the radiologist. 7th edition. Philadelphia: Wolters Kluwer Health/Lippincott Williams & Wilkins; 2012. Available at: http://ovidsp.ovid.com/ovidweb.cgi?T=JS&PAGE=booktext&NEWS=N&DF=bookdb&AN=01438882/7th_Edition&XPATH=/PG(0).
3. Rubin P, Johnston CJ, Williams JP, et al. A perpetual cascade of cytokines postirradiation leads to pulmonary fibrosis. Int J Radiat Oncol Biol Phys 1995; 33(1):99–109.
4. Gross NJ. The pathogenesis of radiation-induced lung damage. Lung 1981;159(3):115–25.
5. Osterreicher J, Pejchal J, Skopek J, et al. Role of type II pneumocytes in pathogenesis of radiation pneumonitis: dose response of radiation-induced lung changes in the transient high vascular permeability period. Exp Toxicol Pathol 2004;56(3):181–7.
6. Gurley LR, London JE, Tietjen GL, et al. Lung hyperpermeability and changes in biochemical

constituents in bronchoalveolar lavage fluids following X irradiation of the thorax. Radiat Res 1993;134(2):151–9.

7. Penney DP, Rubin P. Specific early fine structural changes in the lung irradiation. Int J Radiat Oncol Biol Phys 1977;2(11–12):1123–32.

8. Merill W. Radiation-induced lung injury. Waltham, MA: UptoDate; 2016.

9. Zhang XJ, Sun JG, Sun J, et al. Prediction of radiation pneumonitis in lung cancer patients: a systematic review. J Cancer Res Clin Oncol 2012;138(12):2103–16.

10. Williams JP, Johnston CJ, Finkelstein JN. Treatment for radiation-induced pulmonary late effects: spoiled for choice or looking in the wrong direction? Curr Drug Targets 2010;11(11):1386–94.

11. NIH. Common toxicity criteria for adverse events v4.03. Available at: http://evs.nci.nih.gov/ftp1/CTCAE/CTCAE_4.03_2010-06-14_QuickReference_8.5x11.pdf. Accessed October 28, 2016.

12. Meric F, Buchholz TA, Mirza NQ, et al. Long-term complications associated with breast-conservation surgery and radiotherapy. Ann Surg Oncol 2002;9(6):543–9.

13. Whelan TJ, Olivotto IA, Parulekar WR, et al. Regional nodal irradiation in early-stage breast cancer. N Engl J Med 2015;373(4):307–16.

14. Rancati T, Ceresoli GL, Gagliardi G, et al. Factors predicting radiation pneumonitis in lung cancer patients: a retrospective study. Radiother Oncol 2003;67(3):275–83.

15. Taghian AG, Assaad SI, Niemierko A, et al. Risk of pneumonitis in breast cancer patients treated with radiation therapy and combination chemotherapy with paclitaxel. J Natl Cancer Inst 2001;93(23):1806–11.

16. Mehta V. Radiation pneumonitis and pulmonary fibrosis in non–small-cell lung cancer: pulmonary function, prediction, and prevention. Int J Radiat Oncol Biol Phys 2005;63(1):5–24.

17. McDonald S, Rubin P, Phillips TL, et al. Injury to the lung from cancer therapy: clinical syndromes, measurable endpoints, and potential scoring systems. Int J Radiat Oncol Biol Phys 1995;31(5):1187–203.

18. Lingos TI, Recht A, Vicini F, et al. Radiation pneumonitis in breast cancer patients treated with conservative surgery and radiation therapy. Int J Radiat Oncol Biol Phys 1991;21(2):355–60.

19. Palma DA, Senan S, Tsujino K, et al. Predicting radiation pneumonitis after chemoradiation therapy for lung cancer: an international individual patient data meta-analysis. Int J Radiat Oncol Biol Phys 2013;85(2):444–50.

20. Mao J, Kocak Z, Zhou S, et al. The impact of induction chemotherapy and the associated tumor response on subsequent radiation-related changes in lung function and tumor response. Int J Radiat Oncol Biol Phys 2007;67(5):1360–9.

21. Wang S, Liao Z, Wei X, et al. Association between systemic chemotherapy before chemoradiation and increased risk of treatment-related pneumonitis in esophageal cancer patients treated with definitive chemoradiotherapy. J Thorac Oncol 2008;3(3):277–82.

22. Koh E-S, Tran TH, Heydarian M, et al. A comparison of mantle versus involved-field radiotherapy for Hodgkin's lymphoma: reduction in normal tissue dose and second cancer risk. Radiat Oncol 2007;2(1):13.

23. Specht L, Yahalom J, Illidge T, et al. Modern radiation therapy for Hodgkin lymphoma: field and dose guidelines from the International Lymphoma Radiation Oncology Group (ILROG). Int J Radiat Oncol Biol Phys 2014;89(4):854–62.

24. Pinnix CC, Smith GL, Milgrom S, et al. Predictors of radiation pneumonitis in patients receiving intensity modulated radiation therapy for Hodgkin and non-Hodgkin lymphoma. Int J Radiat Oncol Biol Phys 2015;92(1):175–82.

25. Graham MV, Purdy JA, Emami B, et al. Clinical dose-volume histogram analysis for pneumonitis after 3D treatment for non-small cell lung cancer (NSCLC). Int J Radiat Oncol Biol Phys 1999;45(2):323–9.

26. Allen AM, Czerminska M, Janne PA, et al. Fatal pneumonitis associated with intensity-modulated radiation therapy for mesothelioma. Int J Radiat Oncol Biol Phys 2006;65(3):640–5.

27. Barriger RB, Forquer JA, Brabham JG, et al. A dose-volume analysis of radiation pneumonitis in non-small cell lung cancer patients treated with stereotactic body radiation therapy. Int J Radiat Oncol Biol Phys 2012;82(1):457–62.

28. Harder EM, Park HS, Chen ZJ, et al. Pulmonary dose-volume predictors of radiation pneumonitis following stereotactic body radiation therapy. Pract Radiat Oncol 2016;6(6):e353–9.

29. Kocak Z, Evans ES, Zhou S-M, et al. Challenges in defining radiation pneumonitis in patients with lung cancer. Int J Radiat Oncol Biol Phys 2005;62(3):635–8.

30. Faria SL, Aslani M, Tafazoli FS, et al. The challenge of scoring radiation-induced lung toxicity. Clin Oncol 2009;21(5):371–5.

31. Ikezoe J, Takashima S, Morimoto S, et al. CT appearance of acute radiation-induced injury in the lung. AJR Am J Roentgenol 1988;150(4):765–70.

32. Arbetter KR, Prakash UB, Tazelaar HD, et al. Radiation-induced pneumonitis in the "nonirradiated" lung. Mayo Clin Proc 1999;74(1):27–36.

33. Martin C, Romero S, Sanchez-Paya J, et al. Bilateral lymphocytic alveolitis: a common reaction after unilateral thoracic irradiation. Eur Respir J 1999;13(4):727.

34. Katayama N, Sato S, Katsui K, et al. Analysis of factors associated with radiation-induced bronchiolitis obliterans organizing pneumonia syndrome after breast-conserving therapy. Int J Radiat Oncol Biol Phys 2009;73(4):1049–54.

35. Borst GR, De Jaeger K, Belderbos JS, et al. Pulmonary function changes after radiotherapy in non-small-cell lung cancer patients with long-term disease-free survival. Int J Radiat Oncol Biol Phys 2005;62(3):639–44.

36. Kharofa J, Cohen EP, Tomic R, et al. Decreased risk of radiation pneumonitis with incidental concurrent use of angiotensin-converting enzyme inhibitors and thoracic radiation therapy. Int J Radiat Oncol Biol Phys 2012;84(1):238–43.

37. Harder EM, Park HS, Nath SK, et al. Angiotensin-converting enzyme inhibitors decrease the risk of radiation pneumonitis after stereotactic body radiation therapy. Pract Radiat Oncol 2015;5(6):e643–9.

38. Ward WF, Kim YT, Molteni A, et al. Radiation-induced pulmonary endothelial dysfunction in rats: modification by an inhibitor of angiotensin converting enzyme. Int J Radiat Oncol Biol Phys 1988;15(1):135–40.

39. Ward WF, Molteni A, Ts'ao CH, et al. Captopril reduces collagen and mast cell accumulation in irradiated rat lung. Int J Radiat Oncol Biol Phys 1990;19(6):1405–9.

40. Johansson S, Bjermer L, Franzen L, et al. Effects of ongoing smoking on the development of radiation-induced pneumonitis in breast cancer and oesophagus cancer patients. Radiother Oncol 1998;49(1):41–7.

41. Vogelius IR, Bentzen SM. A literature-based meta-analysis of clinical risk factors for development of radiation induced pneumonitis. Acta Oncol 2012;51(8):975–83.

42. Magana E, Crowell RE. Radiation pneumonitis successfully treated with inhaled corticosteroids. South Med J 2003;96(5):521–4.

43. McCarty MJ, Lillis P, Vukelja SJ. Azathioprine as a steroid-sparing agent in radiation pneumonitis. Chest 1996;109(5):1397–400.

44. Muraoka T, Bandoh S, Fujita J, et al. Corticosteroid refractory radiation pneumonitis that remarkably responded to Cyclosporin A. Intern Med 2002;41(9):730–3.

45. Antonadou D, Coliarakis N, Synodinou M, et al. Randomized phase III trial of radiation treatment ± amifostine in patients with advanced-stage lung cancer. Int J Radiat Oncol Biol Phys 2001;51(4):915–22.

46. Hensley ML, Hagerty KL, Kewalramani T, et al. American Society of Clinical Oncology 2008 clinical practice guideline update: use of chemotherapy and radiation therapy protectants. J Clin Oncol 2009;27(1):127–45.

47. Ozturk B, Egehan I, Atavci S, et al. Pentoxifylline in prevention of radiation-induced lung toxicity in patients with breast and lung cancer: a double-blind randomized trial. Int J Radiat Oncol Biol Phys 2004;58(1):213–9.

48. Abratt RP, Morgan GW, Silvestri G, et al. Pulmonary complications of radiation therapy. Clin Chest Med 2004;25(1):167–77.

49. Kong F-M, Hayman JA, Griffith KA, et al. Final toxicity results of a radiation-dose escalation study in patients with non–small-cell lung cancer (NSCLC): predictors for radiation pneumonitis and fibrosis. Int J Radiat Oncol Biol Phys 2006;65(4):1075–86.

50. Movsas B, Raffin TA, Epstein AH, et al. Pulmonary radiation injury. Chest 1997;111(4):1061–76.

51. Chen Y, Zhu M, Zhang Z, et al. A NEIL1 single nucleotide polymorphism (rs4462560) predicts the risk of radiation-induced toxicities in esophageal cancer patients treated with definitive radiotherapy. Cancer 2013;119(23):4205–11.

52. Edvardsen H, Landmark-Hoyvik H, Reinertsen KV, et al. SNP in TXNRD2 associated with radiation-induced fibrosis: a study of genetic variation in reactive oxygen species metabolism and signaling. Int J Radiat Oncol Biol Phys 2013;86(4):791–9.

53. He J, Deng L, Na F, et al. The association between TGF-beta1 polymorphisms and radiation pneumonia in lung cancer patients treated with definitive radiotherapy: a meta-analysis. PLoS One 2014;9(3):e91100.

54. Chang JY, Zhang X, Wang X, et al. Significant reduction of normal tissue dose by proton radiotherapy compared with three-dimensional conformal or intensity-modulated radiation therapy in Stage I or Stage III non-small-cell lung cancer. Int J Radiat Oncol Biol Phys 2006;65(4):1087–96.

Pulmonary Toxicities from Conventional Chemotherapy

Paul Leger, MD[a], Andrew H. Limper, MD[b],
Fabien Maldonado, MD[c],*

KEYWORDS

• Chemotherapy • Lung toxicity • Bronchoscopy • Radiation therapy • Interstitial lung disease

KEY POINTS

• Lung toxicity due to cytotoxic chemotherapy is common, variable, and often unpredictable.
• A diagnosis of chemotherapy lung is always one of exclusion. Bronchoscopy is generally needed to exclude infection or lymphangitic carcinomatosis.
• Rechallenge is never recommended to avoid the risk of recurrence.
• Corticosteroids may be effective in hastening resolution of symptoms and radiographic manifestations.

INTRODUCTION

The development of lung infiltrates, shortness of breath, and gas exchange abnormalities in a patient with malignancy treated with conventional cytotoxic chemotherapy often creates a diagnostic and therapeutic dilemma for a clinician faced with the difficult decision to withhold a potentially effective and life-saving treatment, often in the absence of firm diagnosis. Adverse drug reactions are uncommon, and chemotherapy lung is estimated to arise in 3% of treated patients.[1] There should, however, be a low threshold of suspecting the diagnosis, because manifestations are nonspecific and protean, and continuing treatment with the culprit chemotherapy agent may have dramatic consequences. That chemotherapy preferentially affects the lungs is not surprising: the blood-gas barrier at the alveolar level is a thin interface made of a nearly continuous sheet of capillaries bathing an extraordinarily large

alveolar surface area estimated of approximately 75 m[2].[2] This interface processes the entire cardiac output exposing vulnerable alveolar structures to the unintended nontargeted toxicity of conventional cytotoxic agents.

Manifestations of chemotherapy lung vary and are a function of the mechanism of action of the drug and the specific susceptibility of the host. Although most toxicities are cumulative in nature, some are idiosyncratic, and others are triggered by concomitant treatments (eg, radiation therapy or oxygen) or patient characteristics (age or renal failure). The differential diagnosis is typically broad in this patient population, often hindering prompt recognition of these complications. Pulmonary metastases and lymphangitic carcinomatosis, as well as opportunistic infections, need to be excluded. Consequently, a diagnosis of chemotherapy lung is always one of exclusion, and general rules for the identification and management of these complications are difficult to outline.

Conflict of Interest Statement: None for all authors.
[a] Division of Internal Medicine, Vanderbilt University Medical Center, T1218 Medical Center North, Nashville, TN 37232-2650, USA; [b] Division of Pulmonary and Critical Care Medicine, Mayo Clinic, 200 First Street SW, Rochester, MN 55905, USA; [c] Division of Allergy, Pulmonary and Critical Care Medicine, Vanderbilt University Medical Center, T1218 Medical Center North, Nashville, TN 37232-2650, USA
* Corresponding author.
E-mail address: fabien.maldonado@vanderbilt.edu

Clin Chest Med 38 (2017) 209–222
http://dx.doi.org/10.1016/j.ccm.2017.01.002
0272-5231/17/© 2017 Elsevier Inc. All rights reserved.

Because these complications are rare, most recommendations are based on anecdotal evidence. This review, therefore, focuses on the general approach to such cases, highlighting the syndromes associated with specific notorious agents, or common offenders, and their usual respiratory complications.

GENERAL PRINCIPLES OF DIAGNOSIS AND MANAGEMENT

The presentation of conventional chemotherapy-induced pulmonary injury includes variable clinical syndromes, such as acute lung injury, pneumonitis, noncardiogenic pulmonary edema, and acute respiratory distress syndrome (ARDS), among others. Likewise, histologic presentations vary considerably and include distinct entities, such as diffuse alveolar damage, organizing pneumonia, and neutrophilic alveolitis. These toxicities may occur weeks to months after treatment initiation. It is also often challenging to identify a specific culprit when patients are treated with multiple-drug regimens. Patients usually present with cough (typically nonproductive), low-grade fever, hypoxemia, dyspnea, and sometimes weight loss. The physical examination may be normal but often reveals bibasilar crackles. Wheezing may be present in cases of drug-induced hypersensitivity with bronchoconstriction. Occasionally, a morbilliform rash, as seen in drug rash with eosinophilia and systemic symptoms, may be present.

The radiographic presentation of drug-induced pulmonary injury includes unilateral or bilateral reticular markings, ground-glass opacities, or consolidations.[3–5] Pleural effusion and nodular consolidation occasionally are confused with cancer progression. High-resolution CT (HRCT) is sensitive but not specific and its prognostic value is generally unclear. A decrease in diffusing capacity for carbon monoxide (DLCO) is often the first anomaly seen in pulmonary function testing (PFT).[6–10] A restrictive pattern can be seen in advanced cases with decreased total lung capacity and forced vital capacity.

Bronchoscopy and bronchoalveolar lavage (BAL) are crucial to rule out infectious processes, diffuse alveolar hemorrhage, recurrent malignancy, or lymphangitic carcinomatosis. The diagnosis of chemotherapy-induced pulmonary toxicity remains one of exclusion based on a high index of suspicion in the context of a compatible clinical presentation and known exposure to a drug associated with pulmonary toxicity.

The treatment of chemotherapy-induced pulmonary toxicity is largely supportive and includes the discontinuation of the offending agent; treatment with systemic glucocorticoids, depending on the severity of symptoms; and supportive measures, such as oxygen supplementation, bronchodilators, and potentially mechanical ventilatory support as indicated.[3,11,12] Once a diagnosis is established, rechallenge with the same agent is generally not recommended, because recurrences are expected and occasionally are fatal.

ANTIBIOTIC CHEMOTHERAPEUTIC AGENTS
Bleomycin

Bleomycin is in many ways the exemplar of chemotherapeutic agents associated with lung toxicity. It is used in bench research to trigger lung toxicity in murine models of lung fibrosis. It is still used in a variety of malignancies, including lymphoma and testicular cancer, and acts by inducing DNA strand breaks.[13,14] It is inactivated in vivo by an enzyme, bleomycin hydrolase, present in all tissues with the notable exception of skin and lungs, which may account for the specific toxicity in these organs.[13,15,16]

The risk of bleomycin-induced lung injury is cumulative, typically after doses exceeding 400 IU/m^2, beyond which potentially life-threatening interstitial pulmonary fibrosis is thought to occur in 5% to 16% of exposed patients.[17–21] Other manifestations are less common but include acute and often idiosyncratic organizing pneumonia and hypersensitivity pneumonitis. Recent data suggest that the risk may be lower and reversible in most cases.[22] The risk factors for bleomycin-induced lung toxicity are presented in **Table 1**.

Clinical features

Symptoms may occur acutely (within days to weeks) or, in cases of pulmonary fibrosis, after months of treatment. Symptoms are nonspecific and include dyspnea and cough. Chest pain during rapid infusion also is described. Bleomycin-induced hypersensitivity pneumonitis and diffuse alveolar damage may present with more rapidly progressive symptoms, sometimes associated with fever and peripheral eosinophilia. Typical radiographic findings include bibasilar subpleural reticular changes with volume loss (in the classic chronic form) or patchy alveolar infiltrates in the acute presentation (**Fig. 1**). Less common nodular, pseudometastatic presentations with nodular infiltrates also are described. A decline of more than 25% in DLCO is considered an indication to discontinue bleomycin, although it is unclear if monitoring PFTs during the course of treatment should be recommended. A bronchoscopy with BAL and, when safe, transbronchial biopsies are generally

Table 1
Risk factors for acute lung toxicities in patients treated with bleomycin

Risk Factors	Comments	References
Age	2.3-fold higher risk in patients >40 y of age	[147,148]
Renal insufficiency	>80% secreted in kidneys. Avoid bleomycin.	[148–150]
Cumulative bleomycin dose	0%–2% toxicity with cumulative dose 270 IU 6%–18% toxicity with cumulative dose >360 IU	[15,17]
Concomitant gemcitabine, cisplatin, thoracic radiation	Risk may be lower with interval >4 wk between chemotherapy and irradiation	[151]
High Fio$_2$	Conflicting evidence	[152,153]
Cigarette smoking	Conflicting evidence	[22,149,154]
G-CSF	Conflicting evidence	[147,155,156]

Abbreviations: Fio$_2$, fraction of inspired oxygen; G-CSF, granulocyte colony-stimulating factor.

recommended to exclude the presence of infection of neoplastic infiltration.

Management

The mainstay of treatment of bleomycin-induced lung toxicity is immediate and permanent discontinuation of bleomycin. Bleomycin should be discontinued in patients with asymptomatic decline in DLCO greater than 25% and in patients with clinical or radiologic manifestations. Treatment with corticosteroids is reserved for patients with symptoms.

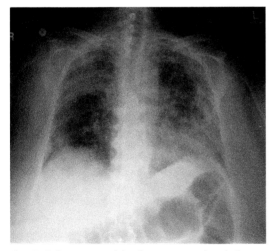

Fig. 1. Pulmonary toxicity from conventional chemotherapy. This is the chest radiograph of a 68-year-old-man with non-Hodgkin lymphoma treated with mechlorethamine, vincristine, procarbazine, and prednisone (MOPP) followed by adriamycin, bleomycin, vinblastine, and dacarbazine (ABVD). He developed bilateral alveolar and interstitial infiltrates with no evidence of infection.

Mitomycin C

Mitomycin C (MMC) is an agent active against a variety of cancers, including bladder, prostate, and breast cancers, although it has largely been replaced by novel agents. The alkyl group of MMC binds to the guanine base of DNA, which leads to irreversible damage and cell death.

The classic pulmonary toxicity of MMC seems dose dependent, typically occurring at doses exceeding 20 mg/m^2, and affects between 2% and 12% of exposed patients.[23–26] Concomitant administration of bleomycin, doxorubicin, cyclophosphamide (CP), and, in particular, vinca alkaloids and prior thoracic irradiation as well as supplemental oxygen may increase the risk of pulmonary toxicity. Four classic presentations are described, including ARDS, bronchospasm, interstitial pneumonitis, and thrombotic microangiopathy. Other, less common manifestations include pulmonary veno-occlusive disease with pulmonary hypertension and exudative pleural effusions.[27–29]

Prevention of pulmonary complications includes pretreatment with corticosteroids, limiting the dose and frequency of MMC treatment, and avoiding association with vinca alkaloids and high fraction of inspired oxygen. In all cases, rechallenge with MMC is discouraged.

Other Antibiotic Antineoplastic Agents

Doxorubicin is an anthracycline characterized by life-threatening, cumulative cardiotoxicity. Few reports of doxorubicin-induced interstitial pneumonitis are described and may present late after treatment in the setting of radiation therapy. Severe cases of noncardiogenic pulmonary edema are described, sometimes exacerbating MMC-induced lung toxicity. Actinomycin D is an antibiotic agent used in the treatment of Wilms tumor and Ewing sarcoma. Some reports suggest that actinomycin D may potentiate radiation pneumonitis.[30]

ALKYLATING AGENTS
Busulfan

Although eclipsed by imatinib as a mainstay of treatment in chronic myelogenous leukemia, busulfan continues to be used in conditioning regimens prior to hematopoietic stem cell transplantation.[31,32] It exerts its action by creating crosslinks between guanine-adenine and guanine-guanine, preventing DNA replication, and promoting cell apoptosis. Busulfan causes direct toxicity to the respiratory epithelium. Destruction of the epithelial liming can lead to diffuse alveolar damage with ARDS, with, occasionally, classic descriptions of pulmonary alveolar proteinosis and diffuse alveolar hemorrhage. Other manifestations include interstitial pneumonitis, organizing pneumonia, and interstitial fibrosis.[1,4,33,34]

Clinical features
Symptomatic pulmonary injury may occur in up to 8% of exposed patients.[33,35–39] Risk factors for pulmonary toxicity include long-term administration (more than 8 months), cumulative exposure of more than 500 mg, and concomitant administration of other chemotherapy drugs associated with lung toxicity and lung irradiation.[40,41] Findings on chest radiograph and HRCT vary and include ground-glass opacities, centrilobular nodules, basilar infiltrates, and peribronchial consolidation. PFTs may reveal reduced DLCO and a restrictive ventilatory pattern.[42,43] Bronchoscopy with BAL is generally recommended to rule out other potential causes of lung injury including infection and metastatic disease.

Management
The management is generally supportive. The role of systemic corticosteroids, even in cases of diffuse alveolar hemorrhage, is unclear. Whole-lung lavage may be considered in severe cases of pulmonary alveolar proteinosis, but its efficacy in this situation is debated.[42,44]

Cyclophosphamide

CP is used in combination chemotherapy for the treatment of hematologic malignancies and some brain tumors; it is more commonly used in the treatment of autoimmune disorders, such as systemic lupus erythematosus, rheumatoid arthritis, and granulomatosis with polyangiitis,[45–48] and is primarily metabolized in the liver into its toxic

metabolites 4-hydroxycyclophosphamide, acrolein, and the alkylating agent phosphoramide mustard.[49]

The risk of lung toxicity from CP seems less than 1%.[50] This risk may increase with concomitant use of substances that activate cytochrome P450, such as alcohol, barbiturates, rifampin, and phenytoin. This risk may also increase with the use of other chemotherapeutic agents, such as bleomycin or busulfan, high inspired oxygen concentration, or radiation therapy.

Clinical features
Two main clinical patterns of lung toxicity are described:

- Early-onset pneumonitis starts within 1 to 6 months of exposure with the onset of fever, cough, shortness of breath, and fatigue.[51,52] Chest radiograph and HRCT reveal reticular infiltrates and ground-glass opacities.
- Late-onset fibrosis occurs after prolonged exposure to CP over several months to years, usually in the context of chronic immunosuppressive therapy.[51,53] This pattern is characterized by an insidious onset with progressive shortness of breath and dry cough. HRCT reveals a fibrotic pattern without basilar predominance (distinguishing it from usual interstitial pneumonia).

Management
Early-onset pneumonitis is typically responsive to discontinuation of CP and initiation of glucocorticoids. Late-onset fibrosis is unlikely, however, to respond to anti-inflammatory agents and may progress despite discontinuation of treatment.

Other Alkylating Agents

Reports of drug-induced lung disease with other alkylating agents are rare or not well characterized. Chlorambucil is associated with acute and chronic interstitial pneumonitis and organizing pneumonia. These manifestations typically occur after 6 months of treatment.[54,55] Melphalan was recently approved in high-dose conditioning regimen before hematopoietic stem cell transplantation in multiple myeloma. Lung toxicity is rare but includes acute interstitial pneumonitis and pulmonary fibrosis with prolonged use. Ifosfamide is an alkylating agent close structurally to CP. Most common side effects include encephalopathy and peripheral neuropathy, but it rarely is associated with early-onset and late-onset pulmonary toxicity.[56,57] Pneumonitis occurring after the second or third cycle of procarbazine also is described.

ANTIMETABOLITES
Methotrexate

Methotrexate (MTX) has antiproliferative, anti-inflammatory, and immunomodulatory properties and is used in a variety of neoplastic and autoimmune conditions. Common toxicities are observed in the bone marrow, lungs, and liver.[58,59] MTX has a similar structure to folic acid and inhibits the enzyme dihydrofolate reductase, thus blocking the conversion of folic acid to tetrahydrofolic acid, hereby interfering with DNA synthesis.[60]

The pulmonary toxicity of MTX may occur insidiously after weeks or months of exposure to low doses for the treatment of rheumatologic disorders in up to 8% of patients. Toxicity may occur more acutely, however, after high doses with intravenous or intrathecal admission for the treatment of malignancies.[61–63] The incidence in patients treated for malignancies is difficult to establish mostly because MTX is generally part of multiple-drug regimens. This toxicity is generally understood to be an idiosyncratic manifestation rather than a dose-related one.

Risk factors include age greater than 60 years old, preexisting pulmonary disease, prior exposure to disease-modifying antirheumatoid drugs, diabetes, hypoalbuminemia, high doses of MTX, more frequent administration of MTX, renal insufficiency, presence of third-space fluid collections (ascites, pleural, and effusion) and, perhaps, genetic susceptibility.[64–67] Baseline chest radiograph and PFTs are recommended before initiation of treatment because of the added risk with preexisting lung diseases.

Clinical features
MTX-induced pulmonary toxicities are generally classified in 2 categories[67–70]:

- Inflammatory lung disease: the classic presentation of MTX-induced pneumonitis is an idiosyncratic hypersensitivity pneumonitis that can occur at any time during the duration of treatment. It is sometimes similar in presentation to sarcoidosis, with evidence of mediastinal and hilar lymphadenopathy, presence of non-necrotizing granulomatous inflammation on transbronchial biopsies, and an elevated CD4/CD8 ratio on BAL. Peripheral eosinophilia is present in 50% of the cases. Organizing pneumonia may also be present and, in chronic cases, pulmonary fibrosis. Exudative pleural effusions are reported.
- Lymphoproliferative disorder: there seems to be an association between the immunosuppression induced by MTX and the occurrence of lymphomas. This is suggested by the

appearance of lymphomas associated with Epstein-Barr virus during MTX treatment (similar to post-transplant lymphoproliferative disorders) and their occasional resolution with discontinuation of MTX.[71–76]

Management
Management strategies follow the general recommendation listed previously. Although there are reported cases of successful rechallenge without recurrence of symptoms, rechallenge is generally avoided. Supplemental folic acid does not seem to prevent lung toxicity.[35,41,69,77,78]

Gemcitabine

Gemcitabine is a highly effective agent in the treatment of non–small cell lung cancer and pancreatic, urothelial, breast, and ovarian cancers. It is a pyrimidine analog that inhibits DNA synthesis.

Clinical features
A large range of pulmonary toxicities is associated with gemcitabine, including interstitial pneumonitis, diffuse alveolar damage, diffuse alveolar hemorrhage, capillary leak syndrome with noncardiogenic pulmonary edema, acute eosinophilic pneumonia, and pleural effusions.[3,79,80]

Although dyspnea has been reported in up to 1 of 4 patients treated with gemcitabine, genuine pulmonary toxicity occurs in 1% to 2% of all treated patients[79,81–86] and may be more common when combined with bleomycin, paclitaxel, or docetaxel (with reports of pulmonary toxicity in up to 20% in these cases).[87,88] This risk is also increased in patients with prior thoracic radiation therapy or preexisting pulmonary fibrosis.[89] Gemcitabine is a potent radiosensitizer, with high risk of lung toxicity when used in combination with radiation therapy. In some instances, prior and distant radiation-induced lung injury may be reactivated during treatment with gemcitabine (radiation recall).[89] More rarely, gemcitabine can also cause bronchoconstriction, thrombotic microangiopathy, and pulmonary veno-occlusive disease.[3,90]

Management
The treatment consists of discontinuation of gemcitabine, and a short course of corticosteroids is often recommended.[82]

Cytosine Arabinoside (Cytarabine)

Cytarabine is a pyrimidine analog and one of the most effective drugs in the treatment of acute leukemia in combination with anthracyclines. The toxicity of cytarabine includes minor side effects, such as fever and rash, and major side effects, such as neurotoxicity, myelosuppression, and gastrointestinal mucosal damage.

Potentially fatal pulmonary toxicity has been reported in 12% to 20% of patients treated with intermediate to high doses of cytarabine after a median duration of treatment of 1 week to 2 weeks (range 1–21 days)[91–93] and is characterized by the acute onset of hypoxemic respiratory failure and ARDS. Histologically, it manifests as diffuse alveolar damage with increased vascular permeability.

This potentially fatal presentation requires immediate discontinuation of the drug and the institution of aggressive supportive measures, such as mechanical ventilation and high-dose corticosteroids. Despite these interventions, the mortality may remain high. In a series of 103 patients treated with high dose cytarabine, 13 patients (13%) developed acute respiratory failure and among them 9 cases were fatal.[92] Cytarabine also is associated with organizing pneumonia, usually responsive to corticosteroids.[94]

Other Antimetabolite Agents

Fludarabine is another purine analog essentially used in the treatment of chronic lymphocytic leukemia. It is associated with interstitial pneumonitis, which occurs generally within weeks of treatment initiation in approximately 10% of patients.[95–98] Fludarabine is also associated with profound immunosuppression, however, which increases considerably the risk of pulmonary opportunistic infections. Patients presenting with respiratory symptoms while on fludarabine should always be evaluated for opportunistic infection with diagnostic bronchoscopy and BAL. Once opportunistic infections are ruled out, discontinuation of fludarabine and institution of corticosteroids usually lead to prompt resolution of symptoms.[99]

6-Mercaptopurine (6-MP) is used in the treatment of acute lymphocytic leukemia and acute promyelocytic leukemia. Azathioprine and 6-MP are purine antagonists that incorporate into the DNA and RNA to inhibit their synthesis. They have immunosuppressive properties useful for the treatment of inflammatory bowel diseases. Rare cases of organizing pneumonia or nonspecific inflammatory pneumonitis are reported in patients with inflammatory bowel diseases treated with 6-MP or azathioprine.[100]

PODOPHYLLOTOXINS AND TAXANES
Podophyllotoxins: Etoposide and Teniposide

Etoposide (VP-16) and teniposide are largely used in combination therapy for the treatment of lung cancer, testicular cancer, lymphoma and leukemia, Kaposi sarcoma, Ewing sarcoma, and glioblastoma multiforme. They are topoisomerase II inhibitors that induce breaks in DNA strands leading to apoptosis of cancer cells. Pulmonary toxicity from these agents is rare, occurring in 1% to 3% of patients after prolonged use, and may present as interstitial pneumonitis or diffuse alveolar damage.[101–103] These drugs can also be associated with anaphylactic infusion reactions resulting in acute dyspnea with bronchoconstriction and hypotension within 10 to 20 minutes of infusion. Theses acute reactions are thought to be related to the drug vehicle (Kolliphor EL, BASF, Germany) rather than the drug itself. The treatment consists of discontinuation of the drug and initiation of corticosteroids.[101–103]

Taxanes: Paclitaxel and Docetaxel

Paclitaxel and docetaxel are used in a wide variety of malignancies, including breast, ovarian, and lung cancers, among others. They interfere with the breakdown of microtubules during cell division. The incidence of pulmonary toxicity with taxanes is not well characterized but seems less than 5%.

Clinical features
Three types of pulmonary toxicity are reported:

- Interstitial pneumonitis, which may develop within hours to a few weeks after taxane administration. It is thought to be an immune-mediated delayed hypersensitivity reaction[104] (**Fig. 2**). It occurs in less than 5% of patients exposed to standard dose of taxanes.[105–109] It is more common with higher dose of paclitaxel or docetaxel.[110,111] Some data suggest a higher incidence of pulmonary toxicity with weekly administration compared with every 3 weeks,[112] in patients with preexisting lung disease,[113] when combined with other cytotoxic drugs, such as gemcitabine,[114–117] and with concomitant radiotherapy.[118–120]
- Capillary leak syndrome occurs exclusively with docetaxel and can manifest as noncardiogenic pulmonary edema, pleural effusion, and peripheral edema.[121,122] The risk of capillary leak syndrome seems higher at cumulative doses exceeding 400 mg/m^2, particularly when docetaxel is administered without corticosteroid premedication.[123] Diuretics can limit the severity of taxane-induced capillary leakage.
- An acute infusion reaction can occur within 10 to 15 minutes of the first 2 infusions. It is characterized by dyspnea, urticaria, hypotension, or, occasionally, hypertension. It is thought to be mediated by the release of histamine

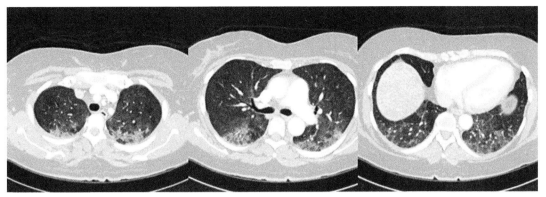

Fig. 2. Pulmonary toxicity from conventional chemotherapy. This is the chest CT scan of a 49-year-old woman with breast cancer treated with paclitaxel. She developed bilateral ground-glass opacities and interstitial infiltration with no evidence of infection.

or histamine-like products, and, similar to the infusion reactions triggered by podophyllotoxins, may be secondary to the vehicle of the drugs (Kolliphor EL, BASF, Germany) rather than the dugs themselves.

Management

The treatment consists of discontinuation of the taxane, systemic corticosteroids, and supportive measures. The role of treatment with corticosteroids once the capillary leak syndrome has occurred is unclear. Mild to moderate infusion reactions can be treated by stopping the infusion for 30 minutes and then restarted at a slower rate. More severe reactions or anaphylaxis require the permanent discontinuation of infusion and administration of epinephrine and antihistamine. New formulations of taxanes have been developed to decrease the frequency of infusion reactions and include nab-paclitaxel and paclitaxel polyglutamate.[124,125]

OTHER MISCELLANEOUS CHEMOTHERAPY AGENTS
Nitrosoureas

Nitrosoureas are alkylating agents used in the treatment of brain tumors, lymphoma, melanoma, and breast cancer. This class includes carmustine (BCNU), lomustine (CCNU), semustine (methyl-CCNU), and chloroethylnitrosourea (SarCNU), with carmustine used most frequently. Carmustine is also used in conditioning regimens with high-dose chemotherapy prior to stem cell transplant in patients with lymphoma.

Clinical features

Carmustine is associated with the development of pulmonary fibrosis in 10% to 30% of patients.[126–128] When used in conditioning regimens,

pulmonary toxicity may happen within a longer time frame.[128–131]

- Acute-onset pneumonitis occurs within weeks to months of treatment or is of late onset occurring many years after discontinuation. Early-onset lung toxicity is associated with higher doses of carmustine ($>$1500 mg/m^2), preexisting lung disease, and prior chest radiation therapy as well as with the concurrent administration of other cytotoxic agents.[126,130]
- Late-onset pulmonary fibrosis is uncommon but may occur many years after discontinuation of treatment and is characterized by progressive upper lobe fibrosis and sometimes apical pleural thickening.

Management

Treatment of early fibrosis consists of discontinuation of carmustine and administration of corticosteroids. Preventive measures include the administration of the lowest possible dose of carmustine, serial monitoring of DLCO, and prompt administration of corticosteroids if a 10% drop or greater in DLCO is noted. Late fibrosis is poorly responsive to anti-inflammatory treatment. The mortality is high, estimated at approximately 50%.[132,133]

Thalidomide and Lenalidomide

Thalidomide and lenalidomide are used in the treatment of multiple myeloma. Both are associated with subjective dyspnea in up to 50% and 15% of patients, respectively. Although case reports of interstitial lung disease are reported in the literature with both agents, the main complication associated with these agents is the risk of thromboembolic disease, thought to occur in 20% of treated patients with multiple myeloma. Venous thromboembolism prophylaxis is

Table 2
Pulmonary toxicities of chemotherapy regimens used in nonthoracic malignancies

Nonthoracic Malignancies	Chemotherapy Regimens	Pulmonary Toxicities
Breast cancer	CMF: CP/MTX/5-fluorouracil	Pneumonitis, PF
	FAC: 5-fluorouracil/doxorubicin/CP	Pneumonitis, PF
	FEC: 5-fluorouracil/epirubicin/CP	Pneumonitis, PF
	FECD: FEC + docetaxel	Pneumonitis, PF, pulmonary edema
	TAC: taxotere/doxorubicin/CP	Pneumonitis, PF, pulmonary edema
Colorectal cancer	FOLFOX: leukovorin/5-fluorouracil/oxaliplatin	Organizing PNA, DAH, pneumonitis
	FOLFiRI: leukovorin/5-fluorouracil/irinotecan	
	FOLFIRINOX: leukovorin/5-fluorouracil/ irinotecan/oxaliplatin	
Pancreatic cancer	FOLFIRINOX: leukovorin/5-fluorouracil/ irinotecan/oxaliplatin	Organizing PNA, DAH
	Gemcitabine/nab-paclitaxel	Interstitial pneumonitis, DAH, eosinophilic pneumonia
Germ cell tumor	BEP: bleomycin/etoposide/platinium-based (cisplatin)	Pneumonitis, DAH, PF

Abbreviations: DAH, diffuse alveolar hemorrhage; PF, pulmonary fibrosis; PNA, pneumonia.

warranted during the duration of treatment.[134–136] The rate of venous thromboembolism reportedly decreases from 20% to less than 10% with administration of prophylaxis.[137,138]

COMBINATION CHEMOTHERAPY

Cytotoxic chemotherapy agents are rarely used in isolation. Their combination with other agents can synergistically increase the risk of pulmonary toxicity and complicate the task of the clinician trying to identify the potential culprit agent. The use of oxaliplatin in combination with 5-fluorouracil and leucovorin (FOLFOX) as adjuvant therapy has improved overall survival and disease-free survival in patients with stage III colorectal cancer.[139–141] Common toxicities of this combination include peripheral neuropathies, gastrointestinal symptoms, and myelosuppression.[142] Oxaliplatin-induced lung injury is rare but can be fatal in 30% of cases.[141] Histopathologic pictures include organizing pneumonia, diffuse alveolar damage, and interstitial pneumonia. The pathophysiology of lung injury is thought related to hypersensitivity reactions, leading to eosinophilia, and glutathione depletion, leading to fibrosis.[143,144] Preexisting lung disease could be predisposing factor. Treatment consists of discontinuation of treatment and institution of high-dose systemic corticosteroids, which leads to variable success rate. In a series of 27 cases of oxaliplatin-induced lung toxicity treated with steroid and reported by Prochilo and colleagues,[145] 8 patients (30%) died. Early initiation of steroids seems associated with more benefit.[141]

Pulmonary toxicities of other combination chemotherapy regimens used in the treatment of nonthoracic malignancies are summarized in **Table 2**.

SUMMARY

The past decade has witnessed unprecedented advances in the understanding of the molecular drivers and alterations leading to the development of metastatic cancer, heralding a new era in the personalized management of many types of malignancies. Yet, despite these advances, conventional chemotherapy and its indiscriminate cytotoxicity remain at the forefront of the majority of first-line chemotherapy regimen in 2017. Toxicities are frequent, variable, difficult to predict, and occasionally life-threatening. Cytotoxic chemotherapy-induced lung toxicity, or chemotherapy lung, remains a major problem in oncology and requires careful assessment by a multidisciplinary team of experts to determine the likelihood of drug-induced lung disease and to evaluate the delicate balance of risks and benefits to the patient associated with the decision to continue or discontinue a life-saving but potentially dangerous chemotherapeutic agent. Because the diagnosis is most often one of exclusion, a high index of suspicion remains paramount, and unreported toxicities should be considered in the absence of satisfactory alternative explanation. Because rare and atypical presentations are possible, readers are invited to consult the database on drug-induced lung diseases developed by Camus[146] (University of Dijon, France) for a comprehensive and updated literature review.

REFERENCES

1. Limper AH. Chemotherapy-induced lung disease. Clin Chest Med 2004;25(1):53–64.
2. West JB. Respiratory physiology: the essentials. 9th edition. Baltimore, MD: Lippincott Williams and Wilkins; 2012.
3. Vahid B, Marik PE. Pulmonary complications of novel antineoplastic agents for solid tumors. Chest 2008;133(2):528–38.
4. Cleverley JR, Screaton NJ, Hiorns MP, et al. Drug-induced lung disease: high-resolution CT and histological findings. Clin Radiol 2002;57(4):292–9.
5. Torrisi JM, Schwartz LH, Gollub MJ, et al. CT findings of chemotherapy-induced toxicity: what radiologists need to know about the clinical and radiologic manifestations of chemotherapy toxicity. Radiology 2011;258(1):41–56.
6. Yerushalmi R, Kramer MR, Rizel S, et al. Decline in pulmonary function in patients with breast cancer receiving dose-dense chemotherapy: a prospective study. Ann Oncol 2009;20(3):437–40.
7. Wardley AM, Hiller L, Howard HC, et al. tAnGo: a randomised phase III trial of gemcitabine in paclitaxel-containing, epirubicin/cyclophosphamide-based, adjuvant chemotherapy for early breast cancer: a prospective pulmonary, cardiac and hepatic function evaluation. Br J Cancer 2008;99(4):597–603.
8. Dimopoulou I, Galani H, Dafni U, et al. A prospective study of pulmonary function in patients treated with paclitaxel and carboplatin. Cancer 2002;94(2):452–8.
9. Leo F, Solli P, Spaggiari L, et al. Respiratory function changes after chemotherapy: an additional risk for postoperative respiratory complications? Ann Thorac Surg 2004;77(1):260–5 [discussion: 265].
10. Bossi G, Cerveri I, Volpini E, et al. Long-term pulmonary sequelae after treatment of childhood Hodgkin's disease. Ann Oncol 1997;8(Suppl 1):19–24.
11. Camus P, Bonniaud P, Fanton A, et al. Drug-induced and iatrogenic infiltrative lung disease. Clin Chest Med 2004;25(3):479–519, vi.
12. Lee C, Gianos M, Klaustermeyer WB. Diagnosis and management of hypersensitivity reactions related to common cancer chemotherapy agents. Ann Allergy Asthma Immunol 2009;102(3):179–87 [quiz: 187–9, 222].
13. Sikic BI. Biochemical and cellular determinants of bleomycin cytotoxicity. Cancer Surv 1986;5(1):81–91.
14. Chandler DB. Possible mechanisms of bleomycin-induced fibrosis. Clin Chest Med 1990;11(1):21–30.
15. Jules-Elysee K, White DA. Bleomycin-induced pulmonary toxicity. Clin Chest Med 1990;11(1):1–20.
16. Lazo JS, Merrill WW, Pham ET, et al. Bleomycin hydrolase activity in pulmonary cells. J Pharmacol Exp Ther 1984;231(3):583–8.
17. Culine S, Kramar A, Théodore C, et al. Randomized trial comparing bleomycin/etoposide/cisplatin with alternating cisplatin/cyclophosphamide/doxorubicin and vinblastine/bleomycin regimens of chemotherapy for patients with intermediate- and poor-risk metastatic nonseminomatous germ cell tumors: Genito-Urinary Group of the French Federation of Cancer Centers Trial T93MP. J Clin Oncol 2008;26(3):421–7.
18. de Wit R, Roberts JT, Wilkinson PM, et al. Equivalence of three or four cycles of bleomycin, etoposide, and cisplatin chemotherapy and of a 3- or 5-day schedule in good-prognosis germ cell cancer: a randomized study of the European Organization for Research and Treatment of Cancer Genitourinary Tract Cancer Cooperative Group and the Medical Research Council. J Clin Oncol 2001;19(6):1629–40.
19. de Wit R, Stoter G, Kaye SB, et al. Importance of bleomycin in combination chemotherapy for good-prognosis testicular nonseminoma: a randomized study of the European Organization for Research and Treatment of Cancer Genitourinary Tract Cancer Cooperative Group. J Clin Oncol 1997;15(5):1837–43.
20. Loehrer PJ Sr, Johnson D, Elson P, et al. Importance of bleomycin in favorable-prognosis disseminated germ cell tumors: an Eastern Cooperative Oncology Group trial. J Clin Oncol 1995;13(2):470–6.
21. Delanoy N, Pécuchet N, Fabre E, et al. Bleomycin-induced pneumonitis in the treatment of ovarian sex cord-stromal tumors: a systematic review and meta-analysis. Int J Gynecol Cancer 2015;25(9):1593–8.
22. Lauritsen J, Kier MG, Bandak M, et al. Pulmonary function in patients with germ cell cancer treated with bleomycin, etoposide, and cisplatin. J Clin Oncol 2016;34(13):1492–9.
23. Verweij J, van Zanten T, Souren T, et al. Prospective study on the dose relationship of mitomycin C-induced interstitial pneumonitis. Cancer 1987;60(4):756–61.
24. Okuno SH, Frytak S. Mitomycin lung toxicity. Acute and chronic phases. Am J Clin Oncol 1997;20(3):282–4.
25. Castro M, Veeder MH, Mailliard JA, et al. A prospective study of pulmonary function in patients receiving mitomycin. Chest 1996;109(4):939–44.
26. Linette DC, McGee KH, McFarland JA. Mitomycin-induced pulmonary toxicity: case report and review of the literature. Ann Pharmacother 1992;26(4):481–4.
27. McCarthy JT, Staats BA. Pulmonary hypertension, hemolytic anemia, and renal failure. A mitomycin-associated syndrome. Chest 1986;89(4):608–11.

28. Gagnadoux F, Capron F, Lebeau B. Pulmonary veno-occlusive disease after neoadjuvant mitomycin chemotherapy and surgery for lung carcinoma. Lung Cancer 2002;36(2):213–5.

29. Waldhorn RE, Tsou E, Smith FP, et al. Pulmonary veno-occlusive disease associated with microangiopathic hemolytic anemia and chemotherapy of gastric adenocarcinoma. Med Pediatr Oncol 1984;12(6):394–6.

30. Cohen IJ, Loven D, Schoenfeld T, et al. Dactinomycin potentiation of radiation pneumonitis: a forgotten interaction. Pediatr Hematol Oncol 1991; 8(2):187–92.

31. Baron F, Labopin M, Peniket A, et al. Reduced-intensity conditioning with fludarabine and busulfan versus fludarabine and melphalan for patients with acute myeloid leukemia: a report from the Acute Leukemia Working Party of the European Group for Blood and Marrow Transplantation. Cancer 2015;121(7):1048–55.

32. Yabe M, Sako M, Yabe H, et al. A conditioning regimen of busulfan, fludarabine, and melphalan for allogeneic stem cell transplantation in children with juvenile myelomonocytic leukemia. Pediatr Transplant 2008;12(8):862–7.

33. Jochelson M, Tarbell NJ, Freedman AS, et al. Acute and chronic pulmonary complications following autologous bone marrow transplantation in non-Hodgkin's lymphoma. Bone Marrow Transplant 1990;6(5):329–31.

34. Vergnon JM, Boucheron S, Riffat J, et al. Interstitial pneumopathies caused by busulfan. Histologic, developmental and bronchoalveolar lavage analysis of 3 cases. Rev Med Interne 1988;9(4): 377–83 [in French].

35. Cooper JA Jr, White DA, Matthay RA. Drug-induced pulmonary disease. Part 1: cytotoxic drugs. Am Rev Respir Dis 1986;133(2):321–40.

36. Smalley RV, Wall RL. Two cases of busulfan toxicity. Ann Intern Med 1966;64(1):154–64.

37. Hankins DG, Sanders S, MacDonald FM, et al. Pulmonary toxicity recurring after a six week course of busulfan therapy and after subsequent therapy with uracil mustard. Chest 1978;73(3): 415–6.

38. Schallier D, Impens N, Warson F, et al. Additive pulmonary toxicity with melphalan and busulfan therapy. Chest 1983;84(4):492–3.

39. Crilley P, Topolsky D, Styler MJ, et al. Extramedullary toxicity of a conditioning regimen containing busulphan, cyclophosphamide and etoposide in 84 patients undergoing autologous and allogenic bone marrow transplantation. Bone Marrow Transplant 1995;15(3):361–5.

40. Ginsberg SJ, Comis RL. The pulmonary toxicity of antineoplastic agents. Semin Oncol 1982;9(1): 34–51.

41. Sostman HD, Matthay RA, Putman CE. Cytotoxic drug-induced lung disease. Am J Med 1977; 62(4):608–15.

42. Lund MB, Kongerud J, Brinch L, et al. Decreased lung function in one year survivors of allogeneic bone marrow transplantation conditioned with high-dose busulphan and cyclophosphamide. Eur Respir J 1995;8(8):1269–74.

43. Bruno B, Souillet G, Bertrand Y, et al. Effects of allogeneic bone marrow transplantation on pulmonary function in 80 children in a single paediatric centre. Bone Marrow Transplant 2004;34(2):143–7.

44. Lund MB, Brinch L, Kongerud J, et al. Lung function 5 yrs after allogeneic bone marrow transplantation conditioned with busulphan and cyclophosphamide. Eur Respir J 2004;23(6):901–5.

45. Steinberg AD, Kaltreider HB, Staples PJ, et al. Cyclophosphamide in lupus nephritis: a controlled trial. Ann Intern Med 1971;75(2):165–71.

46. Townes AS, Sowa JM, Shulman LE. Controlled trial of cyclophosphamide in rheumatoid arthritis. Arthritis Rheum 1976;19(3):563–73.

47. Novack SN, Pearson CM. Cyclophosphamide therapy in Wegener's granulomatosis. N Engl J Med 1971;284(17):938–42.

48. Makhani N, Gorman MP, Branson HM, et al. Cyclophosphamide therapy in pediatric multiple sclerosis. Neurology 2009;72(24):2076–82.

49. Kachel DL, Martin WJ 2nd. Cyclophosphamide-induced lung toxicity: mechanism of endothelial cell injury. J Pharmacol Exp Ther 1994;268(1):42–6.

50. Twohig KJ, Matthay RA. Pulmonary effects of cytotoxic agents other than bleomycin. Clin Chest Med 1990;11(1):31–54.

51. Malik SW, Myers JL, DeRemee RA, et al. Lung toxicity associated with cyclophosphamide use. Two distinct patterns. Am J Respir Crit Care Med 1996;154(6 Pt 1):1851–6.

52. Segura A, Yuste A, Cercos A, et al. Pulmonary fibrosis induced by cyclophosphamide. Ann Pharmacother 2001;35(7–8):894–7.

53. Hamada K, Nagai S, Kitaichi M, et al. Cyclophosphamide-induced late-onset lung disease. Intern Med 2003;42(1):82–7.

54. Kalambokis G, Stefanou D, Arkoumani E, et al. Bronchiolitis obliterans organizing pneumonia following chlorambucil treatment for chronic lymphocytic leukemia. Eur J Haematol 2004;73(2): 139–42.

55. Khong HT, McCarthy J. Chlorambucil-induced pulmonary disease: a case report and review of the literature. Ann Hematol 1998;77(1–2):85–7.

56. Baker WJ, Fistel SJ, Jones RV, et al. Interstitial pneumonitis associated with ifosfamide therapy. Cancer 1990;65(10):2217–21.

57. Elliott TE, Buckner JC, Cascino TL, et al. Phase II study of ifosfamide with mesna in adult patients

with recurrent diffuse astrocytoma. J Neurooncol 1991;10(1):27–30.

58. Lateef O, Shakoor N, Balk RA. Methotrexate pulmonary toxicity. Expert Opin Drug Saf 2005;4(4): 723–30.

59. Imokawa S, Colby TV, Leslie KO, et al. Methotrexate pneumonitis: review of the literature and histopathological findings in nine patients. Eur Respir J 2000;15(2):373–81.

60. Cronstein BN. Molecular therapeutics. Methotrexate and its mechanism of action. Arthritis Rheum 1996;39(12):1951–60.

61. Kinder AJ, Hassell AB, Brand J, et al. The treatment of inflammatory arthritis with methotrexate in clinical practice: treatment duration and incidence of adverse drug reactions. Rheumatology (Oxford) 2005;44(1):61–6.

62. Saravanan V, Kelly C. Drug-related pulmonary problems in patients with rheumatoid arthritis. Rheumatology (Oxford) 2006;45(7):787–9.

63. Rosenow EC 3rd. Drug-induced pulmonary disease. Dis Mon 1994;40(5):253–310.

64. Alarcon GS, Kremer JM, Macaluso M, et al. Risk factors for methotrexate-induced lung injury in patients with rheumatoid arthritis. A multicenter, case-control study. Methotrexate-Lung Study Group. Ann Intern Med 1997;127(5):356–64.

65. Furst DE, Koehnke R, Burmeister LF, et al. Increasing methotrexate effect with increasing dose in the treatment of resistant rheumatoid arthritis. J Rheumatol 1989;16(3):313–20.

66. Golden MR, Katz RS, Balk RA, et al. The relationship of preexisting lung disease to the development of methotrexate pneumonitis in patients with rheumatoid arthritis. J Rheumatol 1995;22(6):1043–7.

67. Hider SL, Bruce IN, Thomson W. The pharmacogenetics of methotrexate. Rheumatology (Oxford) 2007;46(10):1520–4.

68. Bedrossian CW, Miller WC, Luna MA. Methotrexate-induced diffuse interstitial pulmonary fibrosis. South Med J 1979;72(3):313–8.

69. Kremer JM, Alarcón GS, Weinblatt ME, et al. Clinical, laboratory, radiographic, and histopathologic features of methotrexate-associated lung injury in patients with rheumatoid arthritis: a multicenter study with literature review. Arthritis Rheum 1997; 40(10):1829–37.

70. Hilliquin P, Renoux M, Perrot S, et al. Occurrence of pulmonary complications during methotrexate therapy in rheumatoid arthritis. Br J Rheumatol 1996; 35(5):441–5.

71. Kamel OW, van de Rijn M, Weiss LM, et al. Brief report: reversible lymphomas associated with Epstein-Barr virus occurring during methotrexate therapy for rheumatoid arthritis and dermatomyositis. N Engl J Med 1993;328(18): 1317–21.

72. Salloum E, Cooper DL, Howe G, et al. Spontaneous regression of lymphoproliferative disorders in patients treated with methotrexate for rheumatoid arthritis and other rheumatic diseases. J Clin Oncol 1996;14(6):1943–9.

73. Hoshida Y, Xu JX, Fujita S, et al. Lymphoproliferative disorders in rheumatoid arthritis: clinicopathological analysis of 76 cases in relation to methotrexate medication. J Rheumatol 2007; 34(2):322–31.

74. Rizzi R, Curci P, Delia M, et al. Spontaneous remission of "methotrexate-associated lymphoproliferative disorders" after discontinuation of immunosuppressive treatment for autoimmune disease. Review of the literature. Med Oncol 2009;26(1):1–9.

75. Homsi S, Alexandrescu DT, Milojkovic N, et al. Diffuse large B-cell lymphoma with lung involvement in a psoriatic arthritis patient treated with methotrexate. Dermatol Online J 2010;16(5):1.

76. Kamiya Y, Toyoshima M, Suda T. Endobronchial involvement in methotrexate-associated lymphoproliferative disease. Am J Respir Crit Care Med 2016;193(11):1304–6.

77. Lynch JP 3rd, McCune WJ. Immunosuppressive and cytotoxic pharmacotherapy for pulmonary disorders. Am J Respir Crit Care Med 1997;155(2): 395–420.

78. Kremer JM. Methotrexate update. Scand J Rheumatol 1996;25(6):341–4.

79. Boiselle PM, Morrin MM, Huberman MS. Gemcitabine pulmonary toxicity: CT features. J Comput Assist Tomogr 2000;24(6):977–80.

80. Kim YH, Mishima M, Yoshizawa A. Gemcitabine-induced acute eosinophilic pneumonia. J Thorac Oncol 2010;5(8):1308–9.

81. Aapro MS, Martin C, Hatty S. Gemcitabine–a safety review. Anticancer Drugs 1998;9(3):191–201.

82. Roychowdhury DF, Cassidy CA, Peterson P, et al. A report on serious pulmonary toxicity associated with gemcitabine-based therapy. Invest New Drugs 2002;20(3):311–5.

83. Pavlakis N, Bell DR, Millward MJ, et al. Fatal pulmonary toxicity resulting from treatment with gemcitabine. Cancer 1997;80(2):286–91.

84. Linskens RK, Golding RP, van Groeningen CJ, et al. Severe acute lung injury induced by gemcitabine. Neth J Med 2000;56(6):232–5.

85. Marruchella A, Fiorenzano G, Merizzi A, et al. Diffuse alveolar damage in a patient treated with gemcitabine. Eur Respir J 1998;11(2):504–6.

86. Barlesi F, Villani P, Doddoli C, et al. Gemcitabine-induced severe pulmonary toxicity. Fundam Clin Pharmacol 2004;18(1):85–91.

87. Belknap SM, Kuzel TM, Yarnold PR, et al. Clinical features and correlates of gemcitabine-associated lung injury: findings from the RADAR project. Cancer 2006;106(9):2051–7.

88. Friedberg JW, Neuberg D, Kim H, et al. Gemcitabine added to doxorubicin, bleomycin, and vinblastine for the treatment of de novo Hodgkin disease: unacceptable acute pulmonary toxicity. Cancer 2003;98(5):978–82.

89. Umemura S, Yamane H, Suwaki T, et al. Interstitial lung disease associated with gemcitabine treatment in patients with non-small-cell lung cancer and pancreatic cancer. J Cancer Res Clin Oncol 2011;137(10):1469–75.

90. Gupta N, Ahmed I, Steinberg H, et al. Gemcitabine-induced pulmonary toxicity: case report and review of the literature. Am J Clin Oncol 2002; 25(1):96–100.

91. Andersson BS, Cogan BM, Keating MJ, et al. Subacute pulmonary failure complicating therapy with high-dose Ara-C in acute leukemia. Cancer 1985; 56(9):2181–4.

92. Andersson BS, Luna MA, Yee C, et al. Fatal pulmonary failure complicating high-dose cytosine arabinoside therapy in acute leukemia. Cancer 1990; 65(5):1079–84.

93. Kopterides P, Lignos M, Mentzelopoulos S, et al. Cytarabine-induced lung injury: case report. Anticancer Drugs 2005;16(7):743–5.

94. Forghieri F, Luppi M, Morselli M, et al. Cytarabine-related lung infiltrates on high resolution computerized tomography: a possible complication with benign outcome in leukemic patients. Haematologica 2007;92(9):e85–90.

95. Helman DL Jr, Byrd JC, Ales NC, et al. Fludarabine-related pulmonary toxicity: a distinct clinical entity in chronic lymphoproliferative syndromes. Chest 2002;122(3):785–90.

96. Hurst PG, Habib MP, Garewal H, et al. Pulmonary toxicity associated with fludarabine monophosphate. Invest New Drugs 1987;5(2):207–10.

97. Cervantes F, Salgado C, Montserrat E, et al. Fludarabine for prolymphocytic leukaemia and risk of interstitial pneumonitis. Lancet 1990;336(8723):1130.

98. Kane GC, McMichael AJ, Patrick H, et al. Pulmonary toxicity and acute respiratory failure associated with fludarabine monophosphate. Respir Med 1992;86(3):261–3.

99. Levin M, Aziz M, Opitz L. Steroid-responsive interstitial pneumonitis after fludarabine therapy. Chest 1997;111(5):1472–3.

100. Ananthakrishnan AN, Attila T, Otterson MF, et al. Severe pulmonary toxicity after azathioprine/6-mercaptopurine initiation for the treatment of inflammatory bowel disease. J Clin Gastroenterol 2007;41(7):682–8.

101. Gurjal A, An T, Valdivieso M, et al. Etoposide-induced pulmonary toxicity. Lung Cancer 1999; 26(2):109–12.

102. Uchida T, Nakakawaji K, Sakamoto J. Administration of oral etoposide for one year as adjuvant chemotherapy for non-small cell lung cancer-side effect. Gan To Kagaku Ryoho 1996;23(14):1967–70 [in Japanese].

103. Hatakeyama S, Tachibana A, Morita M, et al. Etoposide-induced pneumonitis. Nihon Kyobu Shikkan Gakkai Zasshi 1997;35(2):210–4 [in Japanese].

104. Wang GS, Yang KY, Perng RP. Life-threatening hypersensitivity pneumonitis induced by docetaxel (taxotere). Br J Cancer 2001;85(9):1247–50.

105. Ostoros G, Pretz A, Fillinger J, et al. Fatal pulmonary fibrosis induced by paclitaxel: a case report and review of the literature. Int J Gynecol Cancer 2006;16(Suppl 1):391–3.

106. Dimopoulou I, Bamias A, Lyberopoulos P, et al. Pulmonary toxicity from novel antineoplastic agents. Ann Oncol 2006;17(3):372–9.

107. Graziano SL, Herndon JE 2nd, Socinski MA, et al. Phase II trial of weekly dose-dense paclitaxel in extensive-stage small cell lung cancer: cancer and leukemia group B study 39901. J Thorac Oncol 2008;3(2):158–62.

108. Yasuda K, Igishi T, Kawasaki Y, et al. Phase II study of weekly paclitaxel in patients with non-small cell lung cancer who have failed previous treatments. Oncology 2004;66(5):347–52.

109. Seidman AD, Berry D, Cirrincione C, et al. Randomized phase III trial of weekly compared with every-3-weeks paclitaxel for metastatic breast cancer, with trastuzumab for all HER-2 overexpressors and random assignment to trastuzumab or not in HER-2 nonoverexpressors: final results of Cancer and Leukemia Group B protocol 9840. J Clin Oncol 2008;26(10):1642–9.

110. Stemmer SM, Cagnoni PJ, Shpall EJ, et al. High-dose paclitaxel, cyclophosphamide, and cisplatin with autologous hematopoietic progenitor-cell support: a phase I trial. J Clin Oncol 1996;14(5):1463–72.

111. McNeish IA, Kanfer EJ, Haynes R, et al. Paclitaxel-containing high-dose chemotherapy for relapsed or refractory testicular germ cell tumours. Br J Cancer 2004;90(6):1169–75.

112. Chen YM, Shih JF, Perng RP, et al. A randomized trial of different docetaxel schedules in non-small cell lung cancer patients who failed previous platinum-based chemotherapy. Chest 2006; 129(4):1031–8.

113. Tamiya A, Naito T, Miura S, et al. Interstitial lung disease associated with docetaxel in patients with advanced non-small cell lung cancer. Anticancer Res 2012;32(3):1103–6.

114. Thomas AL, Cox G, Sharma RA, et al. Gemcitabine and paclitaxel associated pneumonitis in non-small cell lung cancer: report of a phase I/II dose-escalating study. Eur J Cancer 2000;36(18):2329–34.

115. Harries M, Moss C, Perren T, et al. A phase II feasibility study of carboplatin followed by sequential weekly paclitaxel and gemcitabine as first-line treatment for ovarian cancer. Br J Cancer 2004; 91(4):627–32.

116. Hensley ML, Blessing JA, Mannel R, et al. Fixed-dose rate gemcitabine plus docetaxel as first-line therapy for metastatic uterine leiomyosarcoma: a Gynecologic Oncology Group phase II trial. Gynecol Oncol 2008;109(3):329–34.

117. Katakami N, Takiguchi Y, Yoshimori K, et al. Docetaxel in combination with either cisplatin or gemcitabine in unresectable non-small cell lung carcinoma: a randomized phase II study by the Japan Lung Cancer Cooperative Clinical Study Group. J Thorac Oncol 2006;1(5):447–53.

118. Nakamura M, Koizumi T, Hayasaka M, et al. Cisplatin and weekly docetaxel with concurrent thoracic radiotherapy for locally advanced stage III non-small-cell lung cancer. Cancer Chemother Pharmacol 2009;63(6):1091–6.

119. Onishi H, Kuriyama K, Yamaguchi M, et al. Concurrent two-dimensional radiotherapy and weekly docetaxel in the treatment of stage III non-small cell lung cancer: a good local response but no good survival due to radiation pneumonitis. Lung Cancer 2003;40(1):79–84.

120. Hanna YM, Baglan KL, Stromberg JS, et al. Acute and subacute toxicity associated with concurrent adjuvant radiation therapy and paclitaxel in primary breast cancer therapy. Breast J 2002;8(3):149–53.

121. Briasoulis E, Froudarakis M, Milionis HJ, et al. Chemotherapy-induced noncardiogenic pulmonary edema related to gemcitabine plus docetaxel combination with granulocyte colony-stimulating factor support. Respiration 2000;67(6):680–3.

122. Amathieu R, Tual L, Fessenmeyer C, et al. Docetaxel-induced acute pulmonary capillary-leak syndrome mimicking cardiogenic oedema. Ann Fr Anesth Reanim 2007;26(2):180–1 [in French].

123. Cortes JE, Pazdur R. Docetaxel. J Clin Oncol 1995; 13(10):2643–55.

124. Edelman MJ. Novel taxane formulations and microtubule-binding agents in non-small-cell lung cancer. Clin Lung Cancer 2009;10(Suppl 1):S30–4.

125. Socinski MA, Manikhas GM, Stroyakovsky DL, et al. A dose finding study of weekly and every-3-week nab-Paclitaxel followed by carboplatin as first-line therapy in patients with advanced non-small cell lung cancer. J Thorac Oncol 2010;5(6):852–61.

126. Weiss RB, Poster DS, Penta JS. The nitrosoureas and pulmonary toxicity. Cancer Treat Rev 1981; 8(2):111–25.

127. Selker RG, Jacobs SA, Moore PB, et al. 1,3-Bis(2-chloroethyl)-1-nitrosourea (BCNU)-induced pulmonary fibrosis. Neurosurgery 1980;7(6):560–5.

128. Durant JR, Norgard MJ, Murad TM, et al. Pulmonary toxicity associated with bischloroethylnitrosourea (BCNU). Ann Intern Med 1979;90(2):191–4.

129. Wadhwa PD, Fu P, Koc ON, et al. High-dose carmustine, etoposide, and cisplatin for autologous stem cell transplantation with or without involved-field radiation for relapsed/refractory lymphoma: an effective regimen with low morbidity and mortality. Biol Blood Marrow Transplant 2005;11(1):13–22.

130. Wong R, Rondon G, Saliba RM, et al. Idiopathic pneumonia syndrome after high-dose chemotherapy and autologous hematopoietic stem cell transplantation for high-risk breast cancer. Bone Marrow Transplant 2003;31(12):1157–63.

131. Frankovich J, Donaldson SS, Lee Y, et al. High-dose therapy and autologous hematopoietic cell transplantation in children with primary refractory and relapsed Hodgkin's disease: atopy predicts idiopathic diffuse lung injury syndromes. Biol Blood Marrow Transplant 2001;7(1):49–57.

132. O'Driscoll BR, Hasleton PS, Taylor PM, et al. Active lung fibrosis up to 17 years after chemotherapy with carmustine (BCNU) in childhood. N Engl J Med 1990;323(6):378–82.

133. O'Driscoll BR, Kalra S, Gattamaneni HR, et al. Late carmustine lung fibrosis. Age at treatment may influence severity and survival. Chest 1995;107(5): 1355–7.

134. Palumbo A, Rajkumar SV, Dimopoulos MA, et al. Prevention of thalidomide- and lenalidomide-associated thrombosis in myeloma. Leukemia 2008;22(2):414–23.

135. Lyman GH, Bohlke K, Falanga A, et al. Venous thromboembolism prophylaxis and treatment in patients with cancer: American Society of Clinical Oncology clinical practice guideline update. J Clin Oncol 2013;31(17):2189–204.

136. Zangari M, Barlogie B, Anaissie E, et al. Deep vein thrombosis in patients with multiple myeloma treated with thalidomide and chemotherapy: effects of prophylactic and therapeutic anticoagulation. Br J Haematol 2004;126(5):715–21.

137. Chen C, Reece DE, Siegel D, et al. Expanded safety experience with lenalidomide plus dexamethasone in relapsed or refractory multiple myeloma. Br J Haematol 2009;146(2):164–70.

138. Richardson PG, Weller E, Lonial S, et al. Lenalidomide, bortezomib, and dexamethasone combination therapy in patients with newly diagnosed multiple myeloma. Blood 2010;116(5):679–86.

139. Andre T, Boni C, Navarro M, et al. Improved overall survival with oxaliplatin, fluorouracil, and leucovorin as adjuvant treatment in stage II or III colon cancer in the MOSAIC trial. J Clin Oncol 2009;27(19): 3109–16.

140. Kuebler JP, Wieand HS, O'Connell MJ, et al. Oxaliplatin combined with weekly bolus fluorouracil and

leucovorin as surgical adjuvant chemotherapy for stage II and III colon cancer: results from NSABP C-07. J Clin Oncol 2007;25(16):2198–204.

141. Watkins J, Slade JH, Phan A, et al. Fatal diffuse alveolar damage associated with oxaliplatin administration. Clin Colorectal Cancer 2011;10(3): 198–202.

142. ELOXATIN prescribing information. 2015. Available at: http://products.sanofi.us/eloxatin/eloxatin.html. Accessed February 8, 2017.

143. Arevalo Lobera S, Sagastibeltza Mariñelarena N, Elejoste Echeberría I, et al. Fatal pneumonitis induced by oxaliplatin. Clin Transl Oncol 2008; 10(11):764–7.

144. Pontes LB, Armentano DP, Soares A, et al. Fatal pneumonitis induced by oxaliplatin: description of three cases. Case Rep Oncol 2012;5(1):104–9.

145. Prochilo T, Abeni C, Bertocchi P, et al. Oxaliplatin-induced lung toxicity. Case report and review of the literature. Curr Drug Saf 2012;7(2):179–82.

146. Camus P. The drug-induced respiratory disease website. 2012. Available at: http://www.pneumotox.com. Accessed February 8, 2017.

147. Martin WG, Ristow KM, Habermann TM, et al. Bleomycin pulmonary toxicity has a negative impact on the outcome of patients with Hodgkin's lymphoma. J Clin Oncol 2005;23(30):7614–20.

148. O'Sullivan JM, Huddart RA, Norman AR, et al. Predicting the risk of bleomycin lung toxicity in patients with germ-cell tumours. Ann Oncol 2003;14(1):91–6.

149. Kawai K, Hinotsu S, Tomobe M, et al. Serum creatinine level during chemotherapy for testicular cancer as a possible predictor of bleomycin-induced pulmonary toxicity. Jpn J Clin Oncol 1998;28(9):546–50.

150. Sleijfer S, van der Mark TW, Schraffordt Koops H, et al. Enhanced effects of bleomycin on pulmonary function disturbances in patients with decreased renal function due to cisplatin. Eur J Cancer 1996;32A(3):550–2.

151. Haugnes HS, Aass N, Fosså SD, et al. Pulmonary function in long-term survivors of testicular cancer. J Clin Oncol 2009;27(17):2779–86.

152. Tryka AF, Skornik WA, Godleski JJ, et al. Potentiation of bleomycin-induced lung injury by exposure to 70% oxygen. Morphologic assessment. Am Rev Respir Dis 1982;126(6): 1074–9.

153. Tryka AF, Godleski JJ, Brain JD. Differences in effects of immediate and delayed hyperoxia exposure on bleomycin-induced pulmonary injury. Cancer Treat Rep 1984;68(5):759–64.

154. Ngeow J, Tan IB, Kanesvaran R, et al. Prognostic impact of bleomycin-induced pneumonitis on the outcome of Hodgkin's lymphoma. Ann Hematol 2011;90(1):67–72.

155. Fossa SD, Kaye SB, Mead GM, et al. Filgrastim during combination chemotherapy of patients with poor-prognosis metastatic germ cell malignancy. European Organization for Research and Treatment of Cancer, Genito-Urinary Group, and the Medical Research Council Testicular Cancer Working Party, Cambridge, United Kingdom. J Clin Oncol 1998;16(2):716–24.

156. Saxman SB, Nichols CR, Einhorn LH. Pulmonary toxicity in patients with advanced-stage germ cell tumors receiving bleomycin with and without granulocyte colony stimulating factor. Chest 1997; 111(3):657–60.

Pulmonary Toxicities from Checkpoint Immunotherapy for Malignancy

Jennifer D. Possick, MD

KEYWORDS

- Pneumonitis • Anti-PD-1 • Anti-CTLA-4 • Checkpoint inhibitors • Immunotherapy
- Immune-related adverse events

KEY POINTS

- Pulmonary toxicity is a rare but clinically significant consequence of anti-PD-1 and anti-CTLA-4 immunotherapy.
- It is particularly important to recognize the variable clinical and radiographic presentations of pulmonary toxicity associated with checkpoint immunotherapy.
- With prompt recognition and intervention, typically with drug cessation ± immunosuppression with corticosteroids, outcomes are generally favorable.
- Toxicity relapses can occur, even in absence of rechallenge with immunotherapy agents, requiring sustained clinical vigilance.
- Re-treatment with immunotherapy agents after immune-related adverse events is variably tolerated; the risk/benefit balance of such decisions but be approached on a case-by-case basis.

INTRODUCTION

The spectrum of treatment-related complications encountered by pulmonologists caring for patients with malignancy is complex, with new challenges arising as novel therapies are developed and introduced. In recent years, advances in the understanding of cancer immunotherapy have permanently altered the therapeutic landscape of oncologic management. The successes of "checkpoint inhibitor" therapies, particularly in metastatic melanoma and advanced non–small cell lung cancer (NSCLC), have precipitated a paradigm shift in therapeutic algorithms for an ever-expanding list of malignancies. As these immunotherapies become more commonplace in the clinical management of patients with many different types of cancer, it is essential to understand immune-related adverse events (IRAEs), to recognize pulmonary toxicities that can arise, and to use existing experience to guide the approach to management. As collective experience with these agents and their complications builds, the hope is to improve identification of individuals at particular risk and to further refine treatment strategies.

IMMUNOLOGY IN THE TUMOR MILIEU

The role for immunotherapies in the treatment of malignancy is based on the intrinsic antitumor immune system response, seeking to either augment or restore these defenses. Therapeutically, this has been explored a variety of ways over time, including cytokine administration, vaccine therapy, cell therapy, and, as in the case of

Section of Pulmonary, Critical Care, and Sleep Medicine, Yale University School of Medicine, 300 Cedar Street, LCI 100, New Haven, CT 06520, USA
E-mail address: Jennifer.possick@yale.edu

Clin Chest Med 38 (2017) 223–232
http://dx.doi.org/10.1016/j.ccm.2016.12.012
0272-5231/17/© 2017 Elsevier Inc. All rights reserved.

LIBRARY
ALLEGANY COLLEGE OF MD LIBRARY
12401 WILLOWBROOK ROAD, SE
CUMBERLAND, MD 21502-2596

checkpoint inhibitor therapies, manipulation of the T-cell regulatory signaling pathways.

The initial immunologic response against a tumor antigen (or any non–self-antigen) requires the concerted effort of innate and adaptive responses across multiple cell types, including B cells, T-cells, and NK cells. This process is mediated by a cascade of cell signaling and release of cytokines, including interleukin-12 (IL-12), interferon-alpha (IFN-alpha), and IFN-gamma. Cytotoxic (CD8+) and helper T-cells (CD4+) respond to antigens presented on the surface of antigen-presenting cells (APCs) such as dendritic cells. This interaction between T-cell receptor complex and APC is complex and highly regulated, but requires binding of the CD4/CD8 protein receptor to the antigen presented by the major histocompatibility complex (MHC) in the presence of costimulatory signals (such as binding of CD28 on naive T-cells to B7-1/B7-2 or CD80/86 on APCs). After an initial phase of immune-mediated destruction, activation of immune checkpoint molecules triggers inhibitory signals to appropriately attenuate the immune response by downregulating or exhausting T-cell function.[1,2]

In the tumor microenvironment, malignant cells may exploit the immune system to evade detection and destruction by a variety of means. Evasive responses can include decreased MHC expression of tumor antigens, direct manipulation of cytokine and cell signal pathways (thus directly or indirectly enhancing Treg activity), or enhanced expression of immune checkpoint molecules themselves.[3]

DEVELOPMENT OF CHECKPOINT INHIBITORS

Appreciation for the role of these checkpoint molecules, including cytotoxic T-lymphocyte associated protein 4 (CTLA-4) and programmed cell death-1 (PD-1), raised their profile as therapeutic targets, particularly as other immunotherapies, such as IL-2, had resulted in frequent incidence of significant systemic toxicity.[4] As these therapies represent a restoration of inherent antitumor response, checkpoint inhibition also has the potential to provide durable therapeutic benefit beyond the duration of treatment, independent of tumor subtype or mutation status, expanding application across different types of malignancies.

Monoclonal antibodies directed against checkpoint molecules have transformed the landscape of oncologic treatment, providing safe, effective, and durable responses in many individuals with advanced stage malignancy.[5,6] Outside of NSCLC, these therapies have been most comprehensively examined and widely used in metastatic melanoma, but the applications of these therapies are continually expanding; at present, these agents are approved in the treatment of certain patients with squamous cell cancer of the head and neck, urothelial carcinoma, renal cell carcinoma, and Hodgkin lymphoma (**Table 1**).

Cytotoxic T-Lymphocyte-Associated Protein 4

CTLA-4 was first explored as an inhibitory mediator of T-cell activation in the 1980s to 1990s. When present on the surface of T-cells, it demonstrates greater affinity for the costimulatory B7-1/B7-2 or CD80/86 receptors than CD-28, leading to downregulation of T-cell activity (**Fig. 1**). CTLA-4 expression itself is upregulated by T-cell receptor activation, IL-12, and IFN-gamma, and therefore, provides feedback inhibition for the T-cell activation pathway.[7] Early murine models of CTLA-4 blockade demonstrated profound decrease in tumor burden in sarcoma and colon cancer, resulting in the development of the monoclonal antibody ipilimumab (see **Table 1**).[8] Ipilimumab has demonstrated dramatic responses in subsets of patients with metastatic melanoma and is now a front-line therapy in the treatment of this disease.[9,10] In contrast, studies of tremelimumab, another anti-CTLA-4 antibody, have not demonstrated survival benefit compared with conventional chemotherapy.[11] As is discussed, the number of individuals treated with ipilimumab in the context of large-scale clinical trials has greatly enhanced the understanding of pulmonary IRAE, which are generally low frequency events.

Programmed Cell Death Protein and Ligand

PD-1 is another inhibitory molecule that is expressed on T-cells, B cells, and NK cells. Like CTLA-4, expression is upregulated in the setting of IL-12 and IFN-gamma, providing a negative feedback control on T-cell effector function. It binds to 2 ligands (PD-L1 and PD-L2) that are expressed on a variety of cells, including tumor cells (see **Fig. 1**).[12] The PD-1/PD-L1 interaction has many effects in the tumor milieu: it prevents tumor cell apoptosis, downregulates T-cell activity, and promotes Treg activity.[1,13]

The anti-PD-1 antibodies nivolumab and pembrolizumab (see **Table 1**) have been extensively studied, particularly in metastatic melanoma and advanced-stage NSCLC, and have significant survival advantage over conventional chemotherapy in both patient populations.[5,14–16] Both agents are approved for use in metastatic melanoma and select patients with metastatic squamous cell carcinoma of the head and neck; nivolumab is also approved for use in all NSCLC,

Table 1
Current US Food and Drug Administration–approved indications for checkpoint immunotherapy agents

Agent	Target	Indications
Ipilimumab	CTLA-4	• Metastatic melanoma • Adjuvant therapy for stage III melanoma
Pembrolizumab	PD-1	• Metastatic melanoma • Stage IV NSCLC without EGFR or ALK mutation and ≥50% PD-L1+ TPS • Stage IV NSCLC and ≥1% PD-L1+ TPS after progression on platinum-based chemotherapy (and EGFR/ALK-directed therapy if mutation present) • Recurent or metastatic head and neck SCC after progression on platinum-based chemotherapy
Nivolumab	PD-1	• Stage IV NSCLC with progression after platinum-based chemotherapy (and EGFR/ALK-directed therapy if mutation present) • Metastatic melanoma (in combination with ipilimumab) • Advanced RCC with progression after anti-angiogenic therapy • Hodgkin lymphoma with relapse or progression after auto-HSCT and brentuximab vedotin • Head and neck SCC with progression after platinum based chemotherapy
Atezolizumab	PDL1	• Stage IV NSCLC with progression after platinum-based chemotherapy (and EGFR/ALK-directed therapy if mutation present) • Locally advanced or metastatic urothelial carcinoma with progression after platinum based chemotherapy

Abbreviations: ALK, anaplastic lymphoma kinase; auto-HSCT, autologous hematopoietic stem cell transplant; EGFR, epidermal growth factor receptor; RCC, renal cell carcinoma; SCC, squamous cell carcinoma; TPS, tumor proportion score.

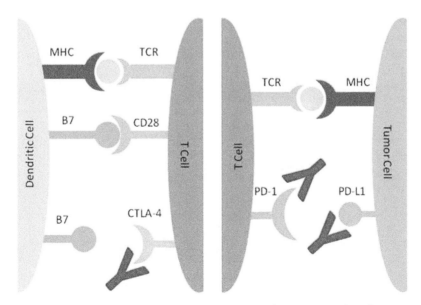

Fig. 1. T-cell regulatory "checkpoints" in the antitumor response. (*left*) Activation of T-cell response requires presentation of an antigen by the MHC of the dendritic cell/APC to the T-cell receptor (TCR) as well as the interaction of costimulatory molecules such as CD-28/B7. The subsequent expression of CTLA-4, which has high affinity for CD-28, provides a downregulatory signal that can be targeted by ipilimumab, an anti-CTLA-4 antibody. Blockade of CTLA-4 restores antitumor activity by T-cells. (*right*) After long-term antigen exposure, T-cells upregulate expression of the PD-1 receptor, which dampens ongoing T-cell responses in the presence of appropriate ligands. PD-L1 can be preferentially expressed by cancer cells to evade antitumor immune defenses. Antibodies directed against PD-1 (nivolumab or pembrolizumab) or PD-L1 (atezolizumab) aim to restore this response.

with the role in therapy stratified depending on degree of PD-L1 expression (or tumor proportion score), whereas pembrolizumab is approved for those individuals with NSCLC whose tumors preferentially express PD-L1.[16] Nivolumab is also approved for use in individuals with Hodgkin lymphoma that have relapsed after both autologous stem cell transplant and treatment with brentuximab vedotin, and in individuals with advanced renal cell carcinoma.[17] Atezolizumab (see **Table 1**), an antibody targeting the corresponding PD-L1 ligand, has been recently approved for use in individuals with treatment-refractory, advanced stage urothelial carcinoma and metastatic NSCLC; it is presently under investigation in a variety of additional malignancies, including melanoma, renal cell carcinoma, ovarian cancer, and colorectal cancer.[6]

IMMUNE-RELATED ADVERSE EFFECTS OF CHECKPOINT IMMUNOTHERAPY
Epidemiology

An expected consequence of anti-PD-1 and anti-CTLA-4 therapies is unintended dysregulation of immune responses. IRAEs are a well-described and widely recognized complication of checkpoint inhibition immunotherapies, occurring in up to 90% of patients treated with anti-CTLA-4,[9] and up to 70% of patients treated with anti-PD-1 or anti-PD-L1.[5,6] A broad spectrum of complications has been observed in multiple organ systems, including the lung (**Box 1**).[18] In fact, polymorphisms of the genes encoding CTLA-4 and PD-1 have been associated with autoimmune diseases that share clinical features with toxicities from these therapies.[18,19]

The reported incidence of pneumonitis varied greatly across clinical trials with these agents, perhaps in part because of suboptimal reporting of low-grade and low-frequency IRAE overall,[20] but is generally accepted as being a rare event occurring in less than 10% of patients. However, pneumonitis has represented some of the most severe IRAEs observed in checkpoint immunotherapy trials and accounted for death in some subjects.[5,16,21,22]

In the existing literature, there is still significant variability in the reporting of frequency, timing of onset, disease characteristics, severity, management, and outcome for all IRAEs.[20] Rarer complications, such as pneumonitis, are particularly challenging to accurately characterize. IRAEs in large clinical trials are graded according to the National Cancer Institute's Common Terminology Criteria for Adverse Events version 4.0 (https://evs.nci.nih.gov/ftp1/CTCAE/

Box 1
Selected immune-related adverse events of anti-PD-1 and anti-CTLA-4 therapy

- Skin
  - Vitiligo
  - Maculopapular rash
  - Psoriasis
- Eye
  - Uveitis
  - Conjunctivitis
  - Blepharitis
  - Retinitis
  - Choroiditis
- Lung
  - Pneumonitis
  - Organizing pneumonia
  - Sarcoid-like reaction
- Heart
  - Cardiomyopathy
  - Myocarditis
  - Pericarditis
- Gastrointestinal tract
  - Gastritis
  - Enterocolitis
  - Hepatitis
  - Pancreatitis
- Endocrine system
  - Hypothyroidism or hyperthyroidism
  - Hypophysitis
  - Adrenal insufficiency
  - Diabetes
- Kidney
  - Interstitial nephritis
  - Lupuslike glomerulonephritis
- Nervous system
  - Peripheral neuropathy
  - Aseptic meningitis
  - Guillain-Barre syndrome
  - Encephalopathy
  - Myelitis
  - Myasthenia
- Musculoskeletal system
  - Arthropathy
  - Myositis
- Hematologic system
  - Hemolytic anemia
  - Thrombocytopenia
  - Neutropenia

Data from Champiat S, Lambotte O, Barreau E, et al. Management of immune checkpoint blockade dysimmune toxicities: a collaborative position paper. Ann Oncol 2016;27(4):559–74; and Michot JM, Bigenwald C, Champiat S, et al. Immune-related adverse events with immune checkpoint blockade: a comprehensive review. Eur J Cancer 2016;54:139–48.

CTCAE_4.03_2010-06-14_QuickReference_5x7. pdf); grading for pneumonitis events is outlined in **Table 2**. Parsing the severity of pulmonary IRAEs can be confounded by subjective thresholds for appreciation of symptoms by both patient and provider, by underlying chronic respiratory symptom burden from malignancy and nonmalignant comorbidities, and by other concomitant immunotherapy side effects such as fatigue and endocrinopathies. Thus, the use of consistent terminology in the grading of IRAE severity is essential, particularly as the body of knowledge about toxicity recognition and management grows.

A retrospective analysis of 298 patients with metastatic melanoma treated at Memorial Sloan Kettering Cancer Center with the standard treatment dose of ipilimumab (3 mg/kg) represents the largest body of data with this agent to date outside of clinical trial experience.[23] Overall, the incidence of any grade IRAE was 85% (with 31% grade 3 or higher); hepatotoxicity, dermatitis, and diarrhea were the most commonly IRAE observed. Pneumonitis was rare (<1%), but it accounted for some of the most clinically serious events. Thirty-five percent of individuals with IRAEs required steroid therapy and 10% required additional immunosuppression with either mycophenolate mofetil or infliximab. The investigators noted that the thresholds for initiation of either therapy were both variable and subjective, and some patients were treated for multiple separate IRAEs occurring concurrently. Nineteen percent of patients ultimately required permanent cessation of immunotherapy, including one patient with pneumonitis.

In the case of anti-PD-1 and anti-PD-L1 therapy, the incidence of pneumonitis has been more specifically addressed, as incidence appears higher with anti-PD-1 in particular compared with anti-CTLA-4. A meta-analysis of nearly 4500 patients who received anti-PD-1 immunotherapy in clinical trials for melanoma, NSCLC, and renal cell carcinoma revealed an overall incidence of pneumonitis at less than 3% for monotherapy with high-grade events in less than 1% of patients. The incidence of pneumonitis was more than doubled when anti-PD-1 therapy was combined with anti-CTLA-4.[24] As is anecdotally reported elsewhere, the rate of pneumonitis in clinical practice seems higher than that observed in clinical trials. A recently published multicenter analysis of greater than 900 patients treated outside of a clinical trial setting included individuals with a range of malignancies and immunotherapy regimens, most of whom were on monotherapy with anti-PD-1.[25] In this analysis of real-world experience, pneumonitis occurred in 5% of patients overall, although grade 3 or higher events remained infrequent at 1%. This study also yielded additional insights into clinical presentation, outcomes, and potential risk factors to be discussed later.

Table 2
Severity grading and management recommendations for pulmonary immune-related adverse events from anti–cytotoxic T-lymphocyte associated protein 4 and anti–programmed cell death-1 therapy

CTCAE Grade	Clinical Presentation	Suggested Initial Therapy	Fate of Immunotherapy
1	Asymptomatic, radiographic changes only	Close observation	Cautiously continue
2	Symptomatic, not interfering with ADL	Systemic oral steroids 0.5–1 mg/kg/d	Suspend temporarily
3	Symptomatic, interfering with ADL or with new oxygen requirement	Systemic oral or IV steroids 1–2 mg/kg/d, considering additional immunosuppression if no improvement in 3–5 d	Suspend, and likely discontinue
4	Life-threatening, requiring ventilatory support	Systemic IV steroids 1–2 mg/kg/d, considering additional immunosuppression for severe respiratory failure or if no improvement in 3–5 d	Discontinue permanently
5	Death		

Abbreviations: ADL, activities of daily living; CTCAE, common terminology criteria for adverse events.
Adapted from CTCAE Version 4.0. Available at: https://evs.nci.nih.gov/ftp1/CTCAE/CTCAE_4.03_2010-06-14_QuickReference_5x7.pdf; and Michot JM, Bigenwald C, Champiat S, et al. Immune-related adverse events with immune checkpoint blockade: a comprehensive review. Eur J Cancer 2016;54:139–48.

The experience with anti-PD-L1 agents remains somewhat limited. Three studies of atezolizumab in the treatment of NSCLC, renal cell carcinoma, and urothelial carcinoma reported an overall incidence of all-grade pneumonitis 2% to 3% with incidence of high-grade complications 0% to 1%; no deaths due to pulmonary toxicity have been reported.[26–28]

Timing of Toxicity

Most complications occur within the first 3 months of therapy with anti-CTLA-4 and within the first 6 months of therapy with anti-PD-1 and resolve within an average of 3 months.[29–31] However, considerable variability has been observed,[32] and toxicity has been observed as early as after the first dose of therapy and may emerge or relapse even after therapy has long since been discontinued. Earlier presentation has been specifically observed in patients with NSCLC, although this may be due to either increased tumor burden within the lungs, lower pulmonary reserve, or more frequent chest imaging.[33] Although there appears to be an increased risk for toxicity with higher doses of ipilimumab,[34] no such dose-dependent relationship has been observed with anti-PD-1 therapies.[29]

Features of Pulmonary Toxicity

The most common symptoms reported are dyspnea and nonproductive cough, with fever and chest pain less commonly reported.[25,32] Up to a third of patients with low-grade pneumonitis may be asymptomatic at presentation. The presence of additional extrapulmonary IRAEs is relatively common and should raise the index of suspicion. In general, any new persistent cough or shortness of breath in a patient receiving immunotherapy should be considered suspicious for pneumonitis.

There is considerable phenotypic variability to radiographic presentation on computed tomographic scan (**Fig. 2**), including organizing pneumonia (patchy consolidation usually in a peripheral distribution), interstitial pneumonitis-like patterns (interlobular septal thickening, sometimes with either subpleural reticulation or even honeycombing), hypersensitivity-like patterns (centrilobular nodules), sarcoidosis (pulmonary nodules with or without adenopathy), and nonspecific changes (including ground glass opacities and mixed presentations involving more than one of the above).[25] In clinical trial experience with anti-PD-1 therapies, organizing pneumonia has been cited as the most commonly observed pattern across cancer type and treatment regimens.[32] Rare cases of acute interstitial pneumonia have also been reported in the same meta-analysis. Of note, chest radiographs are not sensitive for detecting subtler abnormalities, and additional imaging should be pursued when index of suspicion is high.

Similarly, tissue abnormality is variable, reflecting the typical findings observed in each of the phenotypic subtypes described above. Bronchoscopy and lung biopsy remain valuable tools in excluding alternative diagnoses such as infection and progression of disease, but there is no single pathologic finding pathognomonic for pulmonary IRAEs from these agents. Lymphocytic infiltrates on bronchoalveolar lavage predominate, but eosinophils may be present, and granulomatous changes on lung biopsy have been reported. Sarcoidlike reactions represent a distinct pattern of pulmonary or multisystem toxicity seen with both anti-CTLA-4 and anti-PD-1 agents.[35–37] This pulmonary IRAE particularly poses diagnostic and

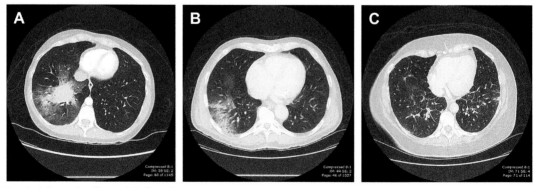

Fig. 2. (*A*) Pembrolizumab-induced pneumonitis in a 39-year-old woman with metastatic breast cancer. (*B*) Pembrolizumab-induced organizing pneumonia in a 78-year-old man with stage IV adenocarcinoma of the lung. (*C*) Ipilimumab/Nivolumab-induced granulomatous interstitial lung disease in a 56-year-old woman with metastatic melanoma who presented with dyspnea, cough, and mild hypoxemia. Note the reticular/nodular changes at the bases. Granulomas were demonstrated on lung biopsy. The patient also had mediastinal and hilar adenopathy (not shown).

management challenges in patients with melanoma, where the presence of new subcutaneous nodules can be mistaken for presumptive metastasis or progression of disease. The appearance of new adenopathy, even PET-avid adenopathy, should also not be presumed to be evidence of disease progression, particularly if accompanied by radiographic changes suggestive of pulmonary sarcoidosis, or if accompanied by dermatologic lesions. Biopsy can be helpful in such cases, acknowledging that granulomatous changes can be seen in association with some malignancies.

At this time, there are no serologic biomarkers that reliably assist in the diagnosis of suspected checkpoint inhibitor toxicity. Although the presence of autoantibodies has been identified in the case of some IRAEs, such as in thyroid endocrinopathies, autoantibodies are not consistently identified in patients with IRAE, making these tests of limited diagnostic utility.[18] Discovery of clinically relevant biomarkers remains a fertile topic for investigation as experience with these therapies expands.

Risk Factors for Toxicity

Rates of pulmonary IRAE vary considerably depending on the type of malignancy treated. Of the 2 diseases studied most extensively, some studies have suggested higher rates in NSCLC versus melanoma, whereas others have not.[24,25] Higher than average rates of pulmonary complications have also been observed in patients with hematologic malignancies and head and neck cancers, although the cohort sizes are too small to draw conclusions.[25]

Underlying pulmonary conditions, including history of smoking, have been more commonly observed in individuals experiencing pulmonary IRAEs, but given small sample sizes, this is a question that requires further investigation. In any case, individuals with underlying lung disease warrant particular vigilance for development of pneumonitis and more aggressive management given their limited pulmonary reserve and, potentially, increased susceptibility to injury.

Concurrent or sequential use of CTLA-4 and PD-1 blockade (particularly concurrent ipilimumab plus nivolumab) has resulted in enhanced clinical response in metastatic melanoma. Unfortunately, the rate of grade 3 or grade 4 IRAEs has been substantially higher than with either agent alone.[24,38] The incidence of pneumonitis in individuals receiving combination checkpoint therapy may be 10% overall.[25] Otherwise, prior non–checkpoint therapies, including multiple lines of chemotherapy and/or radiation therapy, do not appear to be clearly associated with higher rates of pulmonary complications.

Expression of biomarkers on tumor surface, most particularly PD-L1, has been examined in relation to tumor responsiveness with variable results, largely because the thresholds for "PD-L1 positivity" are not consistently defined and methods for staining are unstandardized. Although there is some correlation between PD-L1 expression and therapeutic response,[5] there is as yet no clear correlation between biomarker expression and IRAE, although this relationship has been suggested based on the observation that development of vitiligo is more frequent in melanoma patients with therapeutic response.[39] It is particularly difficult to examine biomarker expression in relation to rarer events, such as pneumonitis. Mechanistically, the development of IRAE in an organ system unaffected by malignancy would only occur if there was cross-reactivity between the anti-PD-1 agent and normal tissue antigens.[40] Therefore, at this point, any clear association between PD-1/PD-L1 expression and pulmonary toxicity remains elusive.

In general, treatment response has not been associated with incidence of IRAE in the case of ipilimumab.[41] In larger cohorts examining pulmonary toxicity with anti-PD-1 and anti-PD-L1 agents, most patients with pneumonitis have been classified as treatment responders; however, the significance of this observation remains unclear because these patients would have been exposed to immunotherapy for longer periods of time and screened for IRAE more extensively. Further investigation is required.[25]

Treatment

In milder cases, cessation of drug alone can be adequate. However, given the mechanism of action of checkpoint inhibitor therapy and the fact that antitumor responses persist long after cessation or completion of therapy, the window of drug-related toxicity may be longer than observed in conventional chemotherapy-related complications.

In cases where individuals are either symptomatic or demonstrate progression of toxicity despite cessation of immunotherapy, current consensus favors the use of corticosteroids.[25,42] Various doses and schedules for systemic steroids have been suggested depending on IRAE severity (see **Table 2**). Most IRAEs are steroid responsive and will resolve within 3 months.[30] An initial course of systemic steroids administered for 2 to 4 weeks, gradually tapered over an additional 4 weeks, serves as a general guide, but must be tailored to the severity of the event and response to initial therapy.[18] For more severe cases of pulmonary toxicity, steroids are initiated at doses of 1 to 2 mg/kg of prednisone or the equivalent until clinical improvement is observed, tapering over a period of 4 weeks or more.

The use of additional immunosuppressive medications, such as azathioprine, mycophenolate mofetil, cyclophosphamide, and infliximab, has been reported in severe, steroid-refractory cases; although impact on survival remains unclear, particularly both azathioprine and mycophenolate have significant delay to effect.[43,44] The suggested use of infliximab is largely extrapolated from the success in treating severe gastrointestinal IRAE, including life-threatening colitis.[45] Larger pooled trials have reported that most patients treated with these additional immunosuppressive agents unfortunately ultimately succumb either to acute respiratory failure from pneumonitis or, more often, secondary opportunistic infections that develop as a consequence of immunosuppression.[25]

Outcomes

The vast majority of patients who develop pulmonary toxicity while on immunotherapy will improve or resolve, either with drug cessation alone or with cessation and corticosteroid treatment.[25] Severity of the initial presentation and rate of response must ultimately guide the duration of steroid taper, and relapses have been reported even in absence of additional drug challenge, making identification of the ideal duration of therapy a challenge.[33] In some cases, subsequent relapses may present with a radiographic phenotype distinct from the initial presentation and may be both more clinically severe and more challenging to effectively treat.[25]

Concerns about the potential negative impact of systemic corticosteroid treatment on antitumor efficacy have been raised, although pooled data have not supported any effect of steroid treatment on overall survival or durability of response.[23] Moreover, in the case of significant IRAE, treatment of the complication takes precedence over impact on therapeutic efficacy.

Resumption of immunotherapy can be safely tolerated in some individuals with grade 1 to 2 pneumonitis once the initial toxicity has resolved, but rechallenge after IRAEs, with either the same or alternative agent, must be approached carefully on a case-by-case basis.[23,32] As with those that relapse without rechallenge, subsequent presentation can be variable, but the IRAE typically responds to repeat treatment with steroids.[25] The risks and benefits of rechallenge should be discussed with the patient and multidisciplinary treatment team, because at present there are no guidelines to differentiate those individuals at risk for recurrent complications from those who may resume therapy safely.

SUMMARY AND FUTURE DIRECTIONS

Real-world experience with immunotherapy, particularly at institutions that have treated large numbers of patients receiving these agents, suggests that the actual incidence of clinically significant IRAE may be higher than suggested by the data. It can therefore be expected that pulmonary toxicity from checkpoint immunotherapy may become more prevalent as use of these agents becomes more ubiquitous.[23,25] As in all cases of suspected drug-related pulmonary toxicity, the decision to discontinue a therapy that may provide substantial clinical benefit in difficult to manage advanced malignancies remains a challenging one. Multidisciplinary collaboration between oncology, pulmonology, radiology, and pathology physicians specializing in this patient population is extremely valuable in expanding the understanding of this phenomenon and developing refined strategies to diagnose and treat these complications with precision. Further investigation into the risk factors and mechanism for IRAE in general, and pneumonitis in particular, will enrich the understanding of these toxicities and the ability to treat patients effectively.

Although current pharmacologic immunotherapy remains squarely focused on the PD-1 and CTLA-4 axes, these are not the only checkpoint inhibitors currently under investigation as therapeutic targets. T-cell immunoglobulin and mucin domain 3 suppress T-cell activation, whereas lymphocyte activation gene 3, which is coexpressed with PD-1, enhances Treg activity and downregulates T-cell differentiation and proliferation; both have antibodies under investigation as clinical targets, particularly in combination with anti-PD-1 therapy.[46,47] Early results are promising, and there are numerous other molecular targets in preclinical stages of investigation.[48] Given the existing experience with IRAEs with checkpoint manipulation, pulmonary toxicities will remain a subject of concern as new therapies are developed in this field.

REFERENCES

1. Harris TJ, Drake CG. Primer on tumor immunology and cancer immunotherapy. J Immunother Cancer 2013;1:12.
2. Schreiber RD, Old LJ, Smyth MJ. Cancer immunoediting: integrating immunity's roles in cancer

suppression and promotion. Science 2011; 331(6024):1565–70.

3. Vinay DS, Ryan EP, Pawelec G, et al. Immune evasion in cancer: mechanistic basis and therapeutic strategies. Semin Cancer Biol 2015;35(Suppl): S185–98.

4. Atkins MB, Lotze MT, Dutcher JP, et al. High-dose recombinant interleukin 2 therapy for patients with metastatic melanoma: analysis of 270 patients treated between 1985 and 1993. J Clin Oncol 1999;17(7):2105–16.

5. Topalian SL, Hodi FS, Brahmer JR, et al. Safety, activity, and immune correlates of anti-PD-1 antibody in cancer. N Engl J Med 2012;366(26):2443–54.

6. Brahmer JR, Tykodi SS, Chow LQ, et al. Safety and activity of anti-PD-L1 antibody in patients with advanced cancer. N Engl J Med 2012;366(26): 2455–65.

7. Chambers CA, Kuhns MS, Egen JG, et al. CTLA-4-mediated inhibition in regulation of T cell responses: mechanisms and manipulation in tumor immunotherapy. Annu Rev Immunol 2001;19:565–94.

8. Leach DR, Krummel MF, Allison JP. Enhancement of antitumor immunity by CTLA-4 blockade. Science 1996;271(5256):1734–6.

9. Hodi FS, O'Day SJ, McDermott DF, et al. Improved survival with ipilimumab in patients with metastatic melanoma. N Engl J Med 2010;363(8):711–23.

10. Robert C, Thomas L, Bondarenko I, et al. Ipilimumab plus dacarbazine for previously untreated metastatic melanoma. N Engl J Med 2011;364(26):2517–26.

11. Ribas A, Kefford R, Marshall MA, et al. Phase III randomized clinical trial comparing tremelimumab with standard-of-care chemotherapy in patients with advanced melanoma. J Clin Oncol 2013;31(5): 616–22.

12. Okazaki T, Honjo T. PD-1 and PD-1 ligands: from discovery to clinical application. Int Immunol 2007; 19(7):813–24.

13. Chen L, Han X. Anti-PD-1/PD-L1 therapy of human cancer: past, present, and future. J Clin Invest 2015;125(9):3384–91.

14. Borghaei H, Paz-Ares L, Horn L, et al. Nivolumab versus docetaxel in advanced nonsquamous non-small-cell lung cancer. N Engl J Med 2015;373(17): 1627–39.

15. Brahmer J, Reckamp KL, Baas P, et al. Nivolumab versus docetaxel in advanced squamous-cell non-small-cell lung cancer. N Engl J Med 2015;373(2): 123–35.

16. Garon EB, Rizvi NA, Hui R, et al. Pembrolizumab for the treatment of non-small-cell lung cancer. N Engl J Med 2015;372(21):2018–28.

17. Ansell SM, Lesokhin AM, Borrello I, et al. PD-1 blockade with nivolumab in relapsed or refractory Hodgkin's lymphoma. N Engl J Med 2015;372(4): 311–9.

18. Michot JM, Bigenwald C, Champiat S, et al. Immune-related adverse events with immune checkpoint blockade: a comprehensive review. Eur J Cancer 2016;54:139–48.

19. Kuehn HS, Ouyang W, Lo B, et al. Immune dysregulation in human subjects with heterozygous germline mutations in CTLA4. Science 2014; 345(6204):1623–7.

20. Chen TW, Razak AR, Bedard PL, et al. A systematic review of immune-related adverse event reporting in clinical trials of immune checkpoint inhibitors. Ann Oncol 2015;26(9):1824–9.

21. Gettinger SN, Horn L, Gandhi L, et al. Overall survival and long-term safety of nivolumab (anti-programmed death 1 antibody, BMS-936558, ONO-4538) in patients with previously treated advanced non-small-cell lung cancer. J Clin Oncol 2015; 33(18):2004–12.

22. Postow MA, Chesney J, Pavlick AC, et al. Nivolumab and ipilimumab versus ipilimumab in untreated melanoma. N Engl J Med 2015;372(21): 2006–17.

23. Horvat TZ, Adel NG, Dang TO, et al. Immune-related adverse events, need for systemic immunosuppression, and effects on survival and time to treatment failure in patients with melanoma treated with ipilimumab at memorial sloan kettering cancer center. J Clin Oncol 2015;33(28):3193–8.

24. Nishino M, Giobbie-Hurder A, Hatabu H, et al. Incidence of programmed cell death 1 inhibitor-related pneumonitis in patients with advanced cancer: a systematic review and meta-analysis. JAMA Oncol 2016;2(12):1607–16.

25. Naidoo J, Wang X, Woo KM, et al. Pneumonitis in patients treated with anti-programmed death-1/programmed death ligand 1 therapy. J Clin Oncol 2016. [Epub ahead of print].

26. Fehrenbacher L, Spira A, Ballinger M, et al. Atezolizumab versus docetaxel for patients with previously treated non-small-cell lung cancer (POPLAR): a multicentre, open-label, phase 2 randomised controlled trial. Lancet 2016;387(10030):1837–46.

27. McDermott DF, Sosman JA, Sznol M, et al. Atezolizumab, an anti-programmed death-ligand 1 antibody, in metastatic renal cell carcinoma: long-term safety, clinical activity, and immune correlates from a phase Ia study. J Clin Oncol 2016;34(8):833–42.

28. Rosenberg JE, Hoffman-Censits J, Powles T, et al. Atezolizumab in patients with locally advanced and metastatic urothelial carcinoma who have progressed following treatment with platinum-based chemotherapy: a single-arm, multicentre, phase 2 trial. Lancet 2016;387(10031):1909–20.

29. Topalian SL, Sznol M, McDermott DF, et al. Survival, durable tumor remission, and long-term safety in patients with advanced melanoma receiving nivolumab. J Clin Oncol 2014;32(10):1020–30.

30. Weber JS, Dummer R, de Pril V, et al. Patterns of onset and resolution of immune-related adverse events of special interest with ipilimumab: detailed safety analysis from a phase 3 trial in patients with advanced melanoma. Cancer 2013;119(9):1675–82.

31. Villadolid J, Amin A. Immune checkpoint inhibitors in clinical practice: update on management of immune-related toxicities. Transl Lung Cancer Res 2015;4(5):560–75.

32. Nishino M, Ramaiya NH, Awad MM, et al. PD-1 inhibitor-related pneumonitis in advanced cancer patients: radiographic patterns and clinical course. Clin Cancer Res 2016;22(24):6051–60.

33. Nishino M, Chambers ES, Chong CR, et al. Anti-PD-1 inhibitor-related pneumonitis in non-small cell lung cancer. Cancer Immunol Res 2016;4(4):289–93.

34. Wolchok JD, Neyns B, Linette G, et al. Ipilimumab monotherapy in patients with pretreated advanced melanoma: a randomised, double-blind, multicentre, phase 2, dose-ranging study. Lancet Oncol 2010; 11(2):155–64.

35. Montaudie H, Pradelli J, Passeron T, et al. Pulmonary sarcoid-like granulomatosis induced by nivolumab. Br J Dermatol 2016. [Epub ahead of print].

36. Cousin S, Toulmonde M, Kind M, et al. Pulmonary sarcoidosis induced by the anti-PD1 monoclonal antibody pembrolizumab. Ann Oncol 2016;27(6): 1178–9.

37. Berthod G, Lazor R, Letovanec I, et al. Pulmonary sarcoid-like granulomatosis induced by ipilimumab. J Clin Oncol 2012;30(17):e156–9.

38. Larkin J, Chiarion-Sileni V, Gonzalez R, et al. Combined nivolumab and ipilimumab or monotherapy in untreated melanoma. N Engl J Med 2015;373(1): 23–34.

39. Robert C, Schachter J, Long GV, et al. Pembrolizumab versus ipilimumab in advanced melanoma. N Engl J Med 2015;372(26):2521–32.

40. Snyder A, Makarov V, Merghoub T, et al. Genetic basis for clinical response to CTLA-4 blockade in melanoma. N Engl J Med 2014;371(23): 2189–99.

41. Ascierto PA, Simeone E, Sileni VC, et al. Clinical experience with ipilimumab 3 mg/kg: real-world efficacy and safety data from an expanded access programme cohort. J Transl Med 2014;12:116.

42. Champiat S, Lambotte O, Barreau E, et al. Management of immune checkpoint blockade dysimmune toxicities: a collaborative position paper. Ann Oncol 2016;27(4):559–74.

43. Nishino M, Sholl LM, Hodi FS, et al. Anti-PD-1-related pneumonitis during cancer immunotherapy. N Engl J Med 2015;373(3):288–90.

44. Friedman CF, Proverbs-Singh TA, Postow MA. Treatment of the immune-related adverse effects of immune checkpoint inhibitors: a review. JAMA Oncol 2016;2(10):1346–53.

45. Johnston RL, Lutzky J, Chodhry A, et al. Cytotoxic T-lymphocyte-associated antigen 4 antibody-induced colitis and its management with infliximab. Dig Dis Sci 2009;54(11):2538–40.

46. Woo SR, Turnis ME, Goldberg MV, et al. Immune inhibitory molecules LAG-3 and PD-1 synergistically regulate T-cell function to promote tumoral immune escape. Cancer Res 2012;72(4):917–27.

47. Sakuishi K, Apetoh L, Sullivan JM, et al. Targeting Tim-3 and PD-1 pathways to reverse T cell exhaustion and restore anti-tumor immunity. J Exp Med 2010;207(10):2187–94.

48. Mandal R, Chan TA. Personalized oncology meets immunology: the path toward precision immunotherapy. Cancer Discov 2016;6(7):703–13.

Early Onset Noninfectious Pulmonary Syndromes after Hematopoietic Cell Transplantation

Lisa K. Vande Vusse, MD, MSc[a,b],*, David K. Madtes, MD[a]

KEYWORDS

- Idiopathic pneumonia syndrome • Cryptogenic organizing pneumonia
- Hematopoietic cell transplantation

KEY POINTS

- Idiopathic pneumonia syndrome (IPS) is an uncommon but deadly complication of transplantation with many clinical phenotypes.
- A better understanding of IPS pathobiology and the role of occult infection is needed to develop effective therapies.
- Some drugs given for conditioning or graft-versus-host disease prevention and treatment have known potential pulmonary toxicities.
- Venous thromboembolism and pulmonary hypertension can cause pulmonary symptoms with normal chest imaging after a hematopoietic cell transplant.

INTRODUCTION

More than a million hematopoietic cell transplants (HCTs) have been performed worldwide to treat a spectrum of benign and malignant diseases.[1,2] Survival rates after HCT are increasing over time because of advances in donor and recipient selection, pretransplant conditioning, infection and graft-versus-host disease (GVHD) prevention and treatment, blood transfusion management, and critical care.[3–6] Nonrelapse mortality within 200 days of allogeneic HCT decreased from 30% to 16% comparing years 1993–1997 to 2003–2007, respectively, at one high-volume US transplant center.[4] Despite improved overall survival, noninfectious lung injuries remain an important cause of morbidity and mortality after HCT. A recent "call to arms"

urges concerted efforts toward identifying effective preventive and therapeutic strategies.[7]

This article focuses on noninfectious pulmonary complications that manifest within the first few months after HCT. The first section reviews epidemiology, pathogenesis, treatment, and outcomes of the diffuse lung injuries collectively referred to as idiopathic pneumonia syndrome (IPS) and its clinically relevant subtypes, including diffuse alveolar hemorrhage (DAH) and cryptogenic organizing pneumonia. The second section reviews pulmonary toxicities of drugs commonly used for conditioning or GVHD prophylaxis and treatment. The final section summarizes the limited knowledge of less common pulmonary syndromes that occur after HCT, including pulmonary alveolar

Disclosures: The authors have no disclosures to report.
[a] Clinical Research Division, Fred Hutchinson Cancer Research Center, 1100 Fairview Avenue North, Mailstop D5-360, Seattle, WA 98109, USA; [b] Division of Pulmonary and Critical Care Medicine, University of Washington, 1959 NE Pacific Street, Seattle, WA 98195, USA
* Corresponding author. Fred Hutchinson Cancer Research Center, 1100 Fairview Avenue North, Mailstop D5-360, Seattle, WA 98109.
E-mail address: lkvandev@u.washington.edu

Clin Chest Med 38 (2017) 233–248
http://dx.doi.org/10.1016/j.ccm.2016.12.007
0272-5231/17/© 2016 Elsevier Inc. All rights reserved.

proteinosis, venous thromboembolism, and pulmonary hypertension.

IDIOPATHIC PNEUMONIA SYNDROME
Definition

The National Institutes of Health sponsored a workshop in 1991 with the goal of unifying research on lung complications of transplantation.[8] The standard IPS definition proposed by this group required evidence of widespread alveolar injury and absence of active lower respiratory tract infection (LRTI). LRTI could be excluded by either nonresponse to broad-spectrum antibiotics or at least one bronchoscopy with bronchoalveolar lavage (BAL) testing negative for an extensive panel of known pulmonary pathogens. Transbronchial biopsy was recommended when clinically permissible. Many clinical syndromes were included in this IPS definition, including acute respiratory distress syndrome (ARDS), acute interstitial pneumonitis, delayed pulmonary toxicity syndrome, peri-engraftment respiratory distress syndrome, DAH, cryptogenic organizing pneumonia, and bronchiolitis obliterans syndrome. The working group acknowledged the clinical heterogeneity within this definition and recommended multidisciplinary investigation to improve our understanding of IPS pathobiology and motivate novel treatments.

The emergence of new diagnostic technologies and newly recognized pulmonary pathogens resulted in updates to the original IPS definition.[9,10] The most recent published revision requires the exclusion of heart failure, acute kidney injury, and iatrogenic fluid overload as cause for the widespread alveolar injury.[11] The modified definition in **Box 1** incorporates an evolved understanding of pulmonary pathogens[12–16] and an appreciation that inflammatory lung injury and hydrostatic pulmonary edema can coexist.[17]

Epidemiology

Our knowledge of IPS epidemiology in the contemporary era is limited by the age of the currently available evidence and heterogeneous definitions used (**Table 1**). Two large retrospective cohort studies applied the standard IPS definition and found results similar to earlier studies of noninfectious interstitial pneumonitis and idiopathic interstitial pneumonitis. Incidence of IPS in these populations that included children and adults was 5.7% after autologous HCT[18] and 8% after allogeneic HCT.[18,19] Median time to IPS onset was 21 days, ranging from 7 to 34 days. Risk factors included high-grade GVHD, age, total-body-irradiation (TBI) dose, and transplant indication.

Box 1
Modified definition of idiopathic pneumonia syndrome

1. Widespread alveolar injury, as evidenced by
   a. Multilobar opacities on chest imaging
   b. Symptoms and signs of pneumonia
   c. Abnormal pulmonary physiology
      i. Increased alveolar to arterial oxygen difference
      ii. New or increased restrictive pulmonary physiology

2. Absence of active LRTI
   a. Negative tests for
      i. *Bacteria*: stains and cultures for bacteria, acid-fast bacilli, *Nocardia*, *Legionella*, *Mycoplasma*
      ii. *Viruses*: culture, DFA, and PCR for respiratory viruses (adenovirus, influenza, parainfluenza, metapneumovirus); shell vial culture (CMV, RSV); DFA for CMV, VZV, HSV; cytopathology for viral inclusions
      iii. *Fungi*: stain and culture; serum and BALF galactomannan ELISA for Aspergillus species; PCR for Zygomycetes and other non-*Aspergillus* invasive molds in some clinical settings
   b. Consider tests for possible pulmonary pathogens: HHV6, rhinovirus, coronavirus
   c. Consider lung biopsy if clinical condition permits and less invasive diagnostics are insufficient

3. No alternate explanatory cause for pulmonary dysfunction, such as heart failure, acute kidney injury, or iatrogenic fluid overload

Abbreviations: BALF, BAL fluid; CMV, cytomegalovirus; DFA, direct fluorescent antibody staining; ELISA, enzyme-linked immunosorbent assay; HHV6, human herpesvirus 6; HSV, herpes simplex virus; PCR, polymerase chain reaction; RSV, respiratory syncytial virus; VZV, varicella zoster virus.

Adapted with permission of the American Thoracic Society. Copyright (c) 2016 American Thoracic Society. Panoskaltsis-Mortari A, Griese M, Madtes DK, et al. An official American Thoracic Society research statement: noninfectious lung injury after hematopoietic stem cell transplantation: idiopathic pneumonia syndrome. Am J Respir Crit Care Med 2011;183(9):1263. The Am J Respir Crit Care Med is an official journal of the American Thoracic Society.

Mechanical ventilation was used in 62% to 69% of IPS cases, and mortality rates were approximately 75% in the hospital or within 30 days of discharge. Recent studies added prior HCT and

Table 1
Idiopathic pneumonia syndrome risk factor studies

First Author, Year	Years	Population	N	IPS Incidence (%)	IPS Risk Factors	Fatality/ Mortality (%)
Meyers et al,[146] 1982	1969–1979	Allo, syn BMT	625	11–12[a]	HM/AA, age, TBI in AA	61
Weiner et al,[147] 1989	1978–1983	Allo BMT	1183	11[a]	Methotrexate, age, severe GVHD, BMT >6 mo after diagnosis, reduced performance status, TBI dose >4 cGy/min	78
Wingard et al,[148] 1988	1976–1985	BMT	382	15[a]	HM	73
Kantrow et al,[18] 1997	1989–1991	First BMT	1165	5.7–7.6	Nonleukemia malignancy, grade IV acute GVHD	74
Bilgrami et al,[149] 2001	1993–1997	Auto PBSCT	271	3.4	—	80
Wong et al,[150] 2003	1992–2000	Auto HCT	164	12	—	15
Fukuda et al,[19] 2003	1997–2001	Allo HCT	1100	2.2–8.4	Age, grade II–IV acute GVHD, acute leukemia or MDS, TBI dose	75
Keates-Baleeiro et al,[23] 2006	1999–2005	Allo HCT[b]	93	11.8	Acute GVHD[c]	64
Zhu et al,[151] 2008	1997–2007	Allo HCT	192	12	HLA matched unrelated donor, grade III–IV acute gut GVHD	87–100
Sakaguchi et al,[24] 2012	1990–2009	Auto, allo HCT[b]	251	8	High-risk disease, busulfan conditioning	15
Sano et al,[20] 2014	1988–2007	Allo HCT[b]	210	6.7	Grade II–IV acute GVHD, prior HCT	79

Abbreviations: AA, aplastic anemia; allo, allogeneic; auto, autologous; BMT, bone marrow transplantation; HM, hematologic malignancy; MDS, myelodysplastic syndrome; PBSCT, peripheral blood stem cell transplantation; syn, syngeneic; TBI, total body irradiation.
[a] Idiopathic interstitial pneumonia considered equivalent to IPS.
[b] Study population included children only.
[c] Univariate analysis.

receipt of blood component transfusions to the list of IPS risk factors.[20–22]

Although IPS definitions, study populations, conditioning regimens, and observation times varied across these studies, there was a consistently high rate of respiratory failure and death. Reported outcomes were better in children than adults.[23,24] Updated studies are needed to better understand potential targets for intervention and inform bedside conversations about prognosis.

Pathogenesis

The histopathology of IPS spans a spectrum that includes diffuse alveolar damage, lymphocytic bronchiolitis, organizing pneumonia, and interstitial pneumonitis (**Fig. 1**).[25] Efforts to elucidate the pathogenesis of IPS are challenged by the heterogeneity of the syndrome and the concurrence of processes that modify biology, such as extrapulmonary GVHD and use of mechanical ventilation. Our current knowledge of IPS pathobiology derives largely from studies using murine models that recapitulate many of the biological features and physiologic changes observed in clinical settings.

In experimental IPS models, cytokine/chemokine-mediated signal transduction cascades orchestrate noninfectious lung inflammation and injury (**Fig. 2**). Tumor necrosis factor (TNF)-α,[26,27] interferon (IFN)-γ,[28,29] and lipopolysaccharide (LPS)[27] are proposed to mediate key pathways that converge in the lung.[30] Early in IPS development, TNF-α released from injured tissues may enhance costimulatory communication between the donor T cells migrating into the lung and radioresistant host monocytes/antigen-presenting cells.[31–35] Through dysregulation of interleukin (IL)-6, low IFN-γ levels promote expansion of alloreactive donor CD4+ cells, including T helper 17 (T$_h$17) cells.[30,31,35,36] Neutrophilic alveolitis is noted in the later stages of experimental IPS.[26,37] It is hypothesized that LPS translocates from intestines that were damaged by conditioning or acute GVHD and circulates to the lung where it activates neutrophils and macrophages.[30] The exact mechanisms of this proposed composite biology and how it ultimately injures host cells are not fully elucidated. In the end, severe pulmonary dysfunction results from capillary leak, pulmonary edema, disruption of pulmonary surfactant, and injury to and in some cases apoptosis of the bronchial epithelium, alveolar epithelium, and/or vascular endothelium.[33,38]

The few clinical studies examining cytokine levels in patients with IPS support some of these experimental findings. Blood and BAL fluid levels of TNF-α signaling and LPS-binding protein are elevated before and during IPS,[39–44] a finding that could be consistent with a "complex interaction of donor cells and recipient macrophages."[41] These studies support the hypothesized model of the dual roles played by TNF-α and LPS in IPS pathogenesis and suggest there is overlapping biology occurring in the systemic and lung compartments. The cytokines IL-2,[42] IL-6,[43] and monocyte chemoattractant protein (MCP)-1 are also elevated in clinical IPS.

Although these studies are important progress toward understanding IPS pathobiology, there remains work to be done. For example, it is not known how biology varies between IPS subtypes. A recent study by Seo and colleagues[45] highlights another important limitation to our understanding of IPS. Using modern molecular diagnostic technologies, the investigators detected occult potential pathogens in 57% of BAL fluid samples taken

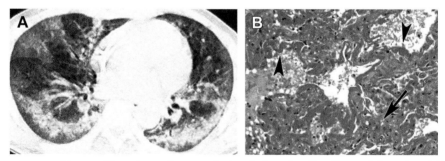

Fig. 1. IPS in 40-year-old man with acute myelogenous leukemia 4 weeks after allogeneic hematopoietic stem cell transplantation. (*A*) High-resolution computed tomography scan obtained at level of lower lung zones shows bilateral patchy areas of consolidation and ground-glass attenuation. (*B*) Photomicrograph of histopathologic specimen shows that alveolar septa are thickened by edema and round cell infiltration (*arrow*). Hyperplasia and desquamation of alveolar lining cells, fibrinous exudation, and hyaline membranes (*arrowheads*) are seen within alveolar spaces (hematoxylin-eosin, original magnification ×250). (*From* Franquet T, Müller NL, Lee KS, et al. Pictorial essay. High-resolution CT and pathologic findings of noninfectious pulmonary complications after hematopoietic stem cell transplantation. Am J Roentgenol 2005;184:629–37. Reprinted with permission from the American Journal of Roentgenology.)

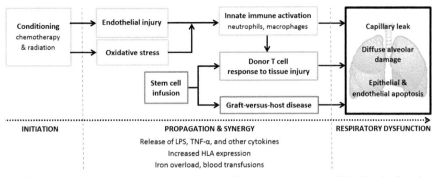

Fig. 2. IPS pathobiology. IPS can result from damage caused by pretransplant conditioning (*yellow boxes*) or from GVHD (*blue boxes*). These two pathways may act simultaneously and synergistically (*green box*) and may be amplified by inflammatory stimuli, such as iron overload and blood transfusions. LPS, lipopolysaccharide; TNF-α, tumor necrosis factor-α.

from clinically diagnosed IPS cases. Patients with occult microorganisms experienced worse outcomes. This study suggests that infection may play unrecognized roles in IPS development, phenotype, or severity. Alternatively, it is possible that clinical research from which the basic understanding of IPS arose was biased because of misclassification of true infectious pneumonia as IPS. Additional research is needed to progress our ability to develop new preventive and therapeutic strategies for IPS.

Predicting the Development and Outcome of Idiopathic Pneumonia Syndrome

Effective methods to identify patients at highest risk for IPS and predict responsiveness to specific immunomodulatory therapies could focus preventive efforts and treatment on those most likely to benefit. Using an unbiased proteomic approach, Schlatzer and colleagues[44] compared profiles of peptides found in blood collected the day of HCT between individuals who subsequently developed IPS and controls. The investigators generated and internally validated high-performing models that used varied combinations of peptides to predict the development of IPS and its response to treatment with etanercept, a soluble TNF-α-binding protein. Several proteins in the acute phase response signaling pathway were selected for inclusion in the prediction models and changed throughout the course of IPS, consistent with dysregulated innate immunity. Although this single study requires validation in an independent population with special attention to the potential role of occult infection, it highlights that biomarkers may be useful to advance our understanding of IPS.

Several other lines of inquiry examined associations between genetic polymorphisms or other biomarkers and the development of end points that overlap with IPS, such as acute lung injury

and GVHD.[46–51] Whether the results of these studies are generalizable to IPS and their potential to identify new therapeutic targets is unknown.

Treatments and Outcomes

High-dose systemic corticosteroids and supportive care are the current standard treatments for IPS. Metcalf and colleagues first reported their observations treating 63 people with DAH following autologous or allogeneic HCT.[52] Survival to hospital discharge was higher in those treated with more than 30 mg of methylprednisolone daily for 4 to 5 days followed by a taper (67% survival vs 10% on lower doses and 0% with supportive therapy alone). The 3 treatment groups experienced similar infection rates. A subsequent cohort study that included 81 IPS cases confirmed better survival with corticosteroids and showed similar outcomes when comparing 2 mg/kg/d prednisolone with 4 mg/kg/d.[19] In these observational studies, corticosteroids may have been withheld from the sickest patients who subsequently died, resulting in an inflated estimate of their benefit. Regardless, survival was unacceptably low at 30% to 33% despite treatment.

In an effort to improve outcomes, a series of studies motivated by preclinical data examined the clinical impact of modulating TNF-α in IPS. In observational studies, coadministration of methylprednisolone 1 to 2 mg/kg/d with *etanercept* 0.4 mg/kg given twice weekly for a maximum of 8 doses resulted in low toxicity, improved pulmonary physiology,[43,53] and increased short-term survival for IPS.[54] In contrast, a randomized placebo-controlled trial of *etanercept/glucocorticoid* combination therapy showed no survival benefit.[55] Importantly, enrollment was terminated early resulting in an increased chance of a false-negative result. In another trial, children receiving *etanercept* experienced higher rates of survival without supplemental oxygen 28 days after enrollment compared with historical controls.[40] Although long-term survival was not studied, 63% of etanercept-treated children remained alive 1 year later, a higher survival rate than seen in prior studies of corticosteroid therapy. The limitations of this trial include the lack of a contemporary control group and potential that participants have different characteristics than the broader population at risk for IPS. Whether *etanercept* improves survival or not and who is most likely to benefit remains unanswered.

A few other agents may meaningfully modify the biology of IPS; however, currently available evidence does not support their routine use. *Keratinocyte growth factor* (KGF) protects against chemoradiation-induced epithelial cell injury and enhances tissue repair, limiting IPS severity in mice and GVHD severity in clinical settings.[56,57] The limited data regarding the potential impact of *antioxidants* on IPS are conflicting.[58] *Antifibrinolytic therapy* may improve outcomes by directly reducing hemorrhage or indirectly by reducing the number of blood component transfusions, though the results of small observational studies are mixed.[59,60] *Defibrotide* is a profibrinolytic therapy that prevents and improves survival from sinusoidal obstruction syndrome,[61,62] a complication of HCT that also arises from endothelial injury.[63] Its use for IPS, however, may be limited by increased risk of hemorrhage. *Macrolides* suppress production of macrophage-derived cytokines implicated in IPS pathogenesis[64] and improve cryptogenic organizing pneumonia in small studies outside HCT settings.[65,66] Macrolides may similarly benefit patients with IPS when administered at doses higher than are commonly used for infection prophylaxis. The recent discovery of Th17 CD4+ T cells[67] and their important role in IPS and GVHD[28,36,68] may lead to new directions using *halofuginone*[69] or other Th17-suppressing therapies for IPS.

CLINICAL SUBTYPES OF IDIOPATHIC PNEUMONIA SYNDROME
Peri-Engraftment Respiratory Distress Syndrome

Engraftment syndrome (ES) is defined as fever or rash occurring within 5 days of neutrophil engraftment.[70] Risk factors for ES include male sex, myeloablative conditioning, high-dose TBI, and non–matched-related stem cell donor.[71] A subset of patients with ES develops the noninfectious pulmonary infiltrates and hypoxemia characteristic of *peri-engraftment respiratory distress syndrome* (PERDS), also known as capillary leak syndrome

(Fig. 3).[72,73] The capillary leak of PERDS results from activation of engrafting neutrophils, possibly in response to conditioning toxicity or T-cell autoreactivity.[72,74] PERDS occurs after 2.5% of autologous HCT. Its reported incidence varies widely after allogeneic HCT, whereby neutrophil activation may be a component of acute GVHD.[75] In the original description of PERDS after autologous HCT, 32% of 19 patients were mechanically ventilated and 26% died.[70] Most severe PERDS cases treated with systemic corticosteroids improved. Whereas ES is associated with transplant-related mortality,[71,75] the better response to corticosteroids and higher survival of PERDS relative to other IPS subtypes highlights the fact that IPS subtypes may have importantly different biology.

Diffuse Alveolar Hemorrhage

DAH is a subtype of IPS defined as BAL showing any of the following[76–78]:

- At least 20% hemosiderin-laden macrophages
- Blood in at least 30% of alveolar surfaces
- Progressively bloodier return on serial lavages

DAH manifests as dyspnea, nonproductive cough or hemoptysis, and hypoxemia with or without fever and may be progressive. Radiographically, diffuse alveolar and interstitial infiltrates in a predominantly central and basilar distribution are particularly suggestive of DAH; however, other patterns of diffuse opacities may

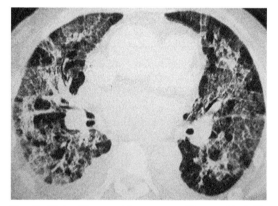

Fig. 3. ES in 46-year-old woman with non-Hodgkin lymphoma 3 weeks after allogeneic hematopoietic stem cell transplantation. High-resolution computed tomography scan shows bilateral areas of consolidation having peribronchovascular and subpleural distribution. Note right pleural effusion. (*From* Franquet T, Müller NL, Lee KS, et al. Pictorial essay. High-resolution CT and pathologic findings of noninfectious pulmonary complications after hematopoietic stem cell transplantation. Am J Roentgenol 2005;184:629–37. Reprinted with permission from the American Journal of Roentgenology.)

be seen (**Fig. 4**).[79] Although proposed to be a biologically distinct subtype of IPS,[80,81] DAH epidemiology and its poor outcomes are similar to those of IPS as a whole. In studies specifically examining DAH in transplant settings, incidence ranges from 1% to 21% with similar rates between autologous and allogeneic HCT.[80] Median onset ranges from 11 to 19 days after HCT.[77,80,82,83] Risk factors for DAH include myeloablative conditioning, TBI, and increased age.[79–81,84] Respiratory failure requiring mechanical ventilation occurs in most cases, and overall mortality ranges from 64% to 100%.[52,82,85,86] High-dose systemic corticosteroids and supportive care that may include platelet transfusions are standard; procoagulant therapies had variable success in small studies and are not routinely used.[59,60,87,88]

Delayed Pulmonary Toxicity Syndrome

Delayed pulmonary toxicity syndrome is a subtype of IPS that only occurs after autologous HCT. It presents with exertional dyspnea, nonproductive cough, often fever, reduced diffusing capacity, and radiographic findings of bilateral ground-glass, linear-nodular, consolidative, or mixed opacities. The incidence is 29% to 64% after receiving pre-HCT conditioning regimens containing carmustine (BCNU), cyclophosphamide, and cisplatin in combination. The median time of onset is 45 days (range, 21–149 days), and treatment with corticosteroids (1 mg/kg/d) results in resolution in up to 92% of cases.[89]

Cryptogenic Organizing Pneumonia/Acute Fibrinous Organizing Pneumonia

Cryptogenic organizing pneumonia (COP), previously called bronchiolitis obliterans-organizing pneumonia, is an idiopathic interstitial pneumonia that occurs after HCT. COP typically manifests as a subacute illness characterized by fever, dyspnea, and nonproductive cough. However, the timing and pace of onset of COP varies; its severity ranges from mild to severe respiratory failure.[90] The median onset is 108 days after HCT.[91] Risk factors include acute and chronic GVHD, female donors for male recipients, and conditioning with combination cyclophosphamide and TBI.[91,92] Radiographs commonly show unilateral or bilateral patchy foci of consolidation and ground-glass opacities with a subpleural, peribronchial, or bandlike pattern (**Fig. 5**).[93] Pulmonary function tests show ventilatory restriction and reduced diffusing capacity with or without obstruction. The definitive diagnosis of COP requires surgical lung biopsy; however, a case presenting with typical clinical features and bronchoscopy excluding infectious pneumonia may justify a treatment trial.[94] Histologic samples are characterized by patchy proliferation of immature fibroblasts called Masson bodies in a matrix of loose connective tissue involving the terminal airways, alveolar ducts, and alveoli with or without bronchiolar intraluminal polyps.[95] COP most often resolves with several months of corticosteroid therapy and frequently relapses with discontinuation of steroids. In one study of 51 COP cases treated with 1 mg/kg/d prednisolone following HCT, 78% resolved or remained stable and 22% progressed resulting in 16% case fatality.[91]

Acute fibrinous organizing pneumonia (AFOP) is a recently recognized, rare, and poorly understood complication of HCT.[96,97] AFOP may be part of the spectrum of nonspecific dysregulated response to lung injury along with diffuse alveolar damage and

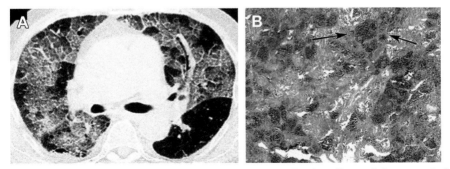

Fig. 4. DAH in 46-year-old woman with non-Hodgkin lymphoma 3 weeks after allogeneic hematopoietic stem cell transplantation. (*A*) High-resolution computed tomography scan obtained at level of carina shows diffuse ground-glass opacity in addition to septal thickening (crazy paving). (*B*) Photomicrograph of histopathologic specimen shows that macrophages containing hemosiderin are present within alveolar spaces (*arrows*) (hematoxylin-eosin, original magnification ×100). (*From* Franquet T, Müller NL, Lee KS, et al. Pictorial essay. High-resolution CT and pathologic findings of noninfectious pulmonary complications after hematopoietic stem cell transplantation. Am J Roentgenol 2005;184:629–37. Reprinted with permission from the American Journal of Roentgenology.)

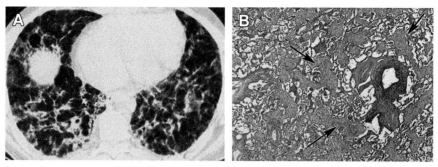

Fig. 5. Organizing pneumonia after hematopoietic stem cell transplantation in 38-year-old man. (*A*) High-resolution computed tomography scan obtained at level of lower lung zones shows bilateral patchy areas of consolidation in predominantly peribronchial distribution. (*B*) Photomicrograph of histopathologic specimen shows presence of fibroblastic tissue in lumina of peribronchial alveoli (*arrows*) (hematoxylin-eosin, original magnification ×100). (*From* Franquet T, Müller NL, Lee KS, et al. Pictorial essay. High-resolution CT and pathologic findings of noninfectious pulmonary complications after hematopoietic stem cell transplantation. Am J Roentgenol 2005;184:629–37. Reprinted with permission from the American Journal of Roentgenology.)

COP.[96] AFOP coexistent with COP marks a worse prognosis.[98] The original series of 17 AFOP cases described an acute to subacute respiratory illness with bibasilar reticular or nodular infiltrates.[99] Histologically, AFOP is characterized by patchy aggregates of intra-alveolar fibrin deposition (fibrin balls) with associated organizing pneumonia and in some cases neutrophilic inflammation of the alveolar walls. The clinical course of AFOP follows one of 2 trajectories: fulminant respiratory failure or subacute disease with recovery after treatment with corticosteroids. Corticosteroids and mycophenolate mofetil dual therapy may be effective for severe cases.[100]

TOXICITIES OF CONDITIONING AND GRAFT-VERSUS-HOST DISEASE PROPHYLAXIS REGIMENS

The patterns of pulmonary toxicity caused by drugs used for pre-HCT conditioning or GVHD are listed in **Table 2**. The drugs are categorized as those with established toxicity in HCT and drugs with toxicities observed outside HCT settings.

Drugs with Known Toxicities in Hematopoietic Cell Transplant

Carmustine, or BCNU, sometimes used alone or in combination before autologous HCT, is associated

Table 2
Pulmonary toxicity of chemotherapeutic and immunosuppressive agents

Agent	Pulmonary Toxicity
Known pulmonary toxicity in HCT	
Carmustine	Acute pneumonitis
Cyclosporine	Capillary leak (noncardiogenic pulmonary edema), ARDS
Sirolimus	Organizing pneumonia, DAH, ARDS, pulmonary alveolar proteinosis
Known pulmonary toxicity in other clinical settings	
Cyclophosphamide	Interstitial pneumonia, organizing pneumonia
Fludarabine	Interstitial pneumonitis, acute eosinophilic pneumonia
Azathioprine	Organizing pneumonia, DAH, interstitial pneumonitis, laryngeal edema, vasculitis
Tacrolimus	Organizing pneumonia
Mycophenolate mofetil	Pulmonary edema, ARDS, pulmonary fibrosis, bronchiectasis
Rituximab anti-CD-20 antibody	ARDS, DAH, interstitial pneumonitis, organizing pneumonia, pulmonary fibrosis, hypersensitivity pneumonitis
Alemtuzumab anti-CD52 antibody	DAH

with acute-onset pneumonitis with an incidence of 4% to 59%. Prior mediastinal radiation therapy, BCNU dose greater than 1000 mg, and age younger than 54 years are risk factors for developing pneumonitis after autologous HCT for lymphoma.[101]

Noncardiogenic pulmonary edema and ARDS have been reported in association with *cyclosporine* after bone marrow transplantation that resolves when the medication is discontinued and is postulated to be an idiosyncratic reaction.[102]

Sirolimus, used for acute GVHD prophylaxis[103] and for primary immunosuppression in active chronic GVHD, causes rare pulmonary toxicities that may be severe and fatal.[104,105] The predominant histologic patterns are organizing pneumonia, pulmonary hemorrhage, diffuse alveolar damage, and in a minority of cases pulmonary alveolar proteinosis.[104,106] The mainstay of treatment is discontinuation of the drug with or without corticosteroids (1 mg/kg/d), which typically results in complete resolution of symptoms within 2 to 4 months.

Drugs with Potential Toxicities in Hematopoietic Cell Transplant

Some chemotherapeutic or immunosuppressive agents used in HCT have known pulmonary toxicities in other clinical settings and should be considered during the evaluation of lung disease following HCT. *Cyclophosphamide,* used in combination with TBI or other chemotherapy agents in preparative regimens for HCT, is associated with interstitial pneumonia.[107] *Fludarabine*, a purine analogue used in nonmyeloablative conditioning regimens before allogeneic HCT, is infrequently associated with pulmonary toxicity in the forms of interstitial pneumonitis or, less commonly, acute eosinophilic pneumonia usually 3 to 14 days after the last dose.[108,109] Most cases respond to systemic corticosteroid therapy (1 mg/kg/d), suggesting an immunologic mechanism in the pathogenesis. Fludarabine-associated pulmonary toxicity can recur during steroid taper with improvement after reinstitution of steroid therapy.[108,110,111]

Monoclonal antibodies used for prophylaxis or treatment of acute GVHD are infrequently associated with pulmonary toxicity. *Rituximab,* a chimeric antibody against CD20, can result in ARDS and DAH developing within hours of administration or interstitial pneumonitis and COP developing within weeks.[112] Most cases resolve completely after discontinuation of therapy with or without corticosteroids.[113] A case series of renal transplant recipients reported DAH after treatment with *Alemtuzumab*, a cytolytic anti-CD52 monoclonal antibody used in reduced-intensity conditioning regimens to decrease the incidence and severity of acute and chronic GVHD and reduce graft rejection.[114]

OTHER NONINFECTIOUS PULMONARY SYNDROMES
Pulmonary Alveolar Proteinosis

In *pulmonary alveolar proteinosis* (PAP), terminal bronchioles and alveoli accumulate pulmonary surfactant and other amorphous periodic acid Schiff (PAS)–positive lipoproteins consequent to macrophage dysfunction.[115,116] PAP presents with cough, dyspnea, hypoxemia, and diffuse alveolar opacities with central mid and lower lung predominance.[117] There are congenital, autoimmune, and secondary forms of PAP. The congenital and autoimmune types arise from malformation of the granulocyte-macrophage colony-stimulating factor (GM-CSF) receptor[118,119] and formation of anti–GM-CSF autoantibody,[120] respectively. Secondary PAP occurs rarely after HCT, possibly from macrophage depletion or anti–GM-CSF alloantibody.[121] The diagnosis is suggested by bronchoscopy yielding opaque/milky BAL fluid and PAS-positive material present within macrophages after exclusion of infectious pneumonia. However, lung biopsy is required for definitive diagnosis. PAP after HCT may be self-limited but can also progress to fatal respiratory failure. Optimal treatment of this rare entity, including the role of GM-CSF therapy, is unknown. As is done in other settings, whole lung lavage should be considered in severe cases to restore alveolar ventilation with repeat lavage considered for recurrences.[122]

Venous Thromboembolism

Venous thromboembolism (VTE) is an underrecognized complication of HCT. In a retrospective study of 1,514 HCT recipients, the incidence of symptomatic VTE within the first 180 days after transplantation was 4.6%, including 0.7% incidence of non–catheter-associated lower extremity deep venous thrombosis (DVT) and 0.6% incidence of pulmonary embolism.[123] The median time after HCT admission to the development of non–catheter-associated lower extremity DVT and pulmonary embolism was 63 and 66 days, respectively. Prior VTE and GVHD were risk factors for the development of VTE after HCT. Thrombocytopenia was only partially protective against the development of VTE. The safety and efficacy of thromboprophylaxis in patients with HCT remains uncertain. In patients with thrombocytopenia, anticoagulant therapy for documented

VTE should be accompanied by platelet transfusions to maintain a platelet count of 5×10^4/L or greater to reduce the risk of bleeding complications.

Pulmonary Cytolytic Thrombus

Pulmonary cytolytic thrombus (PCT) is seen exclusively in allogeneic HCT recipients and almost always in children.[124] The incidence of PCT has been reported to range from 1.2% to 4.0% with a median onset at 3 months (range 1.3–11.3 months) after transplant. Clinical manifestations include fever, cough, and respiratory distress. Radiographic findings range from small, peripheral nodules to diffuse opacities. Diagnosis requires lung biopsy with histology characterized by vascular occlusions in distal pulmonary vessels, entrapment of leukocytes, endothelial disruption, and infarction of adjacent tissue. In a single-center, retrospective study, grades II to IV acute and chronic GVHD were independent risk factors for developing PCT. Treatment of PCT consists of systemic corticosteroids (prednisone 1–2 mg/kg/d) until pulmonary symptoms resolve (typically within 2 weeks) followed by a steroid taper over 2 to 4 weeks. The strong association with acute and chronic GVHD, as well as the response to corticosteroid therapy, suggests that PCT is a manifestation of alloreactive lung injury. The prognosis with PCT is favorable, and there have been no reported deaths attributable to this entity.

Pulmonary Hypertension

Pulmonary hypertension can occur after HCT secondary to a variety of causes that are managed by treating the underlying problem, including VTE, left heart failure, and hypoxemia-inducing diseases of the pulmonary parenchyma and airways.[125] Pulmonary arterial hypertension (PAH) is rarely reported after HCT and is best described in other clinical contexts.[126] This section focuses on *pulmonary venoocclusive disease* (PVOD), a syndrome of increased vascular resistance that is a rare cause of fatigue, dizziness, weakness, and dyspnea after HCT. Because of the overlapping clinical features, PVOD is easily misdiagnosed as PAH and may represent a spectrum of the same process[125]; however, it is important to distinguish from PAH because of the therapeutic implications discussed later.

The true incidence, risk factors, and outcomes of PVOD after HCT are unknown given the lack of prospective studies, nonspecific early manifestations, and heterogeneity of clinical phenotype.[126,127] Reported mortalities are close to 100% 2 years from diagnosis.[128] PVOD is hypothesized to arise from HCT-related vascular endothelial damage[129] and is characterized by pulmonary interstitial edema and capillary congestion due to fibrous occlusion of the postcapillary venules and sometimes larger veins.[130] As a result of elevated capillary pressures, PVOD may be accompanied by radiographic evidence of pulmonary edema and pleural effusions.[131] Elevated pulmonary artery pressures may be detected on echocardiogram; however, cardiac catheterization is recommended to confirm elevated pulmonary vascular resistance.[132] The triad of increased pulmonary vascular resistance with normal left heart filling pressures and radiographic edema is variably present in PVOD[133]; therefore, surgical lung biopsy should be considered if important for prognostication and referral for lung transplantation.[128]

Many therapies used in other clinical settings have been tried for PVOD that develops after HCT. Supplemental oxygen should be prescribed for all patients with hypoxemia.[134] Although there are case reports describing benefits from systemic anticoagulation or immunosuppression, especially in the presence of autoimmune features, the role of these therapies in the contemporary era of pulmonary vasodilator therapies is unknown.[135,136] In some cases, a trial of systemic immunosuppression may be reasonable.[128] Additional potential therapies include diuretics, inotropes, and pulmonary vasodilators (eg, calcium channel blockers, phosphodiesterase-5 inhibitors, endothelin receptor antagonists, prostanoids).[126,128] In contrast to PAH, historical experience with pulmonary vasodilators in PVOD demonstrates mixed results.[137–139] Vasodilators may cause harm and even death in patients with predominantly postcapillary vascular constriction. Alveolar flooding may result from increased perfusion in regions of fixed high postcapillary resistance.[140] Consultation with a pulmonary hypertension specialist is advised before giving vasodilators or inotropes to this population. Therapy may be most safely initialized in closely monitored settings.

Transfusion-Related Acute Lung Injury

Transfusion-related acute lung injury (TRALI) is defined as noncardiogenic pulmonary edema and respiratory failure occurring during or within 6 hours of a blood component transfusion.[141,142] TRALI is likely underrecognized in the highly transfused HCT population.[143] TRALI is caused by activation of pulmonary-sequestered neutrophils in response to passive transfusion of antibodies or other activating substances.[144] TRALI may be mild or result in mechanical ventilation and death.[145] Treatment is supportive care.

SUMMARY

A broad spectrum of noninfectious pulmonary syndromes contributes to morbidity and mortality after HCT. By being aware of the syndromes described in this article, practitioners can diagnose important causes of pulmonary dysfunction and institute appropriate therapies. Research is needed to identify individuals at risk for these syndromes and better elucidate their biology in effort to find more effective therapies.

REFERENCES

1. Gratwohl A, Baldomero H, Aljurf M, et al. Hematopoietic stem cell transplantation: a global perspective. JAMA 2010;303(16):1617–24.
2. Gratwohl A, Pasquini MC, Aljurf M, et al. One million haematopoietic stem-cell transplants: a retrospective observational study. Lancet Haematol 2015;2(3):e91–100.
3. Horan JT, Logan BR, Agovi-Johnson MA, et al. Reducing the risk for transplantation-related mortality after allogeneic hematopoietic cell transplantation: how much progress has been made? J Clin Oncol 2011;29(7):805–13.
4. Gooley TA, Chien JW, Pergan SA, et al. Reduced mortality after allogeneic hematopoietic-cell transplantation. N Engl J Med 2010;363(22):2091–101.
5. Giebel S, Labopin M, Holowiecki J, et al. Outcome of HLA-matched related allogeneic hematopoietic stem cell transplantation for patients with acute leukemia in first complete remission treated in Eastern European centers. Better results in recent years. Ann Hematol 2009;88(10):1005–13.
6. Gratwohl A, Brand R, Frassoni F, et al. Cause of death after allogeneic haematopoietic stem cell transplantation (HSCT) in early leukaemias: an EBMT analysis of lethal infectious complications and changes over calendar time. Bone Marrow Transplant 2005;36(9):757–69.
7. Radhakrishnan SV, Hildebrandt GC. A call to arms: a critical need for interventions to limit pulmonary toxicity in the stem cell transplantation patient population. Stem Cell Transplant 2015;10(1):8–17.
8. Clark JG, Hansen JA, Hertz MI, et al. NHLBI workshop summary. Idiopathic pneumonia syndrome after bone marrow transplantation. Am Rev Respir Dis 1993;147(6 Pt 1):1601–6.
9. Englund JA, Boeckh M, Kuypers J, et al. Brief communications: fatal human metapneumovirus infection in stem-cell transplant recipients. Ann Intern Med 2006;144:344–9.
10. Boeckh M, Erard V, Zerr D, et al. Emerging viral infections after hematopoietic cell transplantation. Pediatr Transplant 2005;9(Suppl 7):48–54.
11. Panoskaltsis-Mortari A, Griese M, Madtes DK, et al. An official American Thoracic Society research statement: noninfectious lung injury after hematopoietic stem cell transplantation: idiopathic pneumonia syndrome. Am J Respir Crit Care Med 2011;183(9):1262–79.
12. Williams JV, Martino R, Rabella N, et al. A prospective study comparing human metapneumovirus with other respiratory viruses in adults with hematologic malignancies and respiratory tract infections. J Infect Dis 2005;192:1061–5.
13. Renaud C, Xie H, Seo S, et al. Mortality rates of human metapneumovirus and respiratory syncytial virus lower respiratory tract infections in hematopoietic cell transplantation recipients. Biol Blood Marrow Transplant 2013;19(8):1220–6.
14. De Pauw B, Walsh TJ, Donnelly JP, et al. Revised definitions of invasive fungal disease from the European Organization for Research and Treatment of Cancer/Invasive Fungal Infections Cooperative Group and the National Institute of Allergy and Infectious Diseases Mycoses Study Group (EORTC/MSG) Consensus Group. Clin Infect Dis 2008;46(12):1813–21.
15. Fisher CE, Stevens AM, Leisenring W, et al. Independent contribution of bronchoalveolar lavage and serum galactomannan in the diagnosis of invasive pulmonary aspergillosis. Transpl Infect Dis 2014;16(3):505–10.
16. Neofytos D, Horn D, Anaissie E, et al. Epidemiology and outcome of invasive fungal infection in adult hematopoietic stem cell transplant recipients: analysis of Multicenter Prospective Antifungal Therapy (PATH) Alliance registry. Clin Infect Dis 2009;48(3):265–73.
17. Ranieri VM, Rubenfeld GD, Thompson BT, et al. Acute respiratory distress syndrome: the Berlin definition. JAMA 2012;307(23):2526–33.
18. Kantrow SP, Hackman RC, Boeckh M, et al. Idiopathic pneumonia syndrome: changing spectrum of lung injury after marrow transplantation. Transplantation 1997;63(8):1079–86.
19. Fukuda T, Hackman RC, Guthrie KA, et al. Risks and outcomes of idiopathic pneumonia syndrome after nonmyeloablative and conventional conditioning regimens for allogeneic hematopoietic stem cell transplantation. Blood 2003;102(8):2777–85.
20. Sano H, Kobayashi R, Iguchi A, et al. Risk factor analysis of idiopathic pneumonia syndrome after allogeneic hematopoietic SCT in children. Bone Marrow Transplant 2014;49(1):38–41.
21. Vande Vusse LK, Madtes DK, Guthrie KA, et al. The association between red blood cell and platelet transfusion and subsequently developing idiopathic pneumonia syndrome after hematopoietic stem cell transplantation. Transfusion 2014;54(4):1071–80.

22. Solh M, Morgan S, McCullough J, et al. Blood transfusions and pulmonary complications after hematopoietic cell transplantation. Transfusion 2016; 56(3):653–61.

23. Keates-Baleeiro J, Moore P, Koyama T, et al. Incidence and outcome of idiopathic pneumonia syndrome in pediatric stem cell transplant recipients. Bone Marrow Transplant 2006;38(4):285–9.

24. Sakaguchi H, Takahashi Y, Watanabe N, et al. Incidence, clinical features, and risk factors of idiopathic pneumonia syndrome following hematopoietic stem cell transplantation in children. Pediatr Blood Cancer 2012;58(5):780–4.

25. Yousem SA. The histological spectrum of pulmonary graft-versus-host disease in bone marrow transplant recipients. Hum Pathol 1995;26(6): 668–75.

26. Hildebrandt GC, Olkiewicz KM, Corrion LA, et al. Donor-derived TNF-alpha regulates pulmonary chemokine expression and the development of idiopathic pneumonia syndrome after allogeneic bone marrow transplantation. Blood 2004;104(2): 586–93.

27. Cooke KR, Hill GR, Gerbitz A, et al. Tumor necrosis factor-alpha neutralization reduces lung injury after experimental allogeneic bone marrow transplantation. Transplantation 2000;70(2):272–9.

28. Mauermann N, Burian J, von Garnier C, et al. Interferon-gamma regulates idiopathic pneumonia syndrome, a Th17+CD4+ T-cell-mediated graft-versus-host disease. Am J Respir Crit Care Med 2008;178(4):379–88.

29. Burman AC, Banovic T, Kuns RD, et al. IFN-gamma differentially controls the development of idiopathic pneumonia syndrome and GVHD of the gastrointestinal tract. Blood 2007;110(3):1064–72.

30. Cooke KR, Yanik G. Acute lung injury after allogeneic stem cell transplantation: is the lung a target of acute graft-versus-host disease? Bone Marrow Transplant 2004;34(9):753–65.

31. Clark JG, Madtes DK, Hackman RC, et al. Lung injury induced by alloreactive Th1 cells is characterized by host-derived mononuclear cell inflammation and activation of alveolar macrohpages. J Immunol 1998;161:1913–20.

32. Panoskaltsis-Mortari A, Taylor PA, Yaeger TM, et al. The critical early proinflammatory events associated with idiopathic pneumonia syndrome in irradiated murine allogeneic recipients are due to donor T cell infusion and potentiated by cyclophosphamide. J Clin Invest 1997;100(5):1015–27.

33. Cooke KR, Krenger W, Hill G, et al. Host reactive donor T cells are associated with lung injury after experimental allogeneic bone marrow transplantation. Blood 1998;92(7):2571–80.

34. Shankar G, Bryson JS, Jennings CD, et al. Idiopathic pneumonia syndrome in mice after allogeneic bone marrow transplantation. Am J Respir Cell Mol Biol 1998;18:235–42.

35. Holt PG, Haining S, Nelson DJ, et al. Origin and steady-state turnover of class II MHC-bearing dendritic cells in the epithelium of the conducting airways. J Immunol 1994;153:256–61.

36. Varelias A, Gartlan KH, Kreijveld E, et al. Lung parenchyma-derived IL-6 promotes IL-17A-dependent acute lung injury after allogeneic stem cell transplantation. Blood 2015;125(15): 2435–44.

37. Bhalla KS, Folz RJ. Idiopathic pneumonia syndrome after syngeneic bone marrow transplant in mice. Am J Respir Crit Care Med 2002; 166(12 Pt 1):1579–89.

38. Gerbitz A, Nickoloff BJ, Olkiewicz K, et al. A role for tumor necrosis factor-α-mediated endothelial apoptosis in the development of experimental idiopathic pneumonia syndrome. Transplantation 2004;78(4):494–502.

39. Holler E, Kolb HJ, Kempeni J, et al. Increased serum levels of tumor necrosis factor alpha precede major complications of bone marrow transplantation. Blood 1990;4:1011–6.

40. Yanik GA, Grupp SA, Pulsipher MA, et al. TNF-receptor inhibitor therapy for the treatment of children with idiopathic pneumonia syndrome. A joint Pediatric Blood and Marrow Transplant Consortium and Children's Oncology Group Study (ASCT0521). Biol Blood Marrow Transplant 2015;21(1):67–73.

41. Hauber HP, Mikkila A, Erich JM, et al. TNF-alpha, interleukin-10 and interleukin-18 expression in cells of the bronchoalveolar lavage in patients with pulmonary complications following bone marrow or peripheral stem cell transplantation: a preliminary study. Bone Marrow Transplant 2002;30(8): 485–90.

42. Clark JG, Madtes DK, Marin TR, et al. Idiopathic pneumonia after bone marrow transplantation: cytokine activation and lipopolysaccharide amplification in the bronchoalveolar compartment. Crit Care Med 1999;27(9):1800–6.

43. Yanik GA, Ho VT, Levine JE, et al. The impact of soluble tumor necrosis factor receptor etanercept on the treatment of idiopathic pneumonia syndrome after allogeneic hematopoietic stem cell transplantation. Blood 2008;112(8):3073–81.

44. Schlatzer DM, Dazard J-E, Ewing RM, et al. Human biomarker discovery and predictive models for disease progression for idiopathic pneumonia syndrome following allogeneic stem cell transplantation. Mol Cell Proteomics 2012;11(6). M111.015479.

45. Seo S, Renaud C, Kuypers JM, et al. Idiopathic pneumonia syndrome after hematopoietic cell transplantation: evidence of occult infectious etiologies. Blood 2015;125(24):3789–97.

46. Kallianpur AR. Genomic screening and complications of hematopoietic stem cell transplantation: has the time come? Bone Marrow Transplant 2005;35(1):1–16.

47. Paczesny S, Raiker N, Brooks S, et al. Graft-versus-host disease biomarkers: omics and personalized medicine. Int J Hematol 2013;98(3):275–92.

48. Dickinson AM, Harrold JL, Cullup H. Haematopoietic stem cell transplantation: can our genes predict clinical outcome? Expert Rev Mol Med 2007;9(29):1–19.

49. Miyamoto M, Onizuka M, Machida S, et al. ACE deletion polymorphism is associated with a high risk of non-infectious pulmonary complications after stem cell transplantation. Int J Hematol 2014; 99(2):175–83.

50. Ueda N, Chihara D, Kohno A, et al. Predictive value of circulating angiopoietin-2 for endothelial damage-related complications in allogeneic hematopoietic stem cell transplantation. Biol Blood Marrow Transplant 2014;20(9):1335–40.

51. Ponce DM, Hilden P, Mumaw C, et al. High day 28 ST2 levels predict for acute graft-versus-host disease and transplant-related mortality after cord blood transplantation. Blood 2015;125(1):199–205.

52. Metcalf JP, Rennard SI, Reed EC, et al. Corticosteroids as adjunctive therapy for diffuse alveolar hemorrhage associated with bone marrow transplantation. Am J Med 1994;96(4):327–34.

53. Yanik G, Hellerstedt B, Custer J, et al. Etanercept (Enbrel) administration for idiopathic pneumonia syndrome after allogeneic hematopoietic stem cell transplantation. Biol Blood Marrow Transplant 2002;8:395–400.

54. Tizon R, Frey N, Heitjan DF, et al. High-dose corticosteroids with or without etanercept for the treatment of idiopathic pneumonia syndrome after allo-SCT. Bone Marrow Transplant 2012;47(10):1332–7.

55. Yanik GA, Horowitz MM, Weisdorf DJ, et al. Randomized, double-blind, placebo-controlled trial of soluble tumor necrosis factor receptor: Enbrel (etanercept) for the treatment of idiopathic pneumonia syndrome after allogeneic stem cell transplantation: blood and marrow transplant clinical trials network protocol. Biol Blood Marrow Transplant 2014;20(6):858–64.

56. Clouthier SG, Cooke KR, Teshima T, et al. Repifermin (keratinocyte growth factor-2) reduces the severity of graft-versus-host disease while preserving a graft-versus-leukemia effect. Biol Blood Marrow Transplant 2003;9:592–603.

57. Panoskaltsis-Mortari A, Taylor PA, Rubin JS, et al. Keratinocyte growth factor facilitates alloengraftment and ameliorates graft-versus-host disease in mice by a mechanism independent of repair of conditioning-induced tissue injury. Blood 2000;96: 4350–6.

58. Haddad IY. Idiopathic pneumonia after marrow transplantation: when are antioxidants effective? Am J Respir Crit Care Med 2002;166(12 Pt 1): 1532–4.

59. Rathi NK, Tanner AR, Dinh A, et al. Low-, medium- and high-dose steroids with or without aminocaproic acid in adult hematopoietic SCT patients with diffuse alveolar hemorrhage. Bone Marrow Transplant 2015;50(3):420–6.

60. Wanko SO, Broadwater G, Folz RJ, et al. Diffuse alveolar hemorrhage: retrospective review of clinical outcome in allogeneic transplant recipients treated with aminocaproic acid. Biol Blood Marrow Transplant 2006;12:949–53.

61. Corbacioglu S, Cesaro S, Faraci M, et al. Defibrotide for prophylaxis of hepatic veno-occlusive disease in paediatric haemopoietic stem-cell transplantation: an open-label, phase 3, randomised controlled trial. Lancet 2012;379(9823):1301–9.

62. Richardson PG, Riches ML, Kernan NA, et al. Phase 3 trial of defibrotide for the treatment of severe veno-occlusive disease and multi-organ failure. Blood 2016;127(13):1656–65.

63. Cooke KR, Jannin A, Ho V. The contribution of endothelial activation and injury to end-organ toxicity following allogeneic hematopoietic stem cell transplantation. Biol Blood Marrow Transplant 2008;14(1 Suppl 1):23–32.

64. Cai M, Bonella F, Dai H, et al. Macrolides inhibit cytokine production by alveolar macrophages in bronchiolitis obliterans organizing pneumonia. Immunobiology 2013;218(6):930–7.

65. Pathak V, Kuhn JM, Durham C, et al. Macrolide use leads to clinical and radiological improvement in patients with cryptogenic organizing pneumonia. Ann Am Thorac Soc 2014;11(1):87–91.

66. Stover DE, Mangino D. Macrolides: a treatment alternative for bronchiolitis obliterans organizing pneumonia? Chest 2005;128(5):3611–7.

67. Weaver CT, Elson CO, Fouser LA, et al. The Th17 pathway and inflammatory diseases of the intestines, lungs, and skin. Annu Rev Pathol 2013;8: 477–512.

68. Carlson MJ, West ML, Coghill JM, et al. In vitro-differentiated Th17 cells mediate lethal acute graft-versus-host disease with severe cutaneous and pulmonary pathologic manifestations. Blood 2009;113(6):1365–74.

69. Sundrud MS, Koralov SB, Feuerer M, et al. Halofuginone inhibits Th17 cell differentiation by activating the amino acid starvation response. Science 2009;324(5932):1334–8.

70. Capizzi SA, Kumar S, Huneke NE, et al. Peri-engraftment respiratory distress syndrome during autologous hematopoietic stem cell transplantation. Bone Marrow Transplant 2001;27: 1299–303.

71. Schmid I, Stachel D, Pagel P, et al. Incidence, predisposing factors, and outcome of engraftment syndrome in pediatric allogeneic stem cell transplant recipients. Biol Blood Marrow Transplant 2008;14(4):438–44.

72. Spitzer TR. Engraftment syndrome following hematopoietic stem cell transplantation. Bone Marrow Transplant 2001;27:893–8.

73. Cahill RA, Spitzer TR, Mazumder A. Marrow engraftment and clinical manifestations of capillary leak syndrome. Bone Marrow Transplant 1996; 18(1):177–84.

74. Afessa B, Abdulai RM, Kremers WK, et al. Risk factors and outcome of pulmonary complications after autologous hematopoietic stem cell transplant. Chest 2012;141(2):442–50.

75. Chang L, Frame D, Braun T, et al. Engraftment syndrome after allogeneic hematopoietic cell transplantation predicts poor outcomes. Biol Blood Marrow Transplant 2014;20(9):1407–17.

76. De Lassence A, Fleury-Feith J, Escudier E, et al. Alveolar hemorrhage. Diagnostic criteria and results in 194 immuncompromised hosts. Am J Respir Crit Care Med 1995;131:157–63.

77. Robbins RA, Linder J, Stahl MG, et al. Diffuse alveolar hemorrhage in autologous bone marrow transplant recipients. Am J Med 1989;87(5):511–8.

78. Agusti C, Ramirez J, Picado A, et al. Diffuse alveolar hemorrhage in allogeneic bone marrow transplantation: a postmortem study. Am J Respir Crit Care Med 1995;151:1006–10.

79. Witte RJ, Gurney JW, Robbins RA, et al. Diffuse pulmonary alveolar hemorrhage after bone marrow transplantation: radiographic findings in 39 patients. AJR Am J Roentgenol 1991;157(3):461–4.

80. Afessa B, Tefferi A, Litzow MR, et al. Diffuse alveolar hemorrhage in hematopoietic stem cell transplant recipients. Am J Respir Crit Care Med 2002; 166(5):641–5.

81. Majhail NS, Parks K, Defor TE, et al. Diffuse alveolar hemorrhage and infection-associated alveolar hemorrhage following hematopoietic stem cell transplantation: related and high-risk clinical syndromes. Biol Blood Marrow Transplant 2006; 12(10):1038–46.

82. Lewis ID, DeFor T, Weisdorf DJ. Increasing incidence of diffuse alveolar hemorrhage following allogeneic bone marrow transplantation: cryptic etiology and uncertain therapy. Bone Marrow Transpl 2000;26:539–43.

83. Raptis A, Marvroudis D, Suffredini AF, et al. High-dose corticosteroid therapy for diffuse alveolar hemorrhage in allogeneic bone marrow stem cell transplant recipients. Bone Marrow Transplant 1999;24:879–83.

84. Sisson JH, Thompson AB, Anderson JR, et al. Airway inflammation predicts diffuse alveolar hemorrhage during bone marrow transplantation in patients with Hodgkin disease. Am Rev Respir Dis 1992; 146:439–43.

85. Nevo S, Swan V, Enger C, et al. Acute bleeding after bone marrow transplantation (BMT) - incidence and effect on survival. A quantitative analysis in 1,402 patients. Blood 1998;91(4):1469–77.

86. Wojno KJ, Vogelsang GB, Beschorner WE, et al. Pulmonary hemorrhage as a cause of death in allogeneic bone marrow recipients with severe acute graft-versus-host disease. Transplantation 1994; 57(1):88–92.

87. Baker MS, Diab KJ, Carlos WG, et al. Intrapulmonary recombinant factor VII as effective treatment for diffuse alveolar hemorrhage. J Bronchology Interv Pulmonol 2016;23(3):255–8.

88. Elinoff JM, Bagci U, Moriyama B, et al. Recombinant human factor VIIa for alveolar hemorrhage following allogeneic stem cell transplantation. Biol Blood Marrow Transplant 2014;20(7):969–78.

89. Wilczynski SW, Erasmus JJ, Petros WP, et al. Delayed pulmonary toxicity syndrome following high-dose chemotherapy and bone marrow transplantation for breast cancer. Am J Respir Crit Care Med 1998;157(2):565–73.

90. American Thoracic Society, European Respiratory Society. American Thoracic Society/European Respiratory Society international multidisciplinary consensus classification of the idiopathic interstitial pneumonias. Am J Respir Crit Care Med 2002; 165(2):277–304.

91. Freudenberger TD, Madtes DK, Curtis JR, et al. Association between acute and chronic graft-versus-host disease and bronchiolitis obliterans organizing pneumonia in recipients of hematopoietic stem cell transplants. Blood 2003;102(10):3822–8.

92. Nakasone H, Onizuka M, Suzuki N, et al. Pre-transplant risk factors for cryptogenic organizing pneumonia/bronchiolitis obliterans organizing pneumonia after hematopoietic cell transplantation. Bone Marrow Transplant 2013;48(10):1317–23.

93. Pipavath SNJ, Chung JH, Chien JW, et al. Organizing pneumonia in recipients of hematopoietic stem cell transplantation: CT features in 16 patients. J Comput Assist Tomogr 2012;36:431–6.

94. Cottin V, Cordier JF. Cryptogenic organizing pneumonia. Semin Respir Crit Care Med 2012;33(5): 462–75.

95. Tabaj GC, Fernandez CF, Sabbagh E, et al. Histopathology of the idiopathic interstitial pneumonias (IIP): a review. Respirology 2015;20(6):873–83.

96. Travis WD, Costabel U, Hansell DM, et al. An official American Thoracic Society/European Respiratory Society statement: update of the international multidisciplinary classification of the idiopathic interstitial pneumonias. Am J Respir Crit Care Med 2013;188(6):733–48.

97. Lee SM, Park JJ, Sung SH, et al. Acute fibrinous and organizing pneumonia following hematopoietic stem cell transplantation. Korean J Intern Med 2009;24(2):156–9.

98. Nishino M, Mathai SK, Schoenfeld D, et al. Clinicopathologic features associated with relapse in cryptogenic organizing pneumonia. Hum Pathol 2014;45(2):342–51.

99. Beasley MB, Franks TJ, Galvin JR, et al. Acute fibrinous and organizing pneumonia: a histological pattern of lung injury and possible variant of diffuse alveolar damage. Arch Pathol Lab Med 2002; 126(9):1064–70.

100. Bhatti S, Hakeem A, Torrealba J, et al. Severe acute fibrinous and organizing pneumonia (AFOP) causing ventilatory failure: successful treatment with mycophenolate mofetil and corticosteroids. Respir Med 2009;103(11):1764–7.

101. Lane AA, Armand P, Feng Y, et al. Risk factors for development of pneumonitis after high-dose chemotherapy with cyclophosphamide, BCNU and etoposide followed by autologous stem cell transplant. Leuk Lymphoma 2012;53(6):1130–6.

102. Madtes DK. Pulmonary complications of stem cell and solid organ transplantation. In: Broaddus VC, editor. Murray and Nadel's textbook of respiratory medicinevol. 2, 6th edition. Philadelphia: Saunders; 2016. p. 1612–23.e8.

103. Cutler C, Logan B, Nakamura R, et al. Tacrolimus/sirolimus vs tacrolimus/methotrexate as GVHD prophylaxis after matched, related donor allogeneic HCT. Blood 2014;124(8):1372–7.

104. Garrod AS, Goyal RK, Weiner DJ. Sirolimus-induced interstitial lung disease following pediatric stem cell transplantation. Pediatr Transplant 2015; 19(3):E75–7.

105. Patel AV, Hahn T, Bogner PN, et al. Fatal diffuse alveolar hemorrhage associated with sirolimus after allogeneic hematopoietic cell transplantation. Bone Marrow Transplant 2010;45(8):1363–4.

106. Champion L, Stern M, Israel-Biet D, et al. Brief communication: sirolimus-associated pneumonitis: 24 cases in renal transplant recipients. Ann Intern Med 2006;144(7):505–9.

107. Malik SW, Myers JL, DeRemee RA, et al. Lung toxicity associated with cyclophosphamide use. Two distinct patterns. Am J Respir Crit Care Med 1996;154(6 Pt 1):1851–6.

108. Helman DL Jr, Byrd JC, Ales NC, et al. Fludarabine-related pulmonary toxicity: a distinct clinical entity in chronic lymphoproliferative syndromes. Chest 2002;122(3):785–90.

109. Trojan A, Meier R, Licht A, et al. Eosinophilic pneumonia after administration of fludarabine for the treatment of non-Hodgkin's lymphoma. Ann Hematol 2002;81:535–7.

110. Hurst PG, Habib MP, Garewal H, et al. Pulmonary toxicity associated with fludarabine monophosphate. Invest New Drugs 1987;5(2):207–10.

111. Disel U, Paydas S, Yavuz S, et al. Severe pulmonary toxicity associated with fludarabine and possible contribution of rituximab. Chemotherapy 2010;56(2):89–93.

112. Liote H, Liote F, Seroussi B, et al. Rituximab-induced lung disease: a systematic literature review. Eur Respir J 2010;35(3):681–7.

113. Hadjinicolaou AV, Nisar MK, Parfrey H, et al. Non-infectious pulmonary toxicity of rituximab: a systematic review. Rheumatology (Oxford) 2012; 51(4):653–62.

114. Sachdeva A, Matuschak GM. Diffuse alveolar hemorrhage following alemtuzumab. Chest 2008; 133(6):1476–8.

115. Rosen SH, Castleman B, Liebow AA, et al. Pulmonary alveolar proteinosis. N Engl J Med 1958;258: 1123–42.

116. Seymour JF, Presneill JJ. Pulmonary alveolar proteinosis: progress in the first 44 years. Am J Respir Crit Care Med 2002;166(2):215–35.

117. Trapnell BC, Whitsett JA, Nakata K. Pulmonary alveolar proteinosis. N Engl J Med 2003;349:2527–39.

118. Dirksen U, Nishinakamura R, Groneck P, et al. Human pulmonary alveolar proteinosis associated with a defect in GM-CSF/IL-3/IL-5 receptor common beta chain expression. J Clin Invest 1997; 100(9):2211–7.

119. Suzuki T, Sakagami T, Rubin BK, et al. Familial pulmonary alveolar proteinosis caused by mutations in CSF2RA. J Exp Med 2008;205(12):2703–10.

120. Sakagumi T, Uchida K, Suzuki T, et al. Human GM-CSF autoantibodies and reproduction of pulmonary alveolar proteinosis. N Engl J Med 2009;361(27): 2679–81.

121. Pidala J, Khalil F, Fernandez H. Pulmonary alveolar proteinosis following allogeneic hematopoietic cell transplantation. Bone Marrow Transplant 2011; 46(11):1480–3.

122. Beccaria M, Luisetti M, Rodi G, et al. Long-term durable benefit after whole lung lavage in pulmonary alveolar proteinosis. Eur Respir J 2004;23(4): 526–31.

123. Gerber DE, Segal JB, Levy MY, et al. The incidence of and risk factors for venous thromboembolism (VTE) and bleeding among 1514 patients undergoing hematopoietic stem cell transplantation: implications for VTE prevention. Blood 2008;112(3):504–10.

124. Woodard JP, Gulbahce E, Shreve M, et al. Pulmonary cytolytic thrombi: a newly recognized complication of stem cell transplantation. Bone Marrow Transplant 2000;25(3):293–300.

125. Simonneau G, Gatzoulis MA, Adatia I, et al. Updated clinical classification of pulmonary hypertension. J Am Coll Cardiol 2013;62(25 Suppl):D34–41.

126. Dandoy CE, Hirsch R, Chima R, et al. Pulmonary hypertension after hematopoietic stem cell transplantation. Biol Blood Marrow Transplant 2013;19(11):1546–56.

127. Bunte MC, Patnaik MM, Pritzker MR, et al. Pulmonary veno-occlusive disease following hematopoietic stem cell transplantation: a rare model of endothelial dysfunction. Bone Marrow Transplant 2008;41(8):677–86.

128. Mandel J, Mark EJ, Hales CA. Pulmonary veno-occlusive disease. Am J Respir Crit Care Med 2000;162:1964–73.

129. Jodele S, Hirsch R, Laskin B, et al. Pulmonary arterial hypertension in pediatric patients with hematopoietic stem cell transplant-associated thrombotic microangiopathy. Biol Blood Marrow Transplant 2013;19(2):202–7.

130. Troussard X, Bernaudin JF, Cordonnier C, et al. Pulmonary veno-occlusive disease after bone marrow transplantation. Thorax 1984;39:956–7.

131. Resten A, Maitre S, Humbert M, et al. Pulmonary hypertension: CT of the chest in pulmonary venoocclusive disease. AJR Am J Roentgenol 2004;183: 65–70.

132. Galie N, Humbert M, Vachiery JL, et al. 2015 ESC/ERS guidelines for the diagnosis and treatment of pulmonary hypertension. Eur Respir J 2015;46: 903–75.

133. Rambihar VS, Fallen EL, Cairns JA. Pulmonary veno-occlusive disease: antemortem diagnosis from roentgenographic and hemodynamic findings. Can Med Assoc J 1979;120:1519–22.

134. Roberts DH, Lepore JJ, Maroo A, et al. Oxygen therapy improves cardiac index and pulmonary vascular resistance in patients with pulmonary hypertension. Chest 2001;120(5):1547–55.

135. Frank H, Ruber K, Mlczoch J, et al. The effect of anticoagulant therapy in primary and anorectic drug-induced pulmonary hypertension. Chest 1997;112(3):714–21.

136. Sanderson JE, Spiro SG, Hendry AT, et al. A case of pulmonary veno-occlusive disease responding to treatment with azathioprine. Thorax 1977;32: 140–8.

137. Kuroda T, Hirota H, Masaki M, et al. Sildenafil as adjunct therapy to high-dose epoprostenol in a patient with pulmonary veno-occlusive disease. Heart Lung Circ 2006;15(2):139–42.

138. Okumura H, Nagaya N, Kyotani S, et al. Effects of continuous IV prostacyclin in a patient with pulmonary veno-occlusive disease. Chest 2002;122(3): 1096–8.

139. Palevsky HI, Pietra GG, Fishman AP. Pulmonary veno-occlusive disease and its response to vasodilator agents. Am Rev Respir Dis 1990;142:426–9.

140. Palmer SM, Robinson LJ, Wang A, et al. Massive pulmonary edema and death after prostacyclin infusion in a patient with pulmonary veno-occlusive disease. Chest 1998;113(1):237–40.

141. Kleinman S, Caulfield T, Chan P, et al. Toward an understanding of transfusion-related acute lung injury: statement of a consensus panel. Transfusion 2004;44:1774–89.

142. Toy P, Popovsky MA, Abraham E, et al. Transfusion-related acute lung injury: definition and review. Crit Care Med 2005;33(4):721–6.

143. Ganguly S, Carrum G, Nizzi F, et al. Transfusion-related acute lung injury (TRALI) following allogeneic stem cell transplant for acute myeloid leukemia. Am J Hematol 2004;75:48–51.

144. Bux J, Sachs UJ. The pathogenesis of transfusion-related acute lung injury (TRALI). Br J Haematol 2007;136(6):788–99.

145. Looney MR, Roubinian N, Gajic O, et al. Prospective study on the clinical course and outcomes in transfusion-related acute lung injury. Crit Care Med 2014;42(7):1676–87.

146. Meyers JD, Flournoy N, Thomas ED. Nonbacterial pneumonia after allogeneic marrow transplantation: a review of ten years' experience. Rev Infect Dis 1982;4(6):1119–32.

147. Weiner RS, Horowitz MM, Gale RP, et al. Risk factors for interstitial pneumonia following bone marrow transplantation for severe aplastic anemia. Br J Haematol 1989;71:535–43.

148. Wingard JR, Mellits ED, Sostrin MB, et al. Interstitial pneumonitis after allogeneic bone marrow transplantation: nine-year experience at a single institution. Medicine 1988;67(3):175–86.

149. Bilgrami SF, Metersky ML, McNally D, et al. Idiopathic pneumonia syndrome following myeloablative chemotherapy and autologous transplantation. Ann Pharmacother 2001;35:196–201.

150. Wong R, Rondon G, Saliba RM, et al. Idiopathic pneumonia syndrome after high-dose chemotherapy and autologous hematopoietic stem cell transplantation for high-risk breast cancer. Bone Marrow Transplant 2003;31:1157–63.

151. Zhu KE, Hu JY, Zhang T, et al. Incidence, risks, and outcome of idiopathic pneumonia syndrome early after allogeneic hematopoietic stem cell transplantation. Eur J Haematol 2008;81(6):461–6.

Late-Onset Noninfectious Pulmonary Complications After Allogeneic Hematopoietic Stem Cell Transplantation

Anne Bergeron, MD, PhD[a,b],*

KEYWORDS

- Bronchiolitis obliterans • Interstitial lung disease • Lung graft-versus-host disease
- Pulmonary vascular disease • Pleural effusion • Organizing pneumonia
- Thoracic air leak syndrome • Pleuroparenchymal fibroelastosis

KEY POINTS

- Late-onset noninfectious pulmonary complications (LONIPCs) occurring after allogeneic hematopoietic stem cell transplantation may involve all anatomic regions of the lung.
- Most instances of LONIPC are associated with extrathoracic graft-versus-host disease.
- Bronchiolitis obliterans syndrome is the most frequently encountered LONIPC. Early diagnostic strategies are needed for the development of a novel treatment options.
- Interstitial lung diseases are overlooked with regard to LONIPCs and include several histologic entities.

INTRODUCTION

Hematologic malignancies are the main clinical indications for allogeneic hematopoietic stem cell transplantation (HSCT). In previous years, the evolution of this procedure—including the reduction of the intensity of conditioning regimen and the development of new stem cell sources—have allowed a growing number of patients to access this type of treatment. Furthermore, advances in the prevention, diagnosis, and treatment of infectious complications have contributed to the reduced early mortality related to infections occurring after allogeneic HSCT. Although patient survival after allogeneic HSCT has increased, late complications involving several organ systems have emerged.

Late-onset noninfectious pulmonary complications (LONIPCs) occur in up to 20% of allogeneic HSCT recipients[1–3] and can involve all lung anatomic regions: bronchi, parenchyma, vessels, and pleura, leading to various clinical entities. LONIPCs are characterized by highly associated mortalities and morbidities.[2,4–6] Each entity of LONIPC is not specific for allogeneic HSCT and can be either idiopathic or diagnosed in other settings, including connective tissue disorders, lung transplantation, and disease due to environmental toxins or drugs. Regardless of the context,

The author declares no conflicts of interest.
[a] Respiratory Medicine Department, AP-HP, Saint-Louis Hospital, 1 Avenue Claude Vellefaux, Paris F-75010, France; [b] Sorbonne Paris Cité, UMR 1153 CRESS, Biostatistics and Clinical Epidemiology Research Team, Univ Paris Diderot, 1 Avenue Claude Vellefaux, Paris F-75010, France
* Respiratory Medicine Department, AP-HP, Saint-Louis Hospital, 1 Avenue Claude Vellefaux, Paris Cedex 10 75475, France.
E-mail address: anne.bergeron-lafaurie@aphp.fr

0272-5231/17/© 2017 Elsevier Inc. All rights reserved.

knowledge of these pulmonary diseases should help clinicians to better understand and manage postallogeneic HSCT patients who develop LONIPCs.

After HSCT, 2 clinical situations lead to the diagnosis of LONIPC: (1) the development of respiratory symptoms (eg, dyspnea, cough, sputum, and wheezing) or (2) the deterioration of lung function based on sequential posttransplant screening pulmonary function tests (PFT). Of note, many events occurring after HSCT such as infection or generalized fatigue may mask dyspnea. A patient who is deconditioned from the HSCT procedure may complain only when resuming a physical activity long after the onset of lung disease. In any case, thoracic imaging (radiograph and lung computed tomography [CT] scan) will guide the diagnosis. Attention should be paid to the fact that abnormalities of the chest wall (eg, subcutaneous tissue, diaphragm, and spine) that may occur after HSCT may be associated with a defect in lung function in the absence of LONIPCs. If an LONIPC is suspected, respiratory infection should be ruled out before retaining the LONIPC diagnosis. Finally, although lung biopsy is the gold standard for classifying LONIPCs, fewer and fewer patients undergo lung surgery due to the associated complications in allogeneic HSCT recipients and the advances in diagnosing and preventing differential infectious diagnoses.[7–9] Lung biopsy should be discussed on a multidisciplinary case-by-case basis. Thus, most LONIPCs diagnoses rely mainly on PFT and CT scan data. In this article, the author reviews the current knowledge about different LONIPCs.

BRONCHIOLITIS OBLITERANS

Postallogeneic HSCT bronchiolitis obliterans (BO) was first described in the early 1980s.[10] It is now recognized as the most frequent LONIPC and the only one that has been definitively linked to pulmonary chronic graft-versus-host disease (cGVHD).[8,11,12]

Diagnostic Criteria for Bronchiolitis Obliterans Syndrome

A diagnosis of bronchiolitis obliterans (BO) relies on histologic analysis of a surgical lung biopsy showing an obliterative bronchiolitis characterized by thickening of the bronchiolar wall via inflammatory fibrosis; this thickening is located between the epithelium and the smooth muscle, narrowing the airway lumen[13,14] (**Fig. 1**). Given the invasiveness of lung biopsy, the diagnosis of bronchiolitis obliterans syndrome (BOS) based on PFT is now endorsed.[8,12]

Clinical signs of BOS are nonspecific and vary among patients. Cough and dyspnea are the most common symptoms; patients may also experience wheezing or repeated lung infections. Lung auscultation may either be normal or reveal wheezing, subcrepitant, or squeaking sounds suggestive of small airway obstruction. Patients may be asymptomatic during the early stages of the disease. Thus, a diagnosis of BOS relies mainly on post-HSCT PFT demonstrating new onset airflow obstruction.

Before 2005, the definition of BOS was variable from one study to another, which explains the wide disparity of the published data.[15–21] In 2005, the National Institutes of Health (NIH) established standardized criteria for the diagnosis of cGVHD in clinical trials.[11] In these consensus guidelines, a diagnosis of BOS required at least one other distinctive manifestation of chronic GVHD in a separate organ system and a workup to rule out an infection in the respiratory tract. The functional diagnosis criteria for BOS were as follows: ratio of forced expiratory volume in 1 second (FEV1)/forced vital capacity (FVC) <0.7 and FEV1 <75% of the predicted value and residual volume (RV) >120% of the predicted volume.[11] The increased RV reflects the air trapping due to the obstruction of the small airways. Air trapping can also be visualized on a high-resolution lung CT

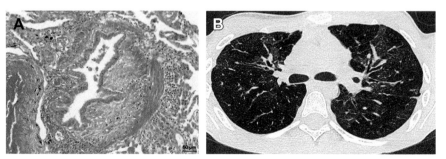

Fig. 1. Histologic features and CT scan of BO. (*A*) The bronchiolar wall is thickened by eccentric fibrosis between the epithelium and the muscle narrowing the bronchiolar lumen (hematoxylin-eosin-saffron, original magnification ×200) (provided by Dr Véronique Meignin). (*B*) High-resolution CT expiratory images of the lung from a patient with a BOS showing mosaic attenuation.

scan showing a mosaic pattern of intensified attenuation on expiratory cuts. Bronchial thickening, bronchiectasis, and centrilobular micronodules have also been associated with a diagnosis of BOS.[22–24]

The publication of these criteria allowed for harmonization of patients included in the clinical trials, but it soon became obvious that these criteria were not satisfactory in clinical practice. New diagnostic criteria were recently published to enhance their sensitivity[8]: FEV1/vital capacity (VC) <0.7 or the fifth percentile of predicted (either FVC or slow VC, whichever is greater), with an FEV1 <75% of predicted with ≥10% decline over less than 2 years. The FEV1 should not correct to greater than 75% of predicted with albuterol, and the patient must present with 1 of the 2 supporting features of BOS:

a. Evidence of either air trapping, as determined by expiratory CT or small airway thickening, or bronchiectasis, as determined by a high-resolution chest CT, or
b. Evidence of air trapping by PFTs as follows: RV greater than 120% of predicted or an RV/total lung capacity (TLC) ratio elevated outside the 90% confidence interval.

Despite the evolution of these criteria, it is likely that a decrease in the FEV1/VC ratio already reflects an advanced stage of the disease, which includes the involvement of numerous bronchioles and an extension to more proximal bronchi. Therefore, these criteria are probably incapable of diagnosing early forms of the disease. Before there was a unified definition of BOS, Chien and colleagues[21] proposed focusing on the decline of posttransplant FEV1 rather than a single posttransplant FEV1 value and showed that a decline of more than 5% per year in percent predicted FEV1 more accurately identified patients who experienced airflow obstruction. Subsequently, delta FEV1 was actually identified as a good predictor of developing later BOS.[5,25] Research is ongoing to improve the current diagnostic criteria to allow for earlier diagnosis. New PFT techniques[26–29] as well as new imaging techniques[30] are being assessed.

Epidemiology

Epidemiologic data concerning BOS depend on the diagnostic criteria used and the frequency of PFT monitoring. Overall, the incidence of BOS varies from 2% to 26% according to retrospective studies.[6,16,18–21,25,31–35] The incidence was the highest in a subpopulation of patients who developed extrathoracic chronic GVHD.[31–33] BOS is usually diagnosed beyond the third month and within the first 2 years after HSCT, although it is infrequently diagnosed outside of these time frames.[31–34]

Recent data suggest that the clinical syndrome of BOS encompass several entities both histologically and functionally. Holbro and colleagues[36] analyzed lung biopsies from patients diagnosed with BOS and found that BOS may reflect either obliterative bronchiolitis or lymphocytic bronchiolitis. Lymphocytic bronchiolitis may represent an earlier stage in the final common pathway toward the development of histologic obliterative bronchiolitis. The clinical and radiological presentations were identical for both histologic types, but the response to treatment was better in patients with lymphocytic bronchiolitis. This study also noted that a significant percentage of patients with biopsy-diagnosed obliterative bronchiolitis did not meet the NIH criteria for BOS.[36] Indeed, although the FEV1/VC ratio is the mainstay for a BOS diagnosis using PFT, it does not detect "restrictive" BOS characterized by a concomitant decrease in both the FEV1 and the VC, resulting in a normal FEV1/VC ratio. In a Danish study, almost 50% of patients with biopsy-proven BO had a normal FEV1/VC ratio.[37] In the author's cohort of patients with BOS, up to one-third of the patients had a decrease in both FEV1 and VC with a normal TLC.[34] Patients with a typical obstructive lung disease pattern including a decreased FEV1/VC ratio also had more severe FEV1 and fewer centrilobular nodules on the CT scan. In the author's retrospective study, the evolution of FEV1 was similar, regardless of the BOS phenotype.[34]

Risk Factors

Numerous risk factors for BOS have been proposed in various retrospective studies with conflicting results. For example, older age of the recipient, sex matching of donor/recipient, acute GVHD, and transplantation procedure (including both the conditioning regimen and the stem cell source) have been implicated in the onset of BOS in some studies.[17,20,32,33,38–40] A busulfan-based conditioning regimen, unrelated transplants, and a peripheral blood stem cell source were associated with the occurrence of the BOS in some studies.[33,39,40] The only association reported in all of these studies was a concomitant extrathoracic chronic GVHD at the time of BOS diagnosis. Patients with cGHVD are more likely to be diagnosed with BOS.[31] However, whether extrathoracic cGVHD precedes the development of BOS remains to be determined. Conversely,

T-cell depletion with antithymocyte globulin administration and cord blood as the stem cell source were identified as protective factors against BOS in other studies.[35,38,40,41]

Pathogenesis of Bronchiolitis Obliterans Syndrome

The pathogenesis of BOS is not well known, but it is hypothesized that the first step in BOS development is bronchiolar epithelium injury by different factors, such as chemotherapy/radiotherapy conditioning, gastroesophageal reflux, or respiratory pathogens followed by an inappropriate inflammatory reaction, resulting in a fibrotic process leading to obstruction of small airways. This process results from an alloimmune response, which is consistent with the absence of BOS development when the graft is T cell depleted.[41–43] Furthermore, the role of innate immunity polymorphisms as well as those of humoral immunity in the development of BOS have been suggested.[44,45] Indeed, in a mouse model of postallogeneic HSCT BO, donor B-cell alloantibody deposition, and germinal center formation are required for the development of BO[46]; furthermore, high levels of soluble B-cell–activating factor are specific to patients with BOS.[47] However, the diverse triggers and clinical course of BOS suggest a multifactorial pathogenesis.[13]

Clinical Course and Outcome

The first studies on BOS have reported different clinical courses. After a diagnosis of BOS, the rate of the decline in FEV1 was highly variable with either quick deterioration, stabilization, or improvement.[16,18,48] More recent studies suggest that a more or less severe and rapid FEV1 decline precedes the NIH diagnosis of BOS and that PFT subsequently stabilizes.[9,27,34] There are currently no reliable predictive markers of the evolution of pulmonary function. The recent identification of different phenotypes of BOS probably explains these various clinical courses, although this issue should be further investigated. Nevertheless, overall BOS is associated with significant morbidity and mortality.[15,16,18,20,31,32] Au and colleagues[31] found that BOS conferred a 1.6-fold increase in the risk for mortality after diagnosis. The prognosis of BOS is even worse if the onset was early after transplantation, particularly within the first year.[20,27,32,34,49] BOS-related deaths are frequently caused by respiratory failure and/or infection resulting from intensified immunosuppression.

Treatment

Until now, no medical treatment has been proven to cure BO. Because BO is considered pulmonary

GVHD, systemic steroids have been the standard therapy for BO despite the lack of evidence for their efficacy and the numerous side effects.[50] Otherwise, several studies have assessed the effect of various immunosuppressive drugs on overall cGVHD, but it is often difficult to find data focused on lung disease in these publications.[51–54] Data that focus on BOS are limited (**Table 1**). Most of these studies conclude that there is treatment efficacy when the PFT stabilizes. The recent improvement in understanding the clinical course of BOS should provide a more critical perspective when reviewing these results.[27,34] Only 3 prospective studies are available; of these, 2 are randomized placebo-controlled studies. One reported the lack of efficacy of azithromycin on both FEV1 and the clinical symptoms of late BOS,[55] and the other reported the beneficial effect of budesonide/formoterol on FEV1 of patients with newly diagnosed BOS with an FEV1 $\geq$ 40% of the predicted value.[56] It was striking that in the latter study, 25% of the patients from the placebo group had an improvement of 200 mL and 12% in FEV1, which provided insights in the natural course of the disease and reinforced the need for placebo-controlled studies.[56] The third study was an open-label study that reported a steroid-sparing effect of the association of fluticasone, azithromycin, and montelukast in the treatment of new-onset BOS.[57]

Currently, the development of a more effective treatment strategy for BOS is needed and should focus on patients with early-stage BOS, who are probably the most responsive to treatment. In addition to these limited treatment options, pulmonary rehabilitation may be an important adjunctive therapy improving patients' quality of life.[58] Finally, lung transplantation is currently a reasonable therapeutic option in selected allogeneic HSCT recipients with post-BOS chronic respiratory failure. Reports from various lung transplant centers are concordant on this matter.[59,60]

Bronchiolitis Obliterans Syndrome Prophylaxis

Given the current poor prognosis for BOS and the limited treatment options, prophylactic strategies are currently under investigation. Two randomized studies found that azithromycin was efficacious in preventing the occurrence of BOS after lung transplantation.[73,74] The question arises whether a similar effect could be observed in allogeneic HSCT recipients. In a murine model of allogeneic HSCT, preventive azithromycin treatment reduced noninfectious lung injury, which supported further investigation in clinical trials.[75] A single retrospective study suggested that prophylactic

Table 1
Clinical studies focused on postallogeneic hematopoietic stem cell transplantation bronchiolitis obliterans syndrome treatment strategies (number of patients >1)

Treatment	Study Design	Results	Reference
High-dose steroids	Case series Case series	FEV1 stabilization in 5/5 patients FEV1 improvement in 7/7 patients	Ratjen et al,[61] 2005 Uhlving et al,[62] 2012
Rituximab	Case series	No response in 3/3 patients	Lorillon et al,[63] 2011
Bortezomib	Prospective open-label, nonrandomized	Ongoing	NCT01163786
Extracorporeal photopheresis	Case series Case series Case series	PFT stabilization in 6/9 patients FEV1 improvement in 10/12 patients FEV1 stabilization at 3 mo in 7/8 patients; FEV1 decline in 6/8 at 1 y	Lucid et al,[64] 2011 Del Fante et al,[65] 2016 Brownback et al,[66] 2016
Imatinib	Prospective, open-label, nonrandomized Case series	FEV1 improvement in 1/9 patients FEV1 stabilization in 2/2	Stadler et al,[67] 2009 Watanabe et al,[68] 2015
Azithromycin	Randomized double blinded placebo-controlled Case series	No change in FEV1 FEV1 improvement in 8/8 patients	Lam et al,[55] 2011 Khalid et al,[69] 2005
Montelukast	Prospective open-label, nonrandomized	Ongoing	NCT00656058
AZD9668, oral neutrophil elastase inhibitor	Prospective, open-label, nonrandomized	Ongoing	NCT02669251
Fluticasone	Retrospective (n = 17)	FEV1 stabilization	Bashoura et al,[70] 2008
Budesonide/formoterol	Retrospective Randomized, double-blinded, placebo-controlled	FEV1 improvement in 7/7 patients FEV1 improvement	Bergeron et al,[71] 2007 Bergeron et al,[56] 2015
Inhaled cyclosporine	Prospective open-label, nonrandomized	Ongoing	NCT01273207
Combination			
Fluticasone plus azithromycin plus montelukast	Case control (n = 8 cases) Prospective open-label, nonrandomized	FEV1 stabilization FEV1 stabilization despite reduction in steroids	Norman et al,[50] 2011 Williams et al,[57] 2016
Budesonide/formoterol plus N-acetyl-cysteine plus montelukast	Retrospective (n = 61)	FEV1 improvement	Kim et al,[72] 2016

azithromycin could not prevent the development of postallogeneic HSCT BOS.[76] The author is currently conducting a phase 3 multicenter randomized placebo-controlled trial to further evaluate the efficacy of azithromycin to prevent BOS after allogeneic HSCT (NCT01959100).

INTERSTITIAL LUNG DISEASES

Although BOS is the only condition recognized as a pulmonary GVHD by the NIH consensus on chronic GVHD,[8,11] several studies suggest that other LONIPCs, such as organizing pneumonia (OP) or other interstitial lung diseases (ILD), can be diagnosed after allogeneic HSCT and are also associated with cGVHD.[3,4,14,48,77–79] These diseases are often overlooked, but they have been found to represent between 12% and more than 60% of LONIPCs in large retrospective studies.[3,4] Various postallogeneic HSCT entities of ILD have been identified according to the classification systems for idiopathic ILD.[14,78,80,81] The author recently reviewed a cohort of 40 patients who were diagnosed with postallogeneic HSCT ILD.[78] The median time from transplant to ILD was 11.3 months. Most of the patients had developed extrathoracic cGVHD at the time of ILD diagnosis. The author identified 2 lung CT scan patterns according to the predominance of either ground glass opacities or alveolar consolidations (**Fig. 2**). A restrictive ventilatory defect was the main pulmonary function pattern. Finally, the median survival rate at 24 months was 61%.[78]

Rarely, post-HSCT ILD has been reported to occur in the context of clinical and biological features of specific autoimmune diseases with extrathoracic symptoms and specific autoantibodies, including Sjögren syndrome, myositis, vasculitis, mixed connective tissue disease or, more recently, anti-MDA5 syndrome.[82,83]

Organizing Pneumonia

OP is the post-HSCT ILD that is best described. OP can be diagnosed early after allogeneic HSCT being part of the spectrum of idiopathic pneumonia syndrome and can also be a significant LONIPC. It is defined histopathologically by intra-alveolar connective tissue plugs of granulation tissue consisting of intermixed myofibroblasts and connective tissue that fill the lumens of the distal airways and extend into the alveolar ducts in association with chronic interstitial inflammation.[84] In a case control study, Freudenberger and colleagues[77] described 49 cases of biopsy-proven OP following allogeneic HSCT and compared them to control subjects from a computerized database of all patients who received an allogeneic transplant. They identified a strong association between OP and previous signs of acute and chronic GVHD, suggesting a causal link between both entities.[8,11,77] The time from HSCT to OP onset ranged from a few days to more than 7 years, with a median time of 108 days. In 22% of these cases, a tapering of immunosuppressive treatments preceded the respiratory symptoms. The clinical presentation was similar to that of cryptogenic OP, mimicking unresolved or subacute infectious pneumonia with unspecific symptoms.[77] Radiological signs were further investigated in dedicated studies.[85,86] Lung abnormalities mainly consisted of ground glass opacities and/or consolidations with a predominant peri-bronchovascular topography.[77,85,86] Unlike cryptogenic OP, opacities were not reported as being migratory.

Freudenberger and colleagues[77] found a normal PFT in 38% of patients with postallogeneic HSCT OP, whereas 43% had a restrictive pattern, 11% had an obstructive ventilatory defect, and 8% had both. In addition, a decrease in the carbon monoxide diffusion capacity was noted in 64% of the patients. Treatment with steroids usually allowed the resolution or stabilization of OP with a risk of relapse when tapering the dose.[77,79]

Pleuroparenchymal Fibroelastosis

Pleuroparenchymal fibroelastosis (PPFE) is a rare entity that has been recently included in the official

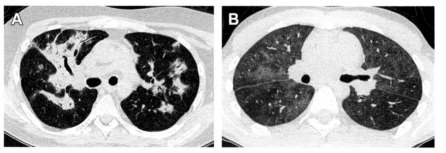

Fig. 2. CT scan patterns of ILD occurring after an allogeneic HSCT showing a predominance of (A) alveolar consolidations or (B) ground glass opacities.

American Thoracic Society/European Respiratory Society statement in 2013 as a group of rare idiopathic interstitial pneumonias.[81] PPFE is characterized by pleural and subpleural parenchymal thickening due to elastic fiber proliferation with minimal inflammation.[81,87] The first 4 cases of post-HSCT PPFE were reported in 2011, including one patient who experienced autologous HSCT.[87] Additional data are still limited; however, the prevalence was recently calculated as 0.28% of HSCT recipients.[88] PPFE can be diagnosed many years after allogeneic HSCT, and its association with cGVHD is inconsistent.[87] The PPFE CT scan pattern is highly suggestive with upper lobe fibrosis, including pleural and subpleural thickening, subpleural reticulations, traction bronchiectasis, and volume reduction subsequently spreading to the lower lobes (**Fig. 3**). PFT showed either a restrictive or a mixed pattern.[88] The clinical course of disease is progressive, and patient prognosis is poor with no therapeutic options other than lung transplantation currently available.

In all cases reported, BO lesions were associated with PPFE based on histology.[87,89,90] Although PPFE was also reported after lung transplantation, whether it is a specific entity of the allogeneic lung or the result of chronic injury is questionable.[91]

Other Interstitial Lung Diseases

In addition to OP and PPFE, a wide spectrum of other ILDs that are frequently associated with extrapulmonary cGVHD has been reported following allogeneic HSCT. This observed association raises the question of whether there are different patterns of lung cGVHD. All these ILDs are characterized by more or less diffuse lung CT scan opacities and are specifically identified on lung biopsy examination. Whether these entities are specific or part of a lesional continuum remains to be determined.

Each ILD entity defined according to the international consensus for idiopathic ILD[81] can be diagnosed after allogeneic HSCT except for usual interstitial pneumonia, which has never been reported in this setting. Therefore, nonspecific interstitial pneumonia, diffuse alveolar damage, and lymphoid interstitial pneumonia have all been associated with pulmonary complications of allogeneic HSCT.[14,78,80,90,92] Furthermore, eosinophilic pneumonia and acute fibrinous organizing pneumonia (AFOP) have also been reported. Acute eosinophilic pneumonia is mainly diagnosed within the first year following HSCT but may occur later (2–41 months).[78,93–95] In the reported cases, peripheral blood eosinophilia was systematically found, and the diagnosis relied either on BAL eosinophilia or histology. All of the patients promptly responded to systemic steroid therapy with improvement of their pulmonary symptoms, imaging, and the resolution of peripheral blood eosinophilia.[93–95]

AFOP is a new and rare histologic entity of acute lung injury characterized by fibrin blocking filling the alveolar spaces without either interstitial infiltrate or fibrosis and ground glass opacities and consolidations on a lung CT scan. A few cases were reported following allogeneic HSCT,[96,97] and the steroid sensitivity was variable.[96,97]

THORACIC AIR LEAK SYNDROME

Thoracic air leak syndrome (ALS) includes pneumothorax, pneumomediastinum, and interstitial emphysema (**Fig. 4**). More than 60 cases were reported in allogeneic HSCT recipients.[98–106] The

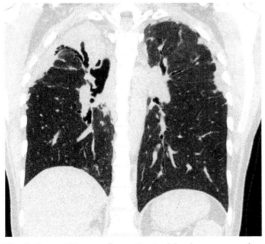

Fig. 3. Lung CT scan of a patient with pleuroparenchymal fibroelastosis characterized by apical fibrosis with traction bronchiectasis, pleural thickening, and reduced lung volumes.

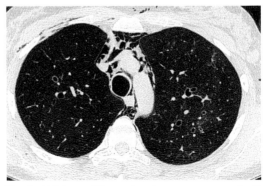

Fig. 4. ALS. Lung CT scan showing a pneumomediastinum in a patient with advanced BO.

prevalence was estimated at 0.83% to 5.7% according to these studies. The median time after HSCT ranged from 202 to 575 days. Between 80% and 100% of patients who developed thoracic ALS after HSCT had an underlying LONIPC of either BO or ILD, particularly PPFE.[87,107] GVHD was the factor most highly associated with ALS.[98] The prognosis of patients who develop ALS is very poor, with a 1-year survival of 45% and a 3-year survival of 15%.[98]

PULMONARY VASCULAR DISEASES

Endothelial dysfunction after allogeneic HSCT, which involves multiple organs, is increasingly recognized and can specifically result in pulmonary vascular diseases. Whether these diseases systematically coexist and whether they are specific entities or part of a lesional continuum is unknown.

Pulmonary Hypertension

According to the pulmonary hypertension (PH) classification,[108] postallogeneic HSCT PH may be a consequence of various conditions such as left heart disease, chronic lung disease/hypoxia, chronic thromboembolic disease, hematological disorders, drug-induced, pulmonary veno-occlusive disease (PVOD), or additional unknown causes. The incidence of PH in patients who undergo allogeneic HSCT is unknown, but 40 cases have been reported in the literature.[109] Although some adults may develop post-HSCT PH, the pediatric population constitutes the largest percentage of these cases.[109] PH can be diagnosed after both myeloablative and nonmyeloablative conditioning regimens and develops in a range of 8 days to 9 months after HSCT.[109,110] Among the 40 patients reported in the literature, 55% died, of whom the vast majority had a cause of death directly related to PH.[109] Histologic analysis found an involvement of only the pulmonary arteries; in 70% of the cases, 23% had PVOD with pulmonary venule involvement and vascular congestion only, and the other patients had a mixed arteriolar-venous abnormality.[109]

Recently, post-HSCT PH was associated with BO; however, no data on the severity of BO and the presence or absence of pre-existing chronic hypoxemia were available.[110,111] PVOD may be a cause of postallogeneic HSCT PH. Most of the patients reported with post-HSCT PVOD were younger than 25 years old. The onset of PVOD occurred between several weeks and several months following transplant.[112,113] The pathogenesis of postallogeneic HSCT PVOD is not elucidated and does not seem to be associated with cGVHD.[112,113] Strikingly, although nontransplant cases of PVOD have a very poor prognosis despite any treatment, half of the HSCT recipients with PVOD responded to steroids.[112,113] Histologically, PVOD and lung transplant-associated thrombotic microangiopathy (TM-TMA) may coexist.[114]

Thrombotic Microangiopathy

For many years, TM-TMA was mostly associated with kidney involvement. Although it is the most frequently affected organ, HSCT-TMA has been recognized in recent years as a multisystem disease involving organs such as the brain, bowel, heart, and lung.[115] The pathophysiology of TA-TMA involves arteriolar thrombi associated with intimal swelling and fibrinoid necrosis of the vessel wall. Its risk factors include high-dose chemotherapy, radiation therapy, an unrelated donor, HLA mismatch, exposure to calcineurin inhibitors with or without concomitant exposure to sirolimus, GVHD, and infection. Notably, contrary to other microangiopathies, TA-TMA has normal levels of ADAMTS-13.[116] Lung TA-TMA has been identified in several situations, such as in patients who presented with acute respiratory distress syndrome or pulmonary edema, with more indolent clinical presentation with isolated hypoxemia, or on autopsy examination.[110,117–119] The diagnosis of TA-TMA ranged from several days to several months after HSCT. Lung TA-TMA may lead to severe PH with a poor prognosis.[110]

Thromboembolic Disease (Venous Thromboembolism and Pulmonary Embolism)

Venous thromboembolic (VTE) disease is a fairly common complication after HSCT and is unrelated to a central venous catheter in 70% of cases.[120] A recent meta-analysis found an overall incidence of VTE after allogeneic HSCT of 4% (range, 2%–6%).[121] The median time from HSCT to a diagnosis of VTE unrelated to a CVC was 9.5 months.[120] VTE was associated with GVHD.[122] In the meta-analysis, the incidence of VTE in chronic GVHD was 35% (range, 20%–54%), whereas in acute GVHD the incidence was 47% (range, 32%–62%).[121] An analysis of the competing factors for venous thrombosis revealed extensive cGVHD to be the only independent prognostic risk factor.[122] The management of post-HSCT VTE is a challenge. Although treatments require anticoagulation, the risk of bleeding is high and is associated with a poor survival.[120,122] Several factors were associated with an increased risk of bleeding: advanced disease, ablative conditioning regimen, umbilical cord blood transplantation, anticoagulation, acute III-IV GVHD, and transplant-associated microangiopathy.[120,122]

Pulmonary Cytolytic Thrombi

Pulmonary cytolytic thrombi (PCT) is an uncommon complication after allogeneic HSCT of unknown origin. This diagnosis is based on the histologic analysis of a pulmonary nodule that reveals hemorrhagic infarcts with occlusive vascular lesions adjacent to but not restricted to the infarcted areas. The clinical picture usually presents as a fever with coughing and chest pain that subsequently leads to the discovery of pulmonary nodules, which are typically peripheral and located at the base of the lungs.[123] In most cases, this LONIPC is observed in children and adolescents, as only 2 cases have been reported in adults over age 18.[124] The condition is often associated with extrathoracic GVHD, and the time before onset after HSCT ranges between 30 and 360 days.[123,124] No deaths have yet been directly attributed to this disorder. The frequency of PCT is likely overlooked because an analysis of the pulmonary nodules biopsied from HSCT recipients over a 5-year period confirmed the diagnosis of PCT in 38% of the cases.[125]

PLEURAL EFFUSION

Although pleural effusion is not distinctive of cGVHD, it is identified as a feature of cGVHD in the NIH consensus.[8,11] A large retrospective study focusing on the occurrence of pleural effusions after allogeneic HSCT was recently published.[126] This study identified 71 patients, leading to a cumulative incidence of pleural effusion of 9.9% at 1 year and 11.8% at 5 years.[126] They found that the distribution of pleural effusion onset demonstrated a bimodal pattern, with a first peak (mainly attributable to infections and volume overload) occurring before the 100 days posttransplant cutoff and a second peak (due to serositis-type cGVHD and OP) occurring after the 100-day cutoff at a median of 334 days (range, 131–869).[126] The pleural effusions were large, moderate, and small in 15%, 42%, and 26% of the patients, respectively. The vast majority of patients had bilateral pleural effusions.[126] Approximately 56% of the patients had exudative effusions, and 36% had transudative effusions. There were 11% of patients with concomitant pericardial effusions or ascites.[126] Pleural effusions associated with cGVHD showed complete resolution following escalation of immunosuppressive therapy in 62% of cases.[126] The occurrence of pleural effusion after allogeneic HSCT was associated with impaired survival.[126,127]

SUMMARY

Late-onset noninfectious pulmonary complications that are mostly associated with cGVHD can involve all anatomic lung regions leading to various clinical entities. BOS is the most frequently encountered LONIPC. Improving the diagnostic specifications of LONIPCs and identifying early risk factors are mandatory for earlier diagnoses and timely treatments. Evaluation of prophylactic strategies for LONIPCs is necessary to improve outcomes in high-risk allogeneic HSCT recipients.

REFERENCES

1. Patriarca F, Poletti V, Costabel U, et al. Clinical presentation, outcome and risk factors of late-onset non-infectious pulmonary complications after allogeneic stem cell transplantation. Curr Stem Cell Res Ther 2009;4(2):161–7.
2. Ueda K, Watadani T, Maeda E, et al. Outcome and treatment of late-onset noninfectious pulmonary complications after allogeneic haematopoietic SCT. Bone Marrow Transplant 2010; 45(12):1719–27.
3. Sakaida E, Nakaseko C, Harima A, et al. Late-onset noninfectious pulmonary complications after allogeneic stem cell transplantation are significantly associated with chronic graft-versus-host disease and with the graft-versus-leukemia effect. Blood 2003;102(12):4236–42.
4. Patriarca F, Skert C, Bonifazi F, et al. Effect on survival of the development of late-onset non-infectious pulmonary complications after stem cell transplantation. Haematologica 2006;91(9): 1268–72.
5. Thompson PA, Lim A, Panek-Hudson Y, et al. Screening with spirometry is a useful predictor of later development of noninfectious pulmonary syndromes in patients undergoing allogeneic stem cell transplantation. Biol Blood Marrow Transplant 2014;20(6):781–6.
6. Solh M, Arat M, Cao Q, et al. Late-onset noninfectious pulmonary complications in adult allogeneic hematopoietic cell transplant recipients. Transplantation 2011;91(7):798–803.
7. Chellapandian D, Lehrnbecher T, Phillips B, et al. Bronchoalveolar lavage and lung biopsy in patients with cancer and hematopoietic stem-cell transplantation recipients: a systematic review and meta-analysis. J Clin Oncol 2015;33(5):501–9.
8. Jagasia MH, Greinix HT, Arora M, et al. National Institutes of Health consensus development project on criteria for clinical trials in chronic graft-versus-host disease: I. The 2014 Diagnosis and Staging Working Group report. Biol Blood Marrow Transplant 2015;21(3):389–401.e1.

9. Cheng GS, Stednick Z, Madtes DK, et al. Decline in the use of surgical biopsy for diagnosis of pulmonary disease in hematopoietic cell transplant recipients in an era of improved diagnostics and empirical therapy. Biol Blood Marrow Transplant 2016;22(12):2243–9.

10. Roca J, Granena A, Rodriguez-Roisin R, et al. Fatal airway disease in an adult with chronic graft-versus-host disease. Thorax 1982;37(1):77–8.

11. Filipovich AH, Weisdorf D, Pavletic S, et al. National Institutes of Health consensus development project on criteria for clinical trials in chronic graft-versus-host disease: I. Diagnosis and staging working group report. Biol Blood Marrow Transplant 2005; 11(12):945–56.

12. Shulman HM, Cardona DM, Greenson JK, et al. NIH consensus development project on criteria for clinical trials in chronic graft-versus-host disease: II. The 2014 Pathology Working Group Report. Biol Blood Marrow Transplant 2015;21(4): 589–603.

13. Barker AF, Bergeron A, Rom WN, et al. Obliterative bronchiolitis. N Engl J Med 2014;370(19):1820–8.

14. Yousem SA. The histological spectrum of pulmonary graft-versus-host disease in bone marrow transplant recipients. Hum Pathol 1995;26(6):668–75.

15. Philit F, Wiesendanger T, Archimbaud E, et al. Post-transplant obstructive lung disease ("bronchiolitis obliterans"): a clinical comparative study of bone marrow and lung transplant patients. Eur Respir J 1995;8(4):551–8.

16. Clark JG, Crawford SW, Madtes DK, et al. Obstructive lung disease after allogeneic marrow transplantation. Clinical presentation and course. Ann Intern Med 1989;111(5):368–76.

17. Marras TK, Chan CK, Lipton JH, et al. Long-term pulmonary function abnormalities and survival after allogeneic marrow transplantation. Bone Marrow Transplant 2004;33(5):509–17.

18. Chan CK, Hyland RH, Hutcheon MA, et al. Small-airways disease in recipients of allogeneic bone marrow transplants. An analysis of 11 cases and a review of the literature. Medicine (Baltimore) 1987;66(5):327–40.

19. Marras TK, Szalai JP, Chan CK, et al. Pulmonary function abnormalities after allogeneic marrow transplantation: a systematic review and assessment of an existing predictive instrument. Bone Marrow Transplant 2002;30(9):599–607.

20. Dudek AZ, Mahaseth H, DeFor TE, et al. Bronchiolitis obliterans in chronic graft-versus-host disease: analysis of risk factors and treatment outcomes. Biol Blood Marrow Transplant 2003;9(10):657–66.

21. Chien JW, Martin PJ, Gooley TA, et al. Airflow obstruction after myeloablative allogeneic hematopoietic stem cell transplantation. Am J Respir Crit Care Med 2003;168(2):208–14.

22. Oh JK, Jung JI, Han DH, et al. Multidetector row computed tomography quantification of bronchiolitis obliterans syndrome after hematopoietic stem cell transplantation: a pilot study. J Thorac Imaging 2013;28(2):114–20.

23. Gunn ML, Godwin JD, Kanne JP, et al. High-resolution CT findings of bronchiolitis obliterans syndrome after hematopoietic stem cell transplantation. J Thorac Imaging 2008;23(4): 244–50.

24. Sargent MA, Cairns RA, Murdoch MJ, et al. Obstructive lung disease in children after allogeneic bone marrow transplantation: evaluation with high-resolution CT. AJR Am J Roentgenol 1995; 164(3):693–6.

25. Abedin S, Yanik GA, Braun T, et al. Predictive value of bronchiolitis obliterans syndrome stage 0p in chronic graft-versus-host disease of the lung. Biol Blood Marrow Transplant 2015;21(6):1127–31.

26. Barisione G, Bacigalupo A, Crimi E, et al. Changes in lung volumes and airway responsiveness following haematopoietic stem cell transplantation. Eur Respir J 2008;32(6):1576–82.

27. Cheng GS, Storer B, Chien JW, et al. Lung function trajectory in bronchiolitis obliterans syndrome after allogeneic hematopoietic cell transplantation. Ann Am Thorac Soc 2016;13(11):1932–9.

28. Lahzami S, Schoeffel RE, Pechey V, et al. Small airways function declines after allogeneic haematopoietic stem cell transplantation. Eur Respir J 2011;38(5):1180–8.

29. Williams KM, Hnatiuk O, Mitchell SA, et al. NHANES III equations enhance early detection and mortality prediction of bronchiolitis obliterans syndrome after hematopoietic SCT. Bone Marrow Transplant 2014;49(4):561–6.

30. Galban CJ, Boes JL, Bule M, et al. Parametric response mapping as an indicator of bronchiolitis obliterans syndrome after hematopoietic stem cell transplantation. Biol Blood Marrow Transplant 2014;20(10):1592–8.

31. Au BK, Au MA, Chien JW. Bronchiolitis obliterans syndrome epidemiology after allogeneic hematopoietic cell transplantation. Biol Blood Marrow Transplant 2011;17(7):1072–8.

32. Vieira AG, Funke VA, Nunes EC, et al. Bronchiolitis obliterans in patients undergoing allogeneic hematopoietic SCT. Bone Marrow Transplant 2014; 49(6):812–7.

33. Ditschkowski M, Elmaagacli AH, Koldehoff M, et al. Bronchiolitis obliterans after allogeneic hematopoietic SCT: further insight–new perspectives? Bone Marrow Transplant 2013;48(9):1224–9.

34. Bergeron A, Godet C, Chevret S, et al. Bronchiolitis obliterans syndrome after allogeneic hematopoietic SCT: phenotypes and prognosis. Bone Marrow Transplant 2013;48(6):819–24.

35. Duque-Afonso J, Ihorst G, Wasch R, et al. Identification of risk factors for bronchiolitis obliterans syndrome after reduced toxicity conditioning before hematopoietic cell transplantation. Bone Marrow Transplant 2013;48(8):1098–103.

36. Holbro A, Lehmann T, Girsberger S, et al. Lung histology predicts outcome of bronchiolitis obliterans syndrome after hematopoietic stem cell transplantation. Biol Blood Marrow Transplant 2013;19(6): 973–80.

37. Uhlving HH, Andersen CB, Christensen IJ, et al. Biopsy-verified bronchiolitis obliterans and other noninfectious lung pathologies after allogeneic hematopoietic stem cell transplantation. Biol Blood Marrow Transplant 2015;21(3):531–8.

38. Nakasone H, Kanda J, Yano S, et al. A case-control study of bronchiolitis obliterans syndrome following allogeneic hematopoietic stem cell transplantation. Transpl Int 2013;26(6):631–9.

39. Santo Tomas LH, Loberiza FR Jr, Klein JP, et al. Risk factors for bronchiolitis obliterans in allogeneic hematopoietic stem-cell transplantation for leukemia. Chest 2005;128(1):153–61.

40. Gazourian L, Rogers AJ, Ibanga R, et al. Factors associated with bronchiolitis obliterans syndrome and chronic graft-versus-host disease after allogeneic hematopoietic cell transplantation. Am J Hematol 2014;89(4):404–9.

41. Dirou S, Malard F, Chambellan A, et al. Stable long-term pulmonary function after fludarabine, antithymocyte globulin and i.v. BU for reduced-intensity conditioning allogeneic SCT. Bone Marrow Transplant 2014;49(5):622–7.

42. Bacigalupo A, Lamparelli T, Barisione G, et al. Thymoglobulin prevents chronic graft-versus-host disease, chronic lung dysfunction, and late transplant-related mortality: long-term follow-up of a randomized trial in patients undergoing unrelated donor transplantation. Biol Blood Marrow Transplant 2006;12(5):560–5.

43. Ditschkowski M, Elmaagacli AH, Trenschel R, et al. T-cell depletion prevents from bronchiolitis obliterans and bronchiolitis obliterans with organizing pneumonia after allogeneic hematopoietic stem cell transplantation with related donors. Haematologica 2007;92(4):558–61.

44. Chien JW, Zhao LP, Hansen JA, et al. Genetic variation in bactericidal/permeability-increasing protein influences the risk of developing rapid airflow decline after hematopoietic cell transplantation. Blood 2006;107(5):2200–7.

45. Hildebrandt GC, Granell M, Urbano-Ispizua A, et al. Recipient NOD2/CARD15 variants: a novel independent risk factor for the development of bronchiolitis obliterans after allogeneic stem cell transplantation. Biol Blood Marrow Transplant 2008;14(1):67–74.

46. Srinivasan M, Flynn R, Price A, et al. Donor B-cell alloantibody deposition and germinal center formation are required for the development of murine chronic GVHD and bronchiolitis obliterans. Blood 2012;119(6):1570–80.

47. Kuzmina Z, Krenn K, Petkov V, et al. CD19(+) CD21(low) B cells and patients at risk for NIH-defined chronic graft-versus-host disease with bronchiolitis obliterans syndrome. Blood 2013; 121(10):1886–95.

48. Palmas A, Tefferi A, Myers JL, et al. Late-onset noninfectious pulmonary complications after allogeneic bone marrow transplantation. Br J Haematol 1998;100(4):680–7.

49. Yoshihara S, Tateishi U, Ando T, et al. Lower incidence of bronchiolitis obliterans in allogeneic hematopoietic stem cell transplantation with reduced-intensity conditioning compared with myeloablative conditioning. Bone Marrow Transplant 2005;35(12):1195–200.

50. Norman BC, Jacobsohn DA, Williams KM, et al. Fluticasone, azithromycin and montelukast therapy in reducing corticosteroid exposure in bronchiolitis obliterans syndrome after allogeneic hematopoietic SCT: a case series of eight patients. Bone Marrow Transplant 2011;46(10):1369–73.

51. Busca A, Locatelli F, Marmont F, et al. Recombinant human soluble tumor necrosis factor receptor fusion protein as treatment for steroid refractory graft-versus-host disease following allogeneic hematopoietic stem cell transplantation. Am J Hematol 2007;82(1):45–52.

52. Olivieri A, Locatelli F, Zecca M, et al. Imatinib for refractory chronic graft-versus-host disease with fibrotic features. Blood 2009;114(3):709–18.

53. Kim SJ, Lee JW, Jung CW, et al. Weekly rituximab followed by monthly rituximab treatment for steroid-refractory chronic graft-versus-host disease: results from a prospective, multicenter, phase II study. Haematologica 2010;95(11): 1935–42.

54. Zeiser R, Burchert A, Lengerke C, et al. Ruxolitinib in corticosteroid-refractory graft-versus-host disease after allogeneic stem cell transplantation: a multicenter survey. Leukemia 2015;29(10):2062–8.

55. Lam DC, Lam B, Wong MK, et al. Effects of azithromycin in bronchiolitis obliterans syndrome after hematopoietic SCT–a randomized double-blinded placebo-controlled study. Bone Marrow Transplant 2011;46(12):1551–6.

56. Bergeron A, Chevret S, Chagnon K, et al. Budesonide/Formoterol for bronchiolitis obliterans after hematopoietic stem cell transplantation. Am J Respir Crit Care Med 2015;191(11):1242–9.

57. Williams KM, Cheng GS, Pusic I, et al. Fluticasone, azithromycin, and montelukast treatment for new-onset bronchiolitis obliterans syndrome after

hematopoietic cell transplantation. Biol Blood Marrow Transplant 2016;22(4):710–6.

58. Tran J, Norder EE, Diaz PT, et al. Pulmonary rehabilitation for bronchiolitis obliterans syndrome after hematopoietic stem cell transplantation. Biol Blood Marrow Transplant 2012;18(8):1250–4.

59. Soubani AO, Kingah P, Alshabani K, et al. Lung transplantation following hematopoietic stem cell transplantation: report of two cases and systematic review of literature. Clin Transplant 2014;28(7): 776–82.

60. Cheng GS, Edelman JD, Madtes DK, et al. Outcomes of lung transplantation after allogeneic hematopoietic stem cell transplantation. Biol Blood Marrow Transplant 2014;20(8):1169–75.

61. Ratjen F, Rjabko O, Kremens B. High-dose corticosteroid therapy for bronchiolitis obliterans after bone marrow transplantation in children. Bone Marrow Transplant 2005;36(2):135–8.

62. Uhlving HH, Buchvald F, Heilmann CJ, et al. Bronchiolitis obliterans after allo-SCT: clinical criteria and treatment options. Bone Marrow Transplant 2012;47(8):1020–9.

63. Lorillon G, Robin M, Meignin V, et al. Rituximab in bronchiolitis obliterans after haematopoietic stem cell transplantation. Eur Respir J 2011;38(2): 470–2.

64. Lucid CE, Savani BN, Engelhardt BG, et al. Extracorporeal photopheresis in patients with refractory bronchiolitis obliterans developing after allo-SCT. Bone Marrow Transplant 2011;46(3):426–9.

65. Del Fante C, Galasso T, Bernasconi P, et al. Extracorporeal photopheresis as a new supportive therapy for bronchiolitis obliterans syndrome after allogeneic stem cell transplantation. Bone Marrow Transplant 2016;51(5):728–31.

66. Brownback KR, Simpson SQ, Pitts LR, et al. Effect of extracorporeal photopheresis on lung function decline for severe bronchiolitis obliterans syndrome following allogeneic stem cell transplantation. J Clin Apher 2016;31(4):347–52.

67. Stadler M, Ahlborn R, Kamal H, et al. Limited efficacy of imatinib in severe pulmonary chronic graft-versus-host disease. Blood 2009;114(17): 3718–9 [author reply: 3719–20].

68. Watanabe S, Waseda Y, Kimura H, et al. Imatinib for bronchiolitis obliterans after allogeneic hematopoietic stem cell transplantation. Bone Marrow Transplant 2015;50(9):1250–2.

69. Khalid M, Al Saghir A, Saleemi S, et al. Azithromycin in bronchiolitis obliterans complicating bone marrow transplantation: a preliminary study. Eur Respir J 2005;25(3):490–3.

70. Bashoura L, Gupta S, Jain A, et al. Inhaled corticosteroids stabilize constrictive bronchiolitis after hematopoietic stem cell transplantation. Bone Marrow Transplant 2008;41(1):63–7.

71. Bergeron A, Belle A, Chevret S, et al. Combined inhaled steroids and bronchodilatators in obstructive airway disease after allogeneic stem cell transplantation. Bone Marrow Transplant 2007;39(9): 547–53.

72. Kim SW, Rhee CK, Kim YJ, et al. Therapeutic effect of budesonide/formoterol, montelukast and N-acetylcysteine for bronchiolitis obliterans syndrome after hematopoietic stem cell transplantation. Respir Res 2016;17(1):63.

73. Vos R, Vanaudenaerde BM, Verleden SE, et al. A randomised controlled trial of azithromycin to prevent chronic rejection after lung transplantation. Eur Respir J 2011;37(1):164–72.

74. Corris PA, Ryan VA, Small T, et al. A randomised controlled trial of azithromycin therapy in bronchiolitis obliterans syndrome (BOS) post lung transplantation. Thorax 2015;70(5):442–50.

75. Radhakrishnan SV, Palaniyandi S, Mueller G, et al. Preventive azithromycin treatment reduces noninfectious lung injury and acute graft-versus-host disease in a murine model of allogeneic hematopoietic cell transplantation. Biol Blood Marrow Transplant 2014;21(1):30–8.

76. Jo KW, Yoon S, Song JW, et al. The efficacy of prophylactic azithromycin on bronchiolitis obliterans syndrome after hematopoietic stem cell transplantation. Int J Hematol 2015;102(3):357–63.

77. Freudenberger TD, Madtes DK, Curtis JR, et al. Association between acute and chronic graft-versus-host disease and bronchiolitis obliterans organizing pneumonia in recipients of hematopoietic stem cell transplants. Blood 2003;102(10):3822–8.

78. Schlemmer F, Chevret S, Lorillon G, et al. Late-onset noninfectious interstitial lung disease after allogeneic hematopoietic stem cell transplantation. Respir Med 2014;108(10):1525–33.

79. Jinta M, Ohashi K, Ohta T, et al. Clinical features of allogeneic hematopoietic stem cell transplantation-associated organizing pneumonia. Bone Marrow Transplant 2007;40(5):465–72.

80. Miyagawa-Hayashino A, Sonobe M, Kubo T, et al. Non-specific interstitial pneumonia as a manifestation of graft-versus-host disease following pediatric allogeneic hematopoietic stem cell transplantation. Pathol Int 2010;60(2):137–42.

81. Travis WD, Costabel U, Hansell DM, et al. An official American Thoracic Society/European Respiratory Society statement: update of the international multidisciplinary classification of the idiopathic interstitial pneumonias. Am J Respir Crit Care Med 2013;188(6):733–48.

82. Lepelletier C, Bengoufa D, Lyes Z, et al. Dermato-pulmonary syndrome associated with anti-MDA5 antibodies after allogeneic hematopoietic stem cell transplantation. JAMA Dermatol 2016. http://dx.doi.org/10.1001/jamadermatol2016.3976.

83. Bergeron A, Bengoufa D, Feuillet S, et al. The spectrum of lung involvement in collagen vascular-like diseases following allogeneic hematopoietic stem cell transplantation: report of 6 cases and review of the literature. Medicine (Baltimore) 2011;90(2):146–57.

84. Cordier JF. Cryptogenic organising pneumonia. Eur Respir J 2006;28(2):422–46.

85. Dodd JD, Muller NL. Bronchiolitis obliterans organizing pneumonia after bone marrow transplantation: high-resolution computed tomography findings in 4 patients. J Comput Assist Tomogr 2005;29(4):540–3.

86. Pipavath SN, Chung JH, Chien JW, et al. Organizing pneumonia in recipients of hematopoietic stem cell transplantation: CT features in 16 patients. J Comput Assist Tomogr 2012;36(4):431–6.

87. von der Thusen JH, Hansell DM, Tominaga M, et al. Pleuroparenchymal fibroelastosis in patients with pulmonary disease secondary to bone marrow transplantation. Mod Pathol 2011;24(12):1633–9.

88. Mariani F, Gatti B, Rocca A, et al. Pleuroparenchymal fibroelastosis: the prevalence of secondary forms in hematopoietic stem cell and lung transplantation recipients. Diagn Interv Radiol 2016;22(5):400–6.

89. Greer M, Riise GC, Hansson L, et al. Dichotomy in pulmonary graft-versus-host disease evident among allogeneic stem-cell transplant recipients undergoing lung transplantation. Eur Respir J 2016;48(6):1807–10.

90. Takeuchi Y, Miyagawa-Hayashino A, Chen F, et al. Pleuroparenchymal fibroelastosis and non-specific interstitial pneumonia: frequent pulmonary sequelae of haematopoietic stem cell transplantation. Histopathology 2015;66(4):536–44.

91. Sato M, Hwang DM, Waddell TK, et al. Progression pattern of restrictive allograft syndrome after lung transplantation. J Heart Lung Transplant 2013;32(1):23–30.

92. Wahla AS, Khan II, Loya A, et al. A new pattern of pulmonary graft vs host disease in a hematopoietic stem cell transplant patient. Clin Respir J 2015;9(4):399–402.

93. Akhtari M, Langston AA, Waller EK, et al. Eosinophilic pulmonary syndrome as a manifestation of GVHD following hematopoietic stem cell transplantation in three patients. Bone Marrow Transplant 2009;43(2):155–8.

94. Yoshimi M, Nannya Y, Watanabe T, et al. Acute eosinophilic pneumonia is a non-infectious lung complication after allogeneic hematopoietic stem cell transplantation. Int J Hematol 2009;89(2):244–8.

95. Wagner T, Dhedin N, Philippe B, et al. Acute eosinophilic pneumonia after allogeneic hematopoietic stem cell transplantation. Ann Hematol 2006;85(3):202–3.

96. Lee SM, Park JJ, Sung SH, et al. Acute fibrinous and organizing pneumonia following hematopoietic stem cell transplantation. Korean J Intern Med 2009;24(2):156–9.

97. Nguyen LP, Ahdoot S, Sriratanaviriyakul N, et al. Acute fibrinous and organizing pneumonia associated with allogenic hematopoietic stem cell transplant successfully treated with corticosteroids: a two-patient case series. J Investig Med High Impact Case Rep 2016;4(2). 2324709616643990.

98. Sakai R, Kanamori H, Nakaseko C, et al. Air-leak syndrome following allo-SCT in adult patients: report from the Kanto Study Group for Cell Therapy in Japan. Bone Marrow Transplant 2011;46(3):379–84.

99. Moon MH, Sa YJ, Cho KD, et al. Thoracic air-leak syndromes in hematopoietic stem cell transplant recipients with graft-versus-host disease: a possible sign for poor response to treatment and poor prognosis. J Korean Med Sci 2010;25(5):658–62.

100. Franquet T, Rodriguez S, Hernandez JM, et al. Air-leak syndromes in hematopoietic stem cell transplant recipients with chronic GVHD: high-resolution CT findings. J Thorac Imaging 2007;22(4):335–40.

101. Toubai T, Tanaka J, Kobayashi N, et al. Mediastinal emphysema and bilateral pneumothoraces with chronic GVHD in patients after allogeneic stem cell transplantation. Bone Marrow Transplant 2004;33(11):1159–63.

102. Vogel M, Brodoefel H, Bethge W, et al. Spontaneous thoracic air-leakage syndrome in patients following allogeneic hematopoietic stem cell transplantation: causes, CT-follow up and patient outcome. Eur J Radiol 2006;60(3):392–7.

103. Iyama S, Sato T, Murase K, et al. Successful treatment by fibrin glue sealant for pneumothorax with chronic GVHD resistant to autologous blood patch pleurodesis. Intern Med 2013;51(15):2011–4.

104. Schneider AE, Talmon GA. Simultaneous bilateral spontaneous pneumothorax following high-dose chemotherapy and bone marrow transplantation for mantle cell lymphoma without evidence of pulmonary disease. Int J Clin Oncol 2010;15(6):635–7.

105. Shin HJ, Park CY, Park YH, et al. Spontaneous pneumothorax developed in patients with bronchiolitis obliterans after unrelated hematopoietic stem cell transplantation: case report and review of the literature. Int J Hematol 2004;79(3):298–302.

106. Chadwick C, Marven SM, Vora AJ. Autologous blood pleurodesis for pneumothorax complicating graft-versus-host disease-related bronchiolitis obliterans. Bone Marrow Transplant 2004;33(4):451–3.

107. Matsui T, Maeda T, Kida T, et al. Pleuroparenchymal fibroelastosis after allogenic hematopoietic stem cell transplantation: important histological component of late-onset noninfectious pulmonary complication accompanied with recurrent pneumothorax. Int J Hematol 2016;104(4):525–30.

108. Simonneau G, Robbins IM, Beghetti M, et al. Updated clinical classification of pulmonary hypertension. J Am Coll Cardiol 2009;54(1 Suppl):S43–54.

109. Dandoy CE, Hirsch R, Chima R, et al. Pulmonary hypertension after hematopoietic stem cell transplantation. Biol Blood Marrow Transplant 2013; 19(11):1546–56.

110. Jodele S, Hirsch R, Laskin B, et al. Pulmonary arterial hypertension in pediatric patients with hematopoietic stem cell transplant-associated thrombotic microangiopathy. Biol Blood Marrow Transplant 2013;19(2):202–7.

111. Pate A, Rotz S, Warren M, et al. Pulmonary hypertension associated with bronchiolitis obliterans after hematopoietic stem cell transplantation. Bone Marrow Transplant 2016;51(2):310–2.

112. Bunte MC, Patnaik MM, Pritzker MR, et al. Pulmonary veno-occlusive disease following hematopoietic stem cell transplantation: a rare model of endothelial dysfunction. Bone Marrow Transplant 2008;41(8):677–86.

113. Hosokawa K, Yamazaki H, Nishitsuji M, et al. Pulmonary veno-occlusive disease following reduced-intensity allogeneic bone marrow transplantation for acute myeloid leukemia. Intern Med 2012;51(2):195–8.

114. Seguchi M, Hirabayashi N, Fujii Y, et al. Pulmonary hypertension associated with pulmonary occlusive vasculopathy after allogeneic bone marrow transplantation. Transplantation 2000;69(1):177–9.

115. Jodele S, Laskin BL, Dandoy CE, et al. A new paradigm: diagnosis and management of HSCT-associated thrombotic microangiopathy as multisystem endothelial injury. Blood Rev 2015;29(3): 191–204.

116. Rosenthal J. Hematopoietic cell transplantation-associated thrombotic microangiopathy: a review of pathophysiology, diagnosis, and treatment. J Blood Med 2016;7:181–6.

117. Selby DM, Rudzki JR, Bayever ES, et al. Vasculopathy of small muscular arteries in pediatric patients after bone marrow transplantation. Hum Pathol 1999;30(7):734–40.

118. Nakamura Y, Mitani N, Ishii A, et al. Idiopathic pneumonia syndrome with thrombotic microangiopathy-related changes after allogeneic hematopoietic stem cell transplantation. Int J Hematol 2013;98(4):496–8.

119. Siami K, Kojouri K, Swisher KK, et al. Thrombotic microangiopathy after allogeneic hematopoietic stem cell transplantation: an autopsy study. Transplantation 2008;85(1):22–8.

120. Labrador J, Gonzalez-Rivero J, Monroy R, et al. Management patterns and outcomes in symptomatic venous thromboembolism following allogeneic hematopoietic stem cell transplantation. A 15-years experience at a single center. Thromb Res 2016; 142:52–6.

121. Zahid MF, Murad MH, Litzow MR, et al. Venous thromboembolism following hematopoietic stem cell transplantation-a systematic review and meta-analysis. Ann Hematol 2016;95(9):1457–64.

122. Labrador J, Lopez-Anglada L, Perez-Lopez E, et al. Analysis of incidence, risk factors and clinical outcome of thromboembolic and bleeding events in 431 allogeneic hematopoietic stem cell transplantation recipients. Haematologica 2013;98(3):437–43.

123. Morales IJ, Anderson PM, Tazelaar HD, et al. Pulmonary cytolytic thrombi: unusual complication of hematopoietic stem cell transplantation. J Pediatr Hematol Oncol 2003;25(1):89–92.

124. Woodard JP, Gulbahce E, Shreve M, et al. Pulmonary cytolytic thrombi: a newly recognized complication of stem cell transplantation. Bone Marrow Transplant 2000;25(3):293–300.

125. Gulbahce HE, Manivel JC, Jessurun J. Pulmonary cytolytic thrombi: a previously unrecognized complication of bone marrow transplantation. Am J Surg Pathol 2000;24(8):1147–52.

126. Modi D, Jang H, Kim S, et al. Incidence, etiology, and outcome of pleural effusions in allogeneic hematopoietic stem cell transplantation. Am J Hematol 2016;91(9):E341–7.

127. Ugai T, Hamamoto K, Kimura S, et al. A retrospective analysis of computed tomography findings in patients with pulmonary complications after allogeneic hematopoietic stem cell transplantation. Eur J Radiol 2015;84(12):2663–70.

Pulmonary Infections in Patients with Malignancy

Bacterial Pneumonia in Patients with Cancer
Novel Risk Factors and Management

Justin L. Wong, MD[a], Scott E. Evans, MD[b],*

KEYWORDS

- Bacterial pneumonia • Cancer • Neutropenia • Hematologic malignancy • Stem cell transplant
- Immunocompromised host pneumonia

KEY POINTS

- Bacterial pneumonias in patients with cancer cause significant morbidity and mortality, particularly among those with treatment-induced cytopenias.
- Cancer-related and cancer treatment-related derangements of lung architecture, mucositis, and impaired airway protection/swallow function all contribute to pneumonia risks.
- Neutropenia, cytotoxic chemotherapy, graft-versus host disease and other factors increase the risk of developing life-threatening bacterial pneumonia.
- Chest imaging is often nonspecific, but may aid in diagnosis. Bronchoscopy with bronchoalveolar lavage is recommended for patients with suspected bacterial pneumonia with new infiltrates on chest imaging.
- Early initiation of antibiotic therapy is recommended for those suspected of having bacterial pneumonia, ensuring coverage of pathogens commonly encountered in the health care setting.

INTRODUCTION

Bacterial pneumonias cause disproportionate morbidity and mortality in patients with cancer, despite the current aggressive use of prophylactic antibiotics and environmental hygiene measures in this population.[1–5] Pneumonias are estimated to cause or complicate nearly 10% of hospital admissions among patients with cancer, notably including patients with hematologic malignancies whose estimated risk of pneumonia during the course of treatment exceeds 30%.[3,5–8] In fact, in the transfusion era, pneumonia is the leading cause of death among patients with acute leukemias.[3,9,10] Some investigations suggest that as many as 80% hematopoietic stem cell transplant (HSCT) recipients will experience at least 1 episode of pneumonia, and pneumonia is the proximate cause of death in 20% of HSCT patients.[11–13] Patients with cancer demonstrate unique susceptibility to bacterial pneumonias owing to the complex immune dysfunction caused by the disease and its treatment, reflecting such disparate mechanisms as neutropenia, lung architectural derangements, and malnutrition.[5,14–17] Further, frequent exposure to uncommon or antibiotic-resistant organisms occurs through repeated encounters with the health care system.[15,18,19] In addition to lethality attributable to

Disclosures: Dr J.L. Wong declares no relevant conflicts of interest. S.E. Evans is an author on United States patent 8,883,174 entitled 'Stimulation of Innate Resistance of the Lungs to Infection with Synthetic Ligands.' S.E. Evans owns stock in Pulmotect, Inc, which holds the commercial options on these patent disclosures.
^a Division of Internal Medicine, Department of Pulmonary, Critical Care and Sleep Medicine, The University of Texas Health Sciences Center, 6431 Fannin Street, MSB 1.434, Houston, TX 77030, USA; ^b Division of Internal Medicine, Department of Pulmonary Medicine, The University of Texas MD Anderson Cancer Center, 1515 Holcombe Boulevard, Unit 1100, Houston, TX 77030, USA
* Corresponding author.
E-mail address: seevans@mdanderson.org

Clin Chest Med 38 (2017) 263–277
http://dx.doi.org/10.1016/j.ccm.2016.12.005
0272-5231/17/© 2016 Elsevier Inc. All rights reserved.

the infection, a diagnosis of bacterial pneumonia is associated with poorer overall outcomes in patients with cancer.[7,20,21] In some cases, worsened outcomes result from cancer progression when cytotoxic treatments are deferred in patients suspected of having pneumonia. However, independent of effects on anticancer treatment, a single episode of bacterial pneumonia is associated with an increased frequency and complexity of hospitalization.[22] This review addresses the prevention, diagnosis, and management of bacterial pneumonia in patients with cancer, with an emphasis on the host factors that contribute to susceptibility.

PATHOGENESIS OF CANCER-ASSOCIATED PNEUMONIA

In both healthy and immunocompromised patients, bacteria reach the peripheral lung via inhalation, aspiration, hematogenous spread, or locoregional progression of proximal airway infections. The overwhelming majority of inhaled or aspirated pathogens are expelled via mucociliary escalator function before reaching the alveolar level, with particulates and microbes impacted in the viscoelastic airway lining fluid by turbulent air flow.[23] Those bacteria that reach the peripheral lung must breach the barrier defenses that exclude pathogens from the lower respiratory tract.[24,25]

The barrier defenses of the lower respiratory tract are often thought of as passive barricades to pathogen translocation. However, the lungs are protected by a complex array of dynamic defenses that include both structural impediments to pathogen entry and active antimicrobial effectors. Epithelial cells express effectors such as cationic antimicrobial peptides, reactive oxygen species, and surfactant proteins into the airway lining fluid, reducing pathogen burden through direct microbiocidal effects, activation of leukocyte-mediated immunity, and enhanced pathogen opsonization.[26–28] Alveolar macrophages engulf invading pathogens and promote host response via the complement system and inflammatory mediators.[29–31] Ligation of local epithelial and macrophage pattern recognition receptors by pathogen-associated molecular patterns promotes recruitment and activation of neutrophil responses and sculpts the adaptive response in the lung.[26–28]

In the intact host, these responses are usually successful in eliminating pathogen threats. However, the immunopathology resulting from the robust expression of antimicrobial mediators may result in local tissue injury and systemic inflammation, particularly when the pathogen successfully establishes infection.[32,33] In fact, many of the classical clinical signs that characterize the syndrome of pneumonia are predominantly manifestations of these host responses. These include radiographic pulmonary infiltrates that reflect airspace filling by edema fluid, leukocytes, and debris; systemic signs such as fever and leukocytosis; and mucopurulent cough.[16,34]

Both cancer and its treatment cause derangements of innate and adaptive responses to bacteria in the lungs. As summarized in **Fig. 1**, leukocyte depletion, dysregulated inflammation, mucosal disruptions, impaired pathogen recognition, tumor-related anatomic abnormalities, and graft-versus-host responses all contribute to the tremendous susceptibility of patients with cancer to lower respiratory tract infections.[5,35] Functional and anatomic defects frequently coexist in patients with cancer. Further, recurrent health care encounters that are typical among patients with cancer promote exposure to nosocomial and drug-resistant pathogens.[15]

Thus, not only are patients with cancer uniquely susceptible to bacterial infections, but their dysfunctional immune responses make the diagnosis of bacterial pneumonia challenging. In the absence of a brisk inflammatory response, many of the cardinal features of clinical pneumonia may not be present. This diagnosis may be made even more difficult when the patient has an already abnormal chest radiograph due to the disease or its treatment, or when a patient has competing causes for fever or cough.

HOST SUSCEPTIBILITY FACTORS IN THE CANCER PATIENT

Patients with cancer encounter myriad homeostatic derangements, and susceptibility to bacterial pneumonia among patients with cancer varies according to the type of malignancy, treatment types, and timing and comorbidities.[15]

General debility, as suggested in individual patients by Eastern Cooperative Oncology Group Performance Status scores of 2 or greater, has been identified as a risk factor among patients with lung cancer for the development of bacterial pneumonia.[36] It has been suggested that this may reflect, in part, the catabolic and malnourished states that are common among patients with cancer. In particular, malignancy-related deficiencies of essential fatty acids and polyribonucleotides, have been noted to cause important (but reversible) impairments of inflammatory and cytotoxic responses that contribute to pneumonia susceptibility.[37] Preexisting lung disease, including emphysema or bronchiectasis, are also

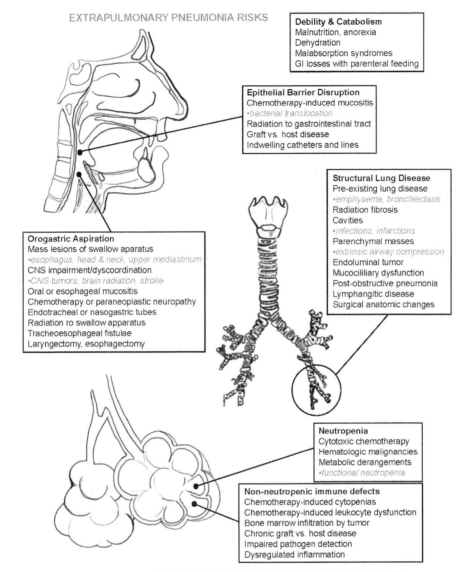

EXTRAPULMONARY PNEUMONIA RISKS

Debility & Catabolism
Malnutrition, anorexia
Dehydration
Malabsorption syndromes
GI losses with parenteral feeding

Epithelial Barrier Disruption
Chemotherapy-induced mucositis
•*bacterial translocation*
Radiation to gastrointestinal tract
Graft vs. host disease
Indwelling catheters and lines

Structural Lung Disease
Pre-existing lung disease
•*emphysema, bronchiectasis*
Radiation fibrosis
Cavities
•*infections, infarctions*
Parenchymal masses
•*extrinsic airway compression*
Endoluminal tumor
Mucocililiary dysfunction
Post-obstructive pneumonia
Lymphangitic disease
Surgical anatomic changes

Orogastric Aspiration
Mass lesions of swallow aparatus
•*esophagus, head & neck, upper mediastinum*
CNS impairment/dyscoordination
•*CNS tumors, brain radiation, stroke*
Oral or esophageal mucositis
Chemotherapy or paraneoplastic neuropathy
Endotracheal or nasogastric tubes
Radiation ro swallow apparatus
Tracheoesophageal fistulae
Laryngectomy, esophagectomy

Neutropenia
Cytotoxic chemotherapy
Hematologic malignancies
Metabolic derangements
•*functional neutropenia*

Non-neutropenic immune defects
Chemotherapy-induced cytopenias
Chemotherapy-induced leukocyte dysfunction
Bone marrow infiltration by tumor
Chronic graft vs. host disease
Impaired pathogen detection
Dysregulated inflammation

IMPAIRED HOST-PATHOGEN INTERACTIONS IN THE AIRSPACES

Fig. 1. Host factors that promote bacterial pneumonia susceptibility in patients with cancer. Although the medical encounters that patients with cancer require expose them to uncommon, virulent, and drug-resistant pathogens, much of the increased risk of pneumonia in this population derives from complex and often concurrent impairments of the host defense. Shown are frequent defects in the pneumonia defenses of patients with cancer, caused by insults both in and outside the lungs. CNS, central nervous system.

associated with increased risk of cancer-related bacterial pneumonia and mortality.[38,39]

Aspiration Events

Poorly coordinated swallow function and impairments of airway protection are frequently observed among patients with cancer. Structural lesions associated with head and neck cancer and neurologic defects associated with central nervous system lesions are well-recognized causes of aspiration of orogastric contents, placing patients at increased risk for pneumonia.[40,41] Similarly, pneumonia risks are increased among patients with esophageal cancers owing to excessive gastric reflux and tracheoesophageal fistulae.[42,43] Unfortunately, these risks may persist after completion of cancer treatment in each of these conditions owing to persistent neuropraxias or permanent anatomic derangements caused by radiation fibrosis, laryngectomy, or esophagectomy.[44–46]

Mass lesions are not the only causes of aspiration-related lower respiratory tract infections in patients with cancer. Oral mucositis and esophagitis commonly affect patients with hematologic malignancies or those receiving stem cell transplantation, also causing impairments of swallow function that result in bacterial pneumonias. Interestingly, although the oral microbial diversity of patients with cancer does not much differ from the general population, the incidence of periodontal disease is significantly greater in those undergoing cancer chemotherapy.[47–49] It has been suggested subsequently that optimized dental care in patients receiving chemotherapy may reduce the incidence of aspiration events and reduce the frequency of fever, productive cough, and positive blood cultures.[50] Relatedly, whereas gut dysbiosis has been associated with such HSCT complications as bloodstream infections and graft-versus-host disease (GVHD), it has been reported recently that altered gut microbiota may also be predictive of pulmonary complications of HSCT, including bacterial pneumonias.[51]

Mucositis and Bacterial Translocation

In addition to the aspiration risk, cancer-related mucositis also facilitates pneumonia caused by hematogenous spread of pathogens that translocate from the upper and lower gastrointestinal tract. Owing to the profound effects on rapidly replicating gastrointestinal epithelial cells, chemotherapy-related mucositis represents a serious threat to mucosal integrity. This has been long observed with the use of drugs that alter DNA synthesis, and has been classically described with such agents as methotrexate, 5-fluoruracil, and cytosine arabinoside. However, the chemotherapeutic agents known to cause mucositis are many and varied in mechanism of action, including melphalan-based regimens,[52–55] cyclophosphamide,[52] docetaxel, and vinorelbine to note a few.[56,57] Repetitive treatment cycles are associated with an increasing risk and severity of mucositis.[58] Even when clinical mucositis scores are low, even the modest degrees of mucositis still represent potentially important breakdowns in the host innate defense barriers.[59]

Unfortunately, although targeted therapies generally have fewer off-target effects than do conventional cytotoxic therapies, mucositis is still widely reported with many tyrosine kinase, mammalian target of rapamycin, epidermal growth factor receptor, and vascular endothelial growth factor receptor inhibitors.[60,61]

Pneumonia-relevant mucositis is also extremely common among patients receiving radiation therapy to the head and neck, mediastinum, esophagus, and to a lesser extent among any patient receiving thoracoabdominal radiation.[62–64]

Anatomic Derangements

As in patients without cancer, distorted lung anatomy owing to preexisting lung disease or prior infections predisposes to colonization and infection with bacterial pathogens.[65–67] Further, architectural changes specific to cancer and its treatment also place patients at increased risk for bacterial pneumonia. Airway obstruction caused by endoluminal disease or extrinsic compression may impede normal mucociliary clearance and promote postobstructive pneumonias.[68–70] Lymphangitic disease may obstruct airways and may impair leukocyte responses to infected lung segments. Similarly, airway distortion caused by prior radiotherapy or surgical intervention may lead to more bacterial infections.

Neutropenia

In 1977, Bodey and colleagues[71] described the inverse association of absolute neutrophil count and risk of infection. Since then, chemotherapy-induced neutropenia has become the most widely recognized risk factor for cancer-associated bacterial pneumonias. Neutrophils are particularly sensitive to nucleoside analogues and alkylating agents, both causing dose-dependent decreases in circulating neutrophil levels. Severe neutropenia (<500 cells/μL) is especially associated with serious lung infections and poor outcomes. Underscoring the relevance of this risk factor, Vento and colleagues[72] estimate that nearly 60% of patients with cancer experiencing chemotherapy-induced neutropenia will develop pulmonary infiltrates on radiographic examination. The rapidity of onset, duration, severity, and underlying physiologic process all further impact susceptibility to neutropenic pneumonia.[18,30,35–39,73] Moreover, impairments of neutrophil phagocytosis and chemotaxis follow common cancer-related insults such as radiation, corticosteroids, hypovolemia, acidosis, and hyperglycemia.[5,40] Thus, functional neutropenia can also contribute to cancer-related pneumonia risk.[3]

Although chemotherapy-induced neutropenia is associated most commonly with treatment of hematologic malignancies and conditioning regimens for HSCT, a number of regimens to treat solid tumors also cause neutropenia.[74–77]

Nonneutropenic Defects

Chemotherapy regimens also cause a wide array of nonneutropenic leukocyte defects that predispose patients to bacterial pneumonias. For example, alkylating agents also cause immune dysfunction through disproportionate depletion of CD4$^+$ T cells, relative to CD8$^+$ T cells.[78–80] Tyrosine kinase inhibitors increase risks for bacterial pneumonia through both neutropenia-dependent and -independent mechanisms, possibly including effects on antibody class switching.[81,82] Anthracyclines, taxanes, topoisomerase inhibitors, and vinca alkaloids all seem to be capable of increasing risk of bacterial pneumonia via nonneutropenic mechanisms during treatment.[83]

There are also a number of nonneutropenic defects that predispose patients to bacterial pneumonia, even after treatment has been completed. For example, agents such as fludarabine and alemtuzumab can cause long-term lymphocyte dysfunction, in some cases lasting years beyond the treatment interval.

In recipients of allogeneic stem cell transplants, GVHD can predispose to bacterial pneumonias both through episodes of mucositis and chronic defects of cell-mediated immunity.[13,84] Moreover, intensification of immunosuppressive therapies in response to GVHD flares notably enhances susceptibility to bacterial pneumonia.

Finally, hematologic malignancies can cause intrinsic immune defects that predispose patients to bacterial pneumonia. Specific defects depend on the cells affected by the malignancy. For example, excessive expansion of clonal leukemia populations can result in deficiencies of functional leukocytes, resulting in immune dysfunction through cytopenias. In contrast, nonmalignant leukocytes may be present at near normal levels in multiple myeloma, but immune defects may exist due to deficiencies of functional immunoglobulins and immunoglobulin class switching.

PREVENTION OF BACTERIAL PNEUMONIA IN PATIENTS WITH CANCER

Minimizing pathogen exposures is foundational to preventing bacterial pneumonia in patients with cancer. Optimized hand hygiene is central to nosocomial spread of pneumonia-causing organisms as well as avoidance of community-acquired pathogens, and no other single intervention has been demonstrated to be more effective.[3] The past 4 decades have also seen reduced pathogen transmission to neutropenic patients through development of protected hospital environments using laminar airflow, ultraviolet light decontamination, and specialized personal protective equipment.

Given the relevance of oropharyngeal aspiration to pneumonia, regular dental care is important in patients with cancer. Periodontal disease after radiation, chemotherapy, or malignancy-related immune dysfunction can all be associated with increased risk of preventable pneumonia.

The role of vaccinations in patients with cancer has been an issue of intensive investigation, given the complex immunologic consequences of malignant diseases, chemotherapy and immunosuppression. The only vaccinations approved by the US Food and Drug Administration available against bacterial pneumonia both target *Streptococcus pneumoniae*. The 23-valent polysaccharide vaccine (PSV23), principally activates mature B-cells, which may be deficient or dysfunctional in patients with cancers such as lymphomas or myelomas. Interestingly, in this population, antibody responses to PSV23 positively correlate with hematologic response to chemotherapy.[85] The conjugated 13-valent pneumococcal vaccination (PCV13) depends more heavily on T-cell responses, and remains more immunogenic in many immunocompromised cancer populations.[86–88]

Two cancer populations of particular note when considering vaccination are those with asplenia and those receiving anti-CD20 therapy, because both generate poor humoral responses to vaccines. Some patients with cancer require therapeutic splenectomy whereas others, including many patients with Hodgkin lymphoma, develop functional asplenia that results in both increased frequency and severity of pneumococcal disease.[89] These patients may generate reduced initial antibody titers to PCV13 vaccination, especially if given during cytoreductive therapy, and even apparently normal initial levels may decline below expected titers years after vaccination.[90] Anti-CD20 therapy such as rituximab disrupts B-cell–mediated antibody production, increasing the risk of invasive pneumococcal disease impairing responses to both PCV13 and PSV23.[87,91]

The current recommendation from the Centers for Disease Control and Prevention is that immunocompromised patients with cancer receive both the PCV13 followed by PSV23 at least 8 weeks later.[92] Where feasible, patients typically initiate vaccination before the initiation of chemotherapy, particularly if rituximab is anticipated. In those not vaccinated before receiving cytotoxic therapy, some experts recommend delaying vaccination up to 6 months after chemotherapy is completed to ensure greater efficacy. The effectiveness of the current recommendations in reducing disease burden remains unclear, potentially owing to the underuse of vaccines in the cancer population resulting from confusion about the usefulness of vaccination in patients who are receiving myeloablative treatments, even in tertiary cancer centers.[93]

The optimized strategy to best protect HSCT patients remains an area of intensive investigation. Multisociety guidelines from 2009[11] recognize that PSV23 elicits inadequately immunogenic responses in the first year after HSCT, so 3 doses of the more immunogenic, but less broad, PCV are recommended in that interval. A fourth vaccination with PSV23 may provide enhanced breadth of coverage, although PCV may be preferred for the fourth dose in patients with chronic GVHD. The timing of the vaccination also remains controversial, because initiation of pneumococcal vaccination 3 months after HSCT may provide confer early protection, but may not provide similarly durable antibody responses or reliable PSV23 boost compared with vaccination started 9 months after HSCT.

DIAGNOSIS OF BACTERIAL PNEUMONIA IN THE PATIENT WITH CANCER

Although the clinical syndrome of pneumonia is well-characterized in the general population, this diagnosis may be challenging in the patients with cancer. Most of the cardinal clinical features of pneumonia represent host response elements that may be impaired or absent in immunocompromised patients with cancer. Conversely, when present, cough, fever, and radiographic infiltrates may be manifestations of the malignancy itself or complications of therapy. Nevertheless, the correct diagnosis of pneumonia and identification of an infecting pathogen are both associated with better outcomes. Thus, a high clinical suspicion and appropriate testing are essential. Further, given the severe immune impairment and frequent health care exposures experienced by patients with cancer, it important to consider the possibility that pneumonias may be caused by uncommon, atypical, or opportunistic organisms.

Imaging Studies

Although plain chest radiographs are often rapidly available and can reveal some lower respiratory tract infections, they are nonspecific and have a poor negative predictive value, particularly in hematologic malignancy and HSCT patients. In 1 recent study, radiologist-interpreted radiographs predicted the correct type of infection in immunocompromised patients with pneumonia only 34% of the time.[94] Computed tomography (CT) scanning is more sensitive than radiography in the detection and characterization of pneumonia. When performed with high-resolution formatting, in particular, CT scanning is better able to discern bilateral and apical disease, and to discriminate

between typical patterns suggestive of bacterial infection than radiographic imaging.[95] In another study of adults with febrile neutropenia, 48% of patients with a CT scan suggestive of pneumonia were found to have a radiograph that was interpreted as normal.[96] Offsetting enthusiasm for early and frequent CT in patients with cancer is the fact that radiographic studies subject patients to radiation exposures, potentially to organs that also receive therapeutic radiation. Ultra–low-dose CT scanning has been investigated as a tool to maintain adequate image quality while reducing radiation dose to patients with cancer. A recent study in patients with febrile neutropenia suggests that this approach may preserve reasonable diagnostic accuracy.[97]

Certain CT patterns, such as lobar consolidation or peribronchial nodules, have been described as characteristic of bacterial pneumonias[98] (**Fig. 2**A–C). However, CT patterns are frequently nonspecific, particularly in patients with impaired immune function, and cannot be relied on for a microbiologic diagnosis.[98,99] Moreover, the patterns observed in patients with cancer with bacterial pneumonia overlap substantially with competing noninfectious diagnoses, as suggested by the CT patterns shown in **Fig. 2**D–F.

PET using fluorine-18 fluorodeoxyglucose has been proposed as a means to predict infection in patients with cancer with infiltrates, although no study has defined clearly the standard uptake values that are confirmatory of infection or changed management.[100–102]

Diagnostic Bronchoscopy

Although CT scanning lacks specificity, it is frequently helpful in directing bronchoscopic investigations. In patients with cancer with suspected pneumonia and from whom high-quality sputum samples cannot be obtained, flexible bronchoscopy with bronchoalveolar lavage (BAL) is the diagnostic tool of choice. Depending on the patient population investigated and the technique used, the diagnostic yield for a pathogen or noninfectious cause of infiltrates (eg, malignant cytology) is reported between 15% and 55%.[103–106] Diagnostic yield may be enhanced by rigorous adherence to BAL protocol.[106] Further, performance of BAL in the first 4 days of symptoms in HSCT patients with suspected pneumonia is associated with improved diagnostic yield and mortality.[107] The role for bronchial washings remains unclear, and the addition of protected specimen brushing and protected BAL has not been shown to improve the diagnosis of pneumonia in patients with hematologic malignancies.[108]

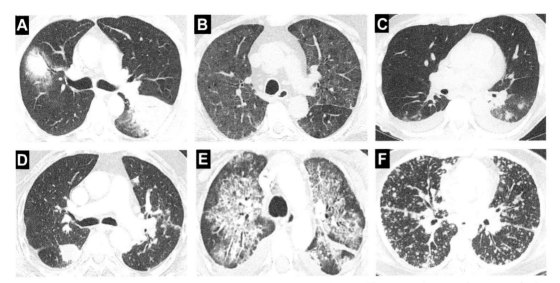

Fig. 2. Radiographic presentations of bacterial pneumonia in patients with cancer. Computed tomography images of patients with cancer with documented bacterial pneumonias. (*A*) Multifocal lobar consolidation in a patient with acute myelogenous leukemia and *Legionella micdadei* pneumonia. (*B*) Diffuse ground-glass infiltrates in a patient with chronic myelomonocytic leukemia and *Raoultella planticola* pneumonia. (*C*) Peribronchial nodules (and small, chronic pleural effusions) in a patient with myelodysplastic syndrome and *Stenotrophomonas maltophilia* pneumonia. (*D*) Multidrug-resistant *Klebsiella pneumoniae* pneumonia presenting as a single mass in a patient with aplastic anemia. (*E*) Diffuse, mixed alveolar and interstitial infiltrates in a patient with myelodysplastic syndrome and *Pseudomonas aeruginosa* pneumonia. (*F*) Methicillin-resistant *Staphylococcus aureus* pneumonia presenting as new nodules on a background of preexisting nodules in a patient with renal cell carcinoma metastatic to the lungs.

Transbronchial biopsy is beneficial principally in aiding the diagnosis of neoplasms or noninfectious pneumonitis.[109] Not only is this procedure often precluded in patients with cancer by thrombocytopenia, but convincing evidence is lacking that culture of biopsy tissue results in reliable culture information. Thus, this intervention is recommended in only select patients with cancer and suspected pneumonia.

Serial dilution culture remains the standard clinical practice for bacterial pathogen detection, owing to the breadth of organisms that can be identified by this strategy, the ability to quantify pathogen burden, and the ability to subculture for antimicrobial susceptibility testing. **Box 1** identifies select bacterial pathogens that are frequently detected in patients with chemotherapy-induced neutropenia by this technique. However, polymerase chain reaction (PCR)-based pathogen detection has the potential to supplement and, theoretically, supplant culture-based methods in patients with cancer. PCR-based strategies obviate the obligate delays for pathogen growth, potentially improving the time to correct antibiotics. Because patients with cancer are typically receiving empiric antimicrobials by the time of BAL, standard growth techniques may be impaired, but PCR assays can detect genomic material even from nonviable bacteria.[110] Further, multiplex detection of resistance cassettes can allow prediction of antibiotic susceptibility and may allow detection of difficult to culture pathogens, including anaerobes.[111] However, the use of standalone PCR detection for bacteria is impeded currently by local laboratory capability and practical challenges of testing sufficiently comprehensive PCR probe sets.

Nonbronchoscopic Diagnostics

Data from general (noncancer) populations indicate that urine antigen testing for bacterial pathogens including *S pneumoniae* and *Legionella* spp. provides enhanced sensitivity for the diagnosis of bacterial pneumonias over culture-only strategies. Moreover, like PCR testing on respiratory secretions, urinary antigen testing can be performed in minutes, potentially improving time to diagnosis and time to correct antibiotics.[112,113] Notably, there seems to be a strong correlation between urine antigen levels and markers of host response, including procalcitonin levels, C-reactive protein levels, and lobar infiltrates on radiographic imaging. Thus, there may be some dependency of urine antigen levels on the host responses, so further testing is required to confirm that the sensitivity

Box 1
Bacterial pneumonia pathogens commonly associated with chemotherapy-induced neutropenia

Gram-positive bacteria

Nocardia spp.

Rhodococcus equi

Streptococcus pneumoniae[a]

Streptococcus pyogenes

Staphylococcus aureus[a,b]

Gram-negative bacteria

Acinetobacter baumannii complex

Alcaligenes/Achromobacter spp.

Burkholderia spp.

Citrobacter spp.[b]

Enterobacter cloacaea[a]

Escherichia coli[b]

Klebsiella pneumonia

Moraxella catarrhalis

Neisseria meningitides

Nontypeable *Haemophilus influenza*[a]

Proteus spp.[b]

Pseudomonas spp.[a,b]

Stenotrophomonas maltophilia[b]

Serretia marcescensa

Atypical bacteria

Chlamydophyla pneumoniae

Legionella spp.

Mycoplasma pneumoniae

[a] Routinely consider in initial selection of antibiotics.
[b] Increased risk for antimicrobial resistance.

is comparable in immunocompromised cancer populations.

Biomarkers to aid in the diagnosis of bacterial pneumonia in immunocompromised patients with cancer have been long sought. Serum concentrations of procalcitonin, interleukin-6, C-reactive protein, serum amyloid proteins, and others have been investigated for their usefulness in the diagnosis of fevers of unknown origin.[114] Although increases in these markers have been observed in critically ill patients, none has demonstrated discriminatory capacity for bacterial pathogens in this population.[115] Procalcitonin levels in pleural fluid may offer some advantage in distinguishing parapneumonic or tuberculous effusions from malignant effusions.[114,116]

MANAGEMENT OF BACTERIAL PNEUMONIA IN THE CANCER PATIENT
Antibiotic Therapy

The value of these diagnostic tests is contingent upon the availability of effective therapies. Because of the broad range of potential pathogens and innumerable host factors, therapeutic strategies must be directed by the patient's immune status and exposure history, both to pathogens and antimicrobials.

Treatment should generally not be withheld while diagnostic interventions are undertaken. Delays in appropriate antimicrobial therapy increase the risk of secondary complications and infection-associated deaths in immunocompromised patients with cancer; thus, it is common practice to initiate empiric or preemptive antibiotic therapy when pneumonia is suspected.[3,18,117,118] No consensus exists for the optimal time to first antibiotic dose, although a recent study suggests that neutropenic fever outcomes are better when antibiotics are delivered within 104 minutes of presentation.[119] Although the earliest possible antibiotic dosing is generally recommended, possible exceptions include when bronchoscopic evaluation is available immediately.[3] In that case, it may be reasonable to hold empiric antibiotic therapy until completion of the brief procedure, potentially enhancing the diagnostic yield of the collected microbiologic cultures. This delay should generally be no longer than 2 hours. Antibiotics should not be held for multiple hours or days in anticipation of bronchoscopy, because the harm from delaying therapy outweighs the benefits of improved test performance.[120–122]

Initial antimicrobial therapy for febrile patients with cancer with pulmonary infiltrates should ensure coverage of multidrug-resistant strains of *Staphylococcus aureus* and *Pseudomonas aeruginosa*.[15,123–126] Coverage for atypical organisms is also appropriate in patients with cancer admitted with community-acquired pneumonia, with the selection of macrolide, fluoroquinolone, or doxycycline therapy largely dependent on the agent(s) chosen for drug-resistant pathogens and on prior prophylactic regimens.[127,128] All antibiotic choices should consider culture data, pneumonia severity, local antibiotic sensitivity profiles, prior antibiotic exposures, and patient immune status.[129] Empiric antibiotics for early hospital-acquired pneumonia (within 7 days of admission) should include coverage of *S pneumoniae*, methicillin-resistant *S aureus*, *Haemophilus influenzae*, and *Enterobacteriaceae*. Initial regimens for patients with late hospital-acquired pneumonia, health care-associated pneumonia, or ventilator-associated pneumonia should ensure enhanced coverage for multidrug resistant Gram-negative bacilli.[117,120,125,130] Secondary antibiotic selections for patients with refractory hospital-acquired pneumonia, health care-associated pneumonia, or ventilator-associated pneumonia should be determined by institutional pathogen susceptibility profiles and on prior patient antimicrobial exposures.[124,125,130,131]

Early deescalation of broad empiric therapy may be considered in patients who demonstrate prompt clinical response and in whom granulocyte recovery has occurred, especially if a susceptible pathogen has been identified.[132,133] Deescalation should be undertaken with caution in patients with poor clinical response to antimicrobial therapy, persistent neutropenia, or ongoing immunosuppressive therapy.[134]

Therapies to Augment Host Defenses

Despite broad-spectrum antibiotic strategies, mortality rates remain unacceptably high in patients with cancer who also have bacterial pneumonia, particularly among neutropenic patients. Often, antibiotic failures arise, at least in part, from the continuing immune defects associated with the primary disease. Consequently, the means to mitigate immune defects of patients with cancer and improve pathogen clearance have become an area of intensive investigation.

A major research focus has been correction of granulocytopenia. Preparations of granulocyte colony stimulating factor (filgrastim, lenograstim, and pegfilgrastim) and granulocyte macrophage colony stimulating factor (sargramostim and molgramostim) are available commercially. Both classes demonstrate efficacy in reducing the duration of neutropenia, although a less favorable side effect profile of granulocyte macrophage colony stimulating factor limits its use primarily to post-HSCT immune reconstitution.[135,136] Although the evidence suggests that colony-stimulating factors may be used safely to prevent some bacterial pneumonias in cancer populations,[137] they are not recommended generally as a treatment of established bacterial infections. Current guidelines recommend the administration of granulocyte colony stimulating factor if the risk of developing febrile neutropenia is greater than 20% based on patient-specific risk factors.[136]

Infusion of donor granulocytes has also been proposed as an adjunct therapy in patients with cancer with febrile neutropenia. Although this strategy holds promise, it remains investigational and interpretation of the associated studies is challenging owing to heterogeneity of the populations and protocols.[138] However, some authors argue that severely ill neutropenic patients may benefit from granulocyte transfusion.[137]

In addition to efforts to increase the absolute number of leukocytes in cytopenic patients, multiple groups have investigated the manipulation of existing leukocytes through the administration of recombinant cytokines. Exogenous interferon-gamma has demonstrated success in reducing some bacterial infections in patients with congenital neutropenia, and more recent studies suggest efficacy in patients with opportunistic infections after HSCT.[139] Postulated mechanisms for this effect include induction of surface molecules such as major histocompatibility complex class II, Fc receptor gamma and integrins, increased phagolysosomal superoxide production, and prolonged half-life of granulocytes. Administration of interleukin-12 has also been proposed as a means to protect against lung infections,[140] potentially via interferon-gamma–dependent and tumor necrosis factor–dependent mechanisms.

Induction of innate antimicrobial responses directly from lung epithelial cells offers a novel alternate strategy to prevent, and possibly treat, pneumonias in patients with cancer. Lung epithelial cells are long lived and relatively resistant to chemotherapy.[141,142] Beyond their well-known barrier function, these cells also demonstrate a substantial capacity to detect pathogens, modulate local immune responses, and generate directly bactericidal responses through the production of antimicrobial peptides and reactive species.[26,143] Advances in the understanding of the molecular mechanisms involved in recognition and signal transduction have allowed development of inhaled therapeutics that induce protective innate immune responses from the lung epithelium in animals. In animal models of pneumonia, this provides protection from lethal pathogens, even when there is concurrent neutropenia.[142,144,145] Preclinical animal studies of one such treatment, PUL-042, demonstrate protection against gram-positive, gram-negative, fungal, and viral pneumonias, and clinical trials are ongoing.[142,145,146] Augmentation of innate immune responses offer several hypothetical advantages in terms of rapidity of effect, breadth of pathogen specificity, and lack of known antimicrobial resistance, but efficacy has not been established in humans.

SUMMARY

Bacterial pneumonias remain a frequent and challenging complication in patients with cancer. The clinical approach requires integration of traditional microbiologic techniques as well as targeted molecular diagnostics. Successful management strategies depend on early recognition, consideration of numerous cancer-related host factors, and prompt initiation of broad-spectrum antibacterial agents. Newer host-directed therapies that help to reconstitute or augment the immune system are under active investigation in clinical trials. These modalities may serve to supplement more traditional approaches in the future.

ACKNOWLEDGMENTS

The authors thank Dr Ahmed Salahudeen for contributing the original art included in this article.

REFERENCES

1. Yoo SS, Cha SI, Shin KM, et al. Bacterial pneumonia following cytotoxic chemotherapy for lung cancer: clinical features, treatment outcome and prognostic factors. Scand J Infect Dis 2010; 42(10):734–40.
2. Hoheisel G, Lange S, Winkler J, et al. Nosocomial pneumonias in haematological malignancies in the medical intensive care unit. Pneumologie 2003;57(2):73–7 [in German].
3. Evans SE, Ost DE. Pneumonia in the neutropenic cancer patient. Curr Opin Pulm Med 2015;21(3): 260–71.
4. Aliberti S, Brock GN, Peyrani P, et al. The pneumonia severity index and the CRB-65 in cancer patients with community-acquired pneumonia. Int J Tuberc Lung Dis 2009;13(12):1550–6.
5. Safdar A, Armstrong D. Infectious morbidity in critically ill patients with cancer. Crit Care Clin 2001; 17(3):531–70, vii–viii.
6. Garcia JB, Lei X, Wierda W, et al. Pneumonia during remission induction chemotherapy in patients with acute leukemia. Ann Am Thorac Soc 2013; 10(5):432–40.
7. Whimbey E, Goodrich J, Bodey GP. Pneumonia in cancer patients. Cancer Treat Res 1995;79: 185–210.
8. Gonzalez C, Johnson T, Rolston K, et al. Predicting pneumonia mortality using CURB-65, PSI, and patient characteristics in patients presenting to the emergency department of a comprehensive cancer center. Cancer Med 2014;3(4):962–70.
9. Chang HY, Rodriguez V, Narboni G, et al. Causes of death in adults with acute leukemia. Medicine (Baltimore) 1976;55(3):259–68.
10. Cannas G, Pautas C, Raffoux E, et al. Infectious complications in adult acute myeloid leukemia: analysis of the Acute Leukemia French Association-9802 prospective multicenter clinical trial. Leuk Lymphoma 2012;53(6):1068–76.
11. Center for International Blood and Marrow Transplant Research, National Marrow Donor Program, European Blood and Marrow Transplant Group, European Blood and Marrow Transplant Group (EBMT), et al. Guidelines for preventing infectious complications among hematopoietic cell transplant recipients: a global perspective. Bone Marrow Transplant 2009;44(8):453–558.
12. Lossos IS, Breuer R, Or R, et al. Bacterial pneumonia in recipients of bone marrow transplantation. A five-year prospective study. Transplantation 1995;60(7):672–8.
13. Aguilar-Guisado M, Jiménez-Jambrina M, Espigado I, et al. Pneumonia in allogeneic stem cell transplantation recipients: a multicenter prospective study. Clin Transplant 2011;25(6):E629–38.
14. Wong A, Marrie TJ, Garg S, et al. Increased risk of invasive pneumococcal disease in haematological and solid-organ malignancies. Epidemiol Infect 2010;138(12):1804–10.
15. Ashour HM, el-Sharif A. Microbial spectrum and antibiotic susceptibility profile of gram-positive aerobic bacteria isolated from cancer patients. J Clin Oncol 2007;25(36):5763–9.
16. Joos L, Tamm M. Breakdown of pulmonary host defense in the immunocompromised host: cancer chemotherapy. Proc Am Thorac Soc 2005;2(5):445–8.
17. Lal A, Bhurgri Y, Rizvi N, et al. Factors influencing in-hospital length of stay and mortality in cancer patients suffering from febrile neutropenia. Asian Pac J Cancer Prev 2008;9(2):303–8.
18. Guinan JL, McGuckin M, Nowell PC. Management of health-care–associated infections in the oncology patient. Oncology (Williston Park) 2003; 17(3):415–20 [discussion: 423–6].
19. Steele RW. Managing infection in cancer patients and other immunocompromised children. Ochsner J 2012;12(3):202–10.
20. Chaoui D, Legrand O, Roche N, et al. Incidence and prognostic value of respiratory events in acute leukemia. Leukemia 2004;18(4):670–5.
21. Kufe DW, Pollock RE, Weichselbaum RR, et al. Cancer medicine 6. 6th edition. Hamilton (Canada): BC Decker; 2003.
22. Kuderer NM, Dale DC, Crawford J, et al. Mortality, morbidity, and cost associated with febrile neutropenia in adult cancer patients. Cancer 2006; 106(10):2258–66.
23. Reynolds HY. Host defense impairments that may lead to respiratory infections. Clin Chest Med 1987;8(3):339–58.
24. Siegel SJ, Weiser JN. Mechanisms of bacterial colonization of the respiratory tract. Annu Rev Microbiol 2015;69:425–44.
25. Scannapieco FA, Mylotte JM. Relationships between periodontal disease and bacterial pneumonia. J Periodontol 1996;67(10 Suppl):1114–22.

26. Bartlett JA, Fischer AJ, McCray PB Jr. Innate immune functions of the airway epithelium. Contrib Microbiol 2008;15:147–63.

27. Evans SE, Xu Y, Tuvim MJ, et al. Inducible innate resistance of lung epithelium to infection. Annu Rev Physiol 2010;72:413–35.

28. Whitsett JA, Alenghat T. Respiratory epithelial cells orchestrate pulmonary innate immunity. Nat Immunol 2015;16(1):27–35.

29. Guzman-Bautista ER, Ramirez-Estudillo MC, Rojas-Gomez OI, et al. Tracheal and bronchial polymeric immunoglobulin secretory immune system (PISIS) development in a porcine model. Dev Comp Immunol 2015;53(2):271–82.

30. Paterson GK, Orihuela CJ. Pneumococci: immunology of the innate host response. Respirology 2010;15(7):1057–63.

31. Kerr AR, Paterson GK, Riboldi-Tunnicliffe A, et al. Innate immune defense against pneumococcal pneumonia requires pulmonary complement component C3. Infect Immun 2005;73(7):4245–52.

32. Sawa T. The molecular mechanism of acute lung injury caused by Pseudomonas aeruginosa: from bacterial pathogenesis to host response. J Intensive Care 2014;2(1):10.

33. Madenspacher JH, Azzam KM, Gowdy KM, et al. p53 Integrates host defense and cell fate during bacterial pneumonia. J Exp Med 2013;210(5):891–904.

34. Yamamoto K, Ahyi AN, Pepper-Cunningham ZA, et al. Roles of lung epithelium in neutrophil recruitment during pneumococcal pneumonia. Am J Respir Cell Mol Biol 2014;50(2):253–62.

35. Wilson R, Cohen JM, Jose RJ, et al. Protection against Streptococcus pneumoniae lung infection after nasopharyngeal colonization requires both humoral and cellular immune responses. Mucosal Immunol 2015;8(3):627–39.

36. Lee JO, Kim DY, Lim JH, et al. Risk factors for bacterial pneumonia after cytotoxic chemotherapy in advanced lung cancer patients. Lung Cancer 2008;62(3):381–4.

37. Heys SD, Gough DB, Khan L, et al. Nutritional pharmacology and malignant disease: a therapeutic modality in patients with cancer. Br J Surg 1996;83(5):608–19.

38. Garcia-Vidal C, Ardanuy C, Tubau F, et al. Pneumococcal pneumonia presenting with septic shock: host- and pathogen-related factors and outcomes. Thorax 2010;65(1):77–81.

39. Lopez-Encuentra A, Astudillo J, Cerezal J, et al. Prognostic value of chronic obstructive pulmonary disease in 2994 cases of lung cancer. Eur J Cardiothorac Surg 2005;27(1):8–13.

40. Smith LH. Preventing aspiration: a common and dangerous problem for patients with cancer. Clin J Oncol Nurs 2009;13(1):105–8.

41. Purkey MT, Levine MS, Prendes B, et al. Predictors of aspiration pneumonia following radiotherapy for head and neck cancer. Ann Otol Rhinol Laryngol 2009;118(11):811–6.

42. Querol JM, Manresa F, Izquierdo J, et al. Lactobacillus pneumonia in a patient with oesophageal carcinoma. Eur Respir J 1989;2(6):589–91.

43. Quint LE. Thoracic complications and emergencies in oncologic patients. Cancer Imaging 2009;9 Spec No A:S75–82.

44. Neoral C, Horakova M, Aujesky R, et al. Infectious complications after esophagectomy. Surg Infect (Larchmt) 2012;13(3):159–62.

45. Hanyu T, Kanda T, Yajima K, et al. Community-acquired pneumonia during long-term follow-up of patients after radical esophagectomy for esophageal cancer: analysis of incidence and associated risk factors. World J Surg 2011;35(11):2454–62.

46. D'Journo XB, Michelet P, Papazian L, et al. Airway colonisation and postoperative pulmonary complications after neoadjuvant therapy for oesophageal cancer. Eur J Cardiothorac Surg 2008;33(3):444–50.

47. Gurgan CA, Özcan M, Karakuş Ö, et al. Periodontal status and post-transplantation complications following intensive periodontal treatment in patients underwent allogenic hematopoietic stem cell transplantation conditioned with myeloablative regimen. Int J Dent Hyg 2013;11(2):84–90.

48. Fernandez-Plata R, Olmedo-Torres D, Martínez-Briseño D, et al. Prevalence of severe periodontal disease and its association with respiratory disease in hospitalized adult patients in a tertiary care center. Gac Med Mex 2015;151(5):608–13 [in Spanish].

49. Bagyi K, Haczku A, Márton I, et al. Role of pathogenic oral flora in postoperative pneumonia following brain surgery. BMC Infect Dis 2009;9:104.

50. Tsuji K, Shibuya Y, Akashi M, et al. Prospective study of dental intervention for hematopoietic malignancy. J Dent Res 2015;94(2):289–96.

51. Harris B, Morjaria SM, Littmann ER, et al. Gut microbiota predict pulmonary infiltrates after allogeneic hematopoietic cell transplantation. Am J Respir Crit Care Med 2016;194(4):450–63.

52. Wardley AM, Jayson GC, Swindell R, et al. Prospective evaluation of oral mucositis in patients receiving myeloablative conditioning regimens and haematopoietic progenitor rescue. Br J Haematol 2000;110(2):292–9.

53. Robien K, Schubert MM, Bruemmer B, et al. Predictors of oral mucositis in patients receiving hematopoietic cell transplants for chronic myelogenous leukemia. J Clin Oncol 2004;22(7):1268–75.

54. Blijlevens N, Schwenkglenks M, Bacon P, et al. Prospective oral mucositis audit: oral mucositis in

patients receiving high-dose melphalan or BEAM conditioning chemotherapy–European Blood and Marrow Transplantation Mucositis Advisory Group. J Clin Oncol 2008;26(9):1519–25.

55. Krishna SG, Zhao W, Grazziutti ML, et al. Incidence and risk factors for lower alimentary tract mucositis after 1529 courses of chemotherapy in a homogenous population of oncology patients: clinical and research implications. Cancer 2011;117(3):648–55.

56. Rodriguez J, Calvo E, Cortes J, et al. Docetaxel plus vinorelbine as salvage chemotherapy in advanced breast cancer: a phase II study. Breast Cancer Res Treat 2002;76(1):47–56.

57. Ibrahim NK, Sahin AA, Dubrow RA, et al. Colitis associated with docetaxel-based chemotherapy in patients with metastatic breast cancer. Lancet 2000;355(9200):281–3.

58. Al-Ansari S, Zecha JA, Barasch A, et al. Oral mucositis induced by anticancer therapies. Curr Oral Health Rep 2015;2(4):202–11.

59. Wuketich S, Hienz SA, Marosi C. Prevalence of clinically relevant oral mucositis in outpatients receiving myelosuppressive chemotherapy for solid tumors. Support Care Cancer 2012;20(1): 175–83.

60. Boers-Doets CB, Epstein JB, Raber-Durlacher JE, et al. Oral adverse events associated with tyrosine kinase and mammalian target of rapamycin inhibitors in renal cell carcinoma: a structured literature review. Oncologist 2012;17(1):135–44.

61. Martins F, de Oliveira MA, Wang Q, et al. A review of oral toxicity associated with mTOR inhibitor therapy in cancer patients. Oral Oncol 2013;49(4):293–8.

62. Trotti A, Bellm LA, Epstein JB, et al. Mucositis incidence, severity and associated outcomes in patients with head and neck cancer receiving radiotherapy with or without chemotherapy: a systematic literature review. Radiother Oncol 2003; 66(3):253–62.

63. Bonomi M, Batt K. Supportive management of mucositis and metabolic derangements in head and neck cancer patients. Cancers (Basel) 2015;7(3): 1743–57.

64. Elting LS, Keefe DM, Sonis ST, et al. Patient-reported measurements of oral mucositis in head and neck cancer patients treated with radiotherapy with or without chemotherapy: demonstration of increased frequency, severity, resistance to palliation, and impact on quality of life. Cancer 2008; 113(10):2704–13.

65. Cabello H, Torres A, Celis R, et al. Bacterial colonization of distal airways in healthy subjects and chronic lung disease: a bronchoscopic study. Eur Respir J 1997;10(5):1137–44.

66. Yamada Y, Sekine Y, Suzuki H, et al. Trends of bacterial colonisation and the risk of postoperative pneumonia in lung cancer patients with chronic obstructive pulmonary disease. Eur J Cardiothorac Surg 2010;37(4):752–7.

67. Sethi S, Evans N, Grant BJ, et al. New strains of bacteria and exacerbations of chronic obstructive pulmonary disease. N Engl J Med 2002;347(7): 465–71.

68. Mohapatra PR, Bhuniya S, Garg S, et al. Endobronchial non-Hodgkin's lymphoma presenting as mass lesion. Indian J Chest Dis Allied Sci 2009;51(2): 107–9.

69. Waheed Z, Irfan M, Fatimi S, et al. Bronchial carcinoid presenting as multiple lung abscesses. J Coll Physicians Surg Pak 2013;23(3):229–30.

70. Gustafsson BI, Kidd M, Chan A, et al. Bronchopulmonary neuroendocrine tumors. Cancer 2008; 113(1):5–21.

71. Bodey GP, Rodriguez V, McCredie KB, et al. Neutropenia and infection following cancer chemotherapy. Int J Radiat Oncol Biol Phys 1976;1(3–4): 301–4.

72. Vento S, Cainelli F, Temesgen Z. Lung infections after cancer chemotherapy. Lancet Oncol 2008; 9(10):982–92.

73. Lopez B, Maisonet TM, Londhe VA. Alveolar NF-kappaB signaling regulates endotoxin-induced lung inflammation. Exp Lung Res 2015;41(2):103–14.

74. Lee HS, Lee YG, Koo DH, et al. Efficacy and safety of ifosfamide in combination with carboplatin and etoposide in small cell lung cancer. Cancer Chemother Pharmacol 2015;76(5):933–7.

75. Nichols CR, Fox EP, Roth BJ, et al. Incidence of neutropenic fever in patients treated with standard-dose combination chemotherapy for small-cell lung cancer and the cost impact of treatment with granulocyte colony-stimulating factor. J Clin Oncol 1994;12(6):1245–50.

76. Rahman Z, Esparza-Guerra L, Yap HY, et al. Chemotherapy-induced neutropenia and fever in patients with metastatic breast carcinoma receiving salvage chemotherapy. Cancer 1997; 79(6):1150–7.

77. do Nascimento TG, de Andrade M, de Oliveira RA, et al. Neutropenia: occurrence and management in women with breast cancer receiving chemotherapy. Rev Lat Am Enfermagem 2014;22(2): 301–8.

78. Steingrimsdottir H, Gruber A, Björkholm M, et al. Immune reconstitution after autologous hematopoietic stem cell transplantation in relation to underlying disease, type of high-dose therapy and infectious complications. Haematologica 2000; 85(8):832–8.

79. Talmadge JE, Jackson JD, Borgeson CD, et al. Differential recovery of polymorphonuclear neutrophils, B and T cell subpopulations in the thymus, bone marrow, spleen and blood of mice following

split-dose polychemotherapy. Cancer Immunol Immunother 1994;39(1):59–67.

80. Garcia Munoz R, Izquierdo-Gil A, Muñoz A, et al. Lymphocyte recovery is impaired in patients with chronic lymphocytic leukemia and indolent non-Hodgkin lymphomas treated with bendamustine plus rituximab. Ann Hematol 2014;93(11):1879–87.

81. de Lavallade H, Khoder A, Hart M, et al. Tyrosine kinase inhibitors impair B-cell immune responses in CML through off-target inhibition of kinases important for cell signaling. Blood 2013;122(2): 227–38.

82. Wang X, Li Y, Yan X. Efficacy and safety of novel agent-based therapies for multiple myeloma: a meta-analysis. Biomed Res Int 2016;2016: 6848902.

83. Hummel M, Hofheinz R, Buchheidt D. Severe Chlamydia pneumoniae infection in a patient with mild neutropenia during treatment of Hodgkin's disease. Ann Hematol 2004;83(7):441–3.

84. Garcia-Cadenas I, Rivera I, Martino R, et al. Patterns of infection and infection-related mortality in patients with steroid-refractory acute graft versus host disease. Bone Marrow Transplant 2017; 52(1):107–13.

85. Hinge M, Ingels HA, Slotved HC, et al. Serologic response to a 23-valent pneumococcal vaccine administered prior to autologous stem cell transplantation in patients with multiple myeloma. APMIS 2012;120(11):935–40.

86. Pasiarski M, Rolinski J, Grywalska E, et al. Antibody and plasmablast response to 13-valent pneumococcal conjugate vaccine in chronic lymphocytic leukemia patients–preliminary report. PLoS One 2014;9(12):e114966.

87. Sangil A, Xercavins M, Rodríguez-Carballeira M, et al. Impact of vaccination on invasive pneumococcal disease in adults with focus on the immunosuppressed. J Infect 2015;71(4):422–7.

88. Robin C, Beckerich F, Cordonnier C. Immunization in cancer patients: where we stand. Pharmacol Res 2015;92:23–30.

89. Chou MY, Brown AE, Blevins A, et al. Severe pneumococcal infection in patients with neoplastic disease. Cancer 1983;51(8):1546–50.

90. Landgren O, Björkholm M, Konradsen HB, et al. A prospective study on antibody response to repeated vaccinations with pneumococcal capsular polysaccharide in splenectomized individuals with special reference to Hodgkin's lymphoma. J Intern Med 2004;255(6):664–73.

91. Berglund A, Willén L, Grödeberg L, et al. The response to vaccination against influenza A(H1N1) 2009, seasonal influenza and Streptococcus pneumoniae in adult outpatients with ongoing treatment for cancer with and without rituximab. Acta Oncol 2014;53(9):1212–20.

92. Centers for Disease Control and Prevention (CDC). Pneumococcal vaccine timing for adults. 2015. Available at: http://www.cdc.gov/vaccines/vpd-vac/pneumo/downloads/adult-vax-clinician-aid.pdf. Accessed January 13, 2017.

93. Toleman MS, Herbert K, McCarthy N, et al. Vaccination of chemotherapy patients-effect of guideline implementation. Support Care Cancer 2016;24(5): 2317–21.

94. Navigante AH, Cerchietti LC, Costantini P, et al. Conventional chest radiography in the initial assessment of adult cancer patients with fever and neutropenia. Cancer Control 2002;9(4):346–51.

95. Syrjala H, Okada F, Mori T, et al. High-resolution computed tomography for the diagnosis of community-acquired pneumonia. Clin Infect Dis 1998;27(2):358–63.

96. Claessens YE, Debray MP, Tubach F, et al. Early chest computed tomography scan to assist diagnosis and guide treatment decision for suspected community-acquired pneumonia. Am J Respir Crit Care Med 2015;192(8):974–82.

97. Kim HJ, Park SY, Lee HY, et al. Ultra-low-dose chest CT in patients with neutropenic fever and hematologic malignancy: image quality and its diagnostic performance. Cancer Res Treat 2014;46(4): 393–402.

98. Nambu A, Ozawa K, Kobayashi N, et al. Imaging of community-acquired pneumonia: roles of imaging examinations, imaging diagnosis of specific pathogens and discrimination from noninfectious diseases. World J Radiol 2014;6(10):779–93.

99. Reynolds JH, Banerjee AK. Imaging pneumonia in immunocompetent and immunocompromised individuals. Curr Opin Pulm Med 2012;18(3):194–201.

100. Wong PS, Lau WF, Worth LJ, et al. Clinically important detection of infection as an 'incidental' finding during cancer staging using FDG-PET/CT. Intern Med J 2012;42(2):176–83.

101. Bleeker-Rovers CP, de Kleijn EM, Corstens FH, et al. Clinical value of FDG PET in patients with fever of unknown origin and patients suspected of focal infection or inflammation. Eur J Nucl Med Mol Imaging 2004;31(1):29–37.

102. Mahfouz T, Miceli MH, Saghafifar F, et al. 18F-fluorodeoxyglucose positron emission tomography contributes to the diagnosis and management of infections in patients with multiple myeloma: a study of 165 infectious episodes. J Clin Oncol 2005;23(31):7857–63.

103. Jain P, Sandur S, Meli Y, et al. Role of flexible bronchoscopy in immunocompromised patients with lung infiltrates. Chest 2004;125(2):712–22.

104. Azoulay E, Mokart D, Rabbat A, et al. Diagnostic bronchoscopy in hematology and oncology patients with acute respiratory failure: prospective multicenter data. Crit Care Med 2008;36(1):100–7.

105. Gilbert CR, Lerner A, Baram M, et al. Utility of flexible bronchoscopy in the evaluation of pulmonary infiltrates in the hematopoietic stem cell transplant population – a single center fourteen year experience. Arch Bronconeumol 2013; 49(5):189–95.

106. Sampsonas F, Kontoyiannis DP, Dickey BF, et al. Performance of a standardized bronchoalveolar lavage protocol in a comprehensive cancer center: a prospective 2-year study. Cancer 2011;117(15): 3424–33.

107. Shannon VR, Andersson BS, Lei X, et al. Utility of early versus late fiberoptic bronchoscopy in the evaluation of new pulmonary infiltrates following hematopoietic stem cell transplantation. Bone Marrow Transplant 2010;45(4):647–55.

108. Boersma WG, Erjavec Z, van der Werf TS, et al. Bronchoscopic diagnosis of pulmonary infiltrates in granulocytopenic patients with hematologic malignancies: BAL versus PSB and PBAL. Respir Med 2007;101(2):317–25.

109. Mulabecirovic A, Gaulhofer P, Auner HW, et al. Pulmonary infiltrates in patients with haematologic malignancies: transbronchial lung biopsy increases the diagnostic yield with respect to neoplastic infiltrates and toxic pneumonitis. Ann Hematol 2004; 83(7):420–2.

110. Abdeldaim GM, Strålin K, Korsgaard J, et al. Multiplex quantitative PCR for detection of lower respiratory tract infection and meningitis caused by Streptococcus pneumoniae, Haemophilus influenzae and Neisseria meningitidis. BMC Microbiol 2010;10:310.

111. Inai K, Iwasaki H, Noriki S, et al. Frequent detection of multidrug-resistant pneumonia-causing bacteria in the pneumonia lung tissues of patients with hematological malignancies. Int J Hematol 2007; 86(3):225–32.

112. Choi MJ, Song JY, Cheong HJ, et al. Clinical usefulness of pneumococcal urinary antigen test, stratified by disease severity and serotypes. J Infect Chemother 2015;21(9):672–9.

113. Molinos L, Zalacain R, Menéndez R, et al. Sensitivity, specificity, and positivity predictors of the pneumococcal urinary antigen test in community-acquired pneumonia. Ann Am Thorac Soc 2015; 12(10):1482–9.

114. San Jose ME, Valdés L, Vizcaíno LH, et al. Procalcitonin, C-reactive protein, and cell counts in the diagnosis of parapneumonic pleural effusions. J Investig Med 2010;58(8):971–6.

115. von Lilienfeld-Toal M, Dietrich MP, Glasmacher A, et al. Markers of bacteremia in febrile neutropenic patients with hematological malignancies: procalcitonin and IL-6 are more reliable than C-reactive protein. Eur J Clin Microbiol Infect Dis 2004;23(7): 539–44.

116. Wang CY, Hsiao YC, Jerng JS, et al. Diagnostic value of procalcitonin in pleural effusions. Eur J Clin Microbiol Infect Dis 2011;30(3):313–8.

117. Carratala J, Rosón B, Fernández-Sevilla A, et al. Bacteremic pneumonia in neutropenic patients with cancer: causes, empirical antibiotic therapy, and outcome. Arch Intern Med 1998; 158(8):868–72.

118. Brun-Buisson C, Lemaire F. Administration of antibiotics for pneumonia during respiratory failure: reaching the target. Am J Respir Crit Care Med 2001;164(9):1554–5.

119. Lynn JJ, Chen KF, Weng YM, et al. Risk factors associated with complications in patients with chemotherapy-induced febrile neutropenia in emergency department. Hematol Oncol 2013; 31(4):189–96.

120. Phillips R, Hancock B, Graham J, et al. Prevention and management of neutropenic sepsis in patients with cancer: summary of NICE guidance. BMJ 2012;345:e5368.

121. Rosa RG, Goldani LZ. Cohort study of the impact of time to antibiotic administration on mortality in patients with febrile neutropenia. Antimicrob Agents Chemother 2014;58(7):3799–803.

122. Mattison G, Bilney M, Haji-Michael P, et al. A nurse-led protocol improves the time to first dose intravenous antibiotics in septic patients post chemotherapy. Support Care Cancer 2016; 24(12):5001–5.

123. Vuotto F, Berthon C, Lemaitre N, et al. Risk factors, clinical features, and outcome of Pseudomonas aeruginosa bacteremia in patients with hematologic malignancies: a case-control study. Am J Infect Control 2013;41(6):527–30.

124. Ghannam DE, Rodriguez GH, Raad II, et al. Inhaled aminoglycosides in cancer patients with ventilator-associated Gram-negative bacterial pneumonia: safety and feasibility in the era of escalating drug resistance. Eur J Clin Microbiol Infect Dis 2009;28(3):253–9.

125. Wunderink RG, Niederman MS, Kollef MH, et al. Linezolid in methicillin-resistant Staphylococcus aureus nosocomial pneumonia: a randomized, controlled study. Clin Infect Dis 2012;54(5):621–9.

126. Schmidt-Ioanas M, de Roux A, Lode H. New antibiotics for the treatment of severe staphylococcal infection in the critically ill patient. Curr Opin Crit Care 2005;11(5):481–6.

127. Mandell LA, Wunderink RG, Anzueto A, et al. Infectious Diseases Society of America/American Thoracic Society consensus guidelines on the management of community-acquired pneumonia in adults. Clin Infect Dis 2007;44(Suppl 2):S27–72.

128. Rabello LS, Azevedo LC, de Souza IAO, et al. Severe pneumonia in critically ill cancer patients: clinical outcomes and a comparison between

healthcare-associated pneumonia and community-acquired pneumonia. Crit Care 2013;
17(Suppl 4):28.

129. Rabello LS, Silva JR, Azevedo LC, et al. Clinical
outcomes and microbiological characteristics of
severe pneumonia in cancer patients: a prospective cohort study. PLoS One 2015;10(3):e0120544.

130. Corey GR, Kollef MH, Shorr AF, et al. Telavancin for
hospital-acquired pneumonia: clinical response
and 28-day survival. Antimicrob Agents Chemother
2014;58(4):2030–7.

131. Kiem S, Schentag JJ. Relationship of minimal inhibitory concentration and bactericidal activity to
efficacy of antibiotics for treatment of ventilator-
associated pneumonia. Semin Respir Crit Care
Med 2006;27(1):51–67.

132. Maschmeyer G, Carratalà J, Buchheidt D, et al.
Diagnosis and antimicrobial therapy of lung infil-
trates in febrile neutropenic patients (allogeneic
SCT excluded): updated guidelines of the Infec-
tious Diseases Working Party (AGIHO) of the
German Society of Hematology and Medical
Oncology (DGHO). Ann Oncol 2015;26(1):21–33.

133. Nesher L, Tverdek FP, Mahajan SN, et al. Ertape-
nem usage in cancer patients with and without
neutropenia: a report on 97 cases from a comprehensive cancer center. Infection 2015;43(5):
545–50.

134. Miedema KG, Tissing WJ, Abbink FC, et al. Risk-
adapted approach for fever and neutropenia in
paediatric cancer patients–a national multicentre
study. Eur J Cancer 2016;53:16–24.

135. Dale DC. Colony-stimulating factors for the management of neutropenia in cancer patients. Drugs
2002;62(Suppl 1):1–15.

136. Skoetz N, Bohlius J, Engert A, et al. Prophylactic
antibiotics or G(M)-CSF for the prevention of infections and improvement of survival in cancer
patients receiving myelotoxic chemotherapy. Cochrane Database Syst Rev 2015;(12):CD007107.

137. Estcourt LJ, Stanworth SJ, Hopewell S, et al. Granulocyte transfusions for treating infections in people with neutropenia or neutrophil dysfunction.
Cochrane Database Syst Rev 2016;(4):CD005339.

138. Seidel MG, Peters C, Wacker A, et al. Randomized
phase III study of granulocyte transfusions in neutropenic patients. Bone Marrow Transplant 2008;
42(10):679–84.

139. Safdar A, Rodriguez GH, Lichtiger B, et al. Recombinant interferon gamma1b immune enhancement
in 20 patients with hematologic malignancies and
systemic opportunistic infections treated with
donor granulocyte transfusions. Cancer 2006;
106(12):2664–71.

140. Sun K, Salmon SL, Lotz SA, et al. Interleukin-12
promotes gamma interferon-dependent neutrophil
recruitment in the lung and improves protection
against respiratory Streptococcus pneumoniae
infection. Infect Immun 2007;75(3):1196–202.

141. Rawlins EL, Hogan BL. Ciliated epithelial cell life-
span in the mouse trachea and lung. Am J Physiol
Lung Cell Mol Physiol 2008;295(1):L231–4.

142. Leiva-Juarez MM, Ware HH, Kulkarni VV, et al.
Inducible epithelial resistance protects mice
against leukemia-associated pneumonia. Blood
2016;128(7):982–92.

143. Evans SE, Scott BL, Clement CG, et al. Stimulated
innate resistance of lung epithelium protects mice
broadly against bacteria and fungi. Am J Respir
Cell Mol Biol 2010;42(1):40–50.

144. Munoz N, Van Maele L, Marqués JM, et al. Mucosal
administration of flagellin protects mice from Streptococcus pneumoniae lung infection. Infect Immun
2010;78(10):4226–33.

145. Cleaver JO, You D, Michaud DR, et al. Lung epithelial
cells are essential effectors of inducible resistance to
pneumonia. Mucosal Immunol 2014;7(1):78–88.

146. Duggan JM, You D, Cleaver JO, et al. Synergistic
interactions of TLR2/6 and TLR9 induce a high level
of resistance to lung infection in mice. J Immunol
2011;186(10):5916–26.

Fungal Pneumonia in Patients with Hematologic Malignancies and Hematopoietic Cell Transplantation

 CrossMark

Steven A. Pergam, MD, MPH, FIDSA[a,b,c,d],*

KEYWORDS

- Fungal • Pneumonia • Aspergillosis • Mucorales • Zygomycoses • Filamentous • Antifungal
- Prophylaxis

KEY POINTS

- Fungal pneumonias are a common cause of morbidity and mortality among patients with hematologic malignancies.
- Common risk factors for fungal pneumonia include the type of hematologic malignancy, level of immunosuppression, and length of neutropenia.
- *Aspergillus* spp are the most frequent cause of fungal pneumonia during therapy for hematologic malignancies.
- Antifungal prophylaxis should be considered for all high-risk patients to prevent the development of invasive fungal infections.

INTRODUCTION

Over the past few decades advancements in hematologic malignancies (HMs) and in hematopoietic cell transplantation (HCT) have expanded treatment options and prolonged survival.[1–4] Immunosuppression, either from the primary disease and or the therapies used to control these maladies, is associated with an increase in the risk for infections. Invasive fungal infections (IFIs), which occur primarily as a consequence of prolonged neutropenia and immunosuppression, are among the most serious infectious complications seen among these patient populations.

Although use of prophylaxis, enhanced diagnostics, and expanded treatment options have led to improvements in the care of fungal pneumonias, IFIs remain a major cause of morbidity and mortality for patients undergoing treatment (including HCT) for an underlying HM.[5–10]

EPIDEMIOLOGY

Multicenter studies and clinical trials have helped to characterize both incidence and outcomes,[7,11–16] but data are influenced by the specific disease or treatment modality. Reported prevalence varies from 4% to 23% in allogeneic HCT,[6–8,13,17,18] 1%

Disclosures: S.A. Pergam has received research support and been a consultant for Merck, Sharp and Dohme, Corp. and Optimer/Cubist Pharmaceuticals.
[a] Vaccine & Infectious Disease Division, Fred Hutchinson Cancer Research Center, 1100 Fairview Avenue North, E4-100, Seattle, WA 98109, USA; [b] Clinical Research Division, Fred Hutchinson Cancer Research Center, 1100 Fairview Avenue North, E4-100, Seattle, WA 98109, USA; [c] Department of Medicine, University of Washington, 1959 NE Pacific Street, Seattle, WA 98195, USA; [d] Infection Prevention, Seattle Cancer Care Alliance, 825 Eastlake Avenue East, Seattle, WA 98109, USA
* Fred Hutchinson Cancer Research Center, 1100 Fairview Avenue North, E4-100, Seattle, WA 98109.
E-mail address: spergam@fhcrc.org

Clin Chest Med 38 (2017) 279–294
http://dx.doi.org/10.1016/j.ccm.2016.12.006
0272-5231/17/© 2017 Elsevier Inc. All rights reserved.

to 4% in autologous HCT,[7,13,19] 6% to 24% in acute myelogenous leukemia (AML)/myelodysplastic syndrome (MDS),[5,12,18,20,21] 3% to 7% in aplastic anemia (AA),[22,23] 2% to 4% in acute lymphoblastic leukemia (ALL),[12,15] and 2% to 3% chronic myelogenous leukemia.[12] Data are limited among other HMs, but the rate is likely to be less than 2%.[12] Characterizing the overall contribution to mortality of fungal pneumonia is challenging but this has been estimated to be from 30% to 70%, depending on risk factors, specific fungal pathogens, level of immunosuppression, and age of the patient, among other issues.[12,13,24,25]

Timing of IFIs is highly variable depending on the population of interest, with fungal infections occurring during periods of postchemotherapy neutropenia among patients with AML/MDS, and later events among HCT recipients more closely linked to patients with graft-versus-host disease (GVHD).[12,13,26] Published data on IFIs in HMs also vary by study population, geographic location, chemotherapy and transplant practices, use of antifungal prophylaxis, and availability of diagnostic modalities, making comparisons challenging.[7] Although large multicenter studies have helped to address some of these concerns, many important populations, such as pediatric patients with cancer and unique transplant populations (eg, umbilical cord blood), make up only small proportions in these more comprehensive cohorts.[7,10,14]

Fungal Pathogens

Aspergillus spp are the most common fungal pathogens identified, led primarily by *Aspergillus fumigatus* (**Box 1**). Other *Aspergillus* spp, such as *Aspergillus flavus*, *Aspergillus niger*, and *Aspergillus ustus*, are reported at much lower frequencies. Invasive aspergillosis (IA) is thought to make up from 70% to 90% of all fungal pneumonias in HMs.[7,12] Mucorales species are the second most frequent, making up 3% to 12% of reported IFIs in these high-risk patients[7,12]; *Rhizopus* spp are the most commonly identified.[27] *Fusarium*

Box 1
Fungal pneumonia pathogens

Aspergillus spp
  Aspergillus flavus
  Aspergillus fumigatus
  Aspergillus lentulus

  Aspergillus nidulans
  Aspergillus niger
  Aspergillus terreus

Cryptococcus spp
  Cryptococcus gattii
  Cryptococcus neoformans

Endemic mycoses
  Blastomyces dermatitidis
  Coccidioides immitis

  Histoplasma capsulatum
  Paracoccidioides brasiliensis

Fusarium spp[a]
  Fusarium solani complex
  Fusarium oxysporum complex

Mucorales species
  Apophysomyces spp
  Cunninghamella bertholletiae
  Lichtheimia corymbifera
  Mucor spp
    Mucor circinelloides
    Mucor hiemalis
    Mucor racemosus

  Rhizomucor spp
    Rhizomucor pusillus
    Rhizomucor mehei
  Rhizopus spp
    Rhizopus azygosporus
    Rhizopus microsporus
    Rhizopus orzyae

Paecilomyces spp (eg, *Paecilomyces variotii*)
  Purpureocillium lilacinum[b]

Scedosporium spp
  Scedosporium apiospermum
  Scedosporium prolificans

Scopularopsis spp (eg, *Scopularopsis brevicaulis*)

This list represents common and uncommon fungal pathogens associated with pneumonia in patients with hematologic malignancies, including the most frequent *Aspergillus* and *Mucor* spp that cause disease, but is not comprehensive.
  [a] Multiple other *Fusarium* spp are associated with pneumonia; see Ref.[117]
  [b] Formerly *Paecilomyces lilacinum*.

spp are the third most frequent in most studies, followed by other rare molds, such as *Scedosporium* spp, *Paecilomyces* spp, among numerous others.[28] Some molds, such as the dematiaceous molds (phaeohyphomycosis) rarely cause pulmonary infections.[29] Dual infections may represent up to 13% in some studies.[30] Endemic molds are infrequently reported.[31] *Pneumocystis*, a common fungal pathogen, is not discussed in this article because it has been reviewed elsewhere.[32] *Candida* spp are colonizers of the aerodigestive airway, and are not discussed as causal agents of pneumonia in this article.[33]

RISK FACTORS FOR FUNGAL PNEUMONIA

There are several risk factors that have been linked to fungal disease in patients with cancer (**Table 1**). Factors that increase immunosuppression and weaken host defenses, particularly those that lead to the development of neutropenia and T-cell depression, are associated with fungal pneumonias. Many risk factors should be considered when choosing empiric therapy and/or antifungal prophylaxis.

Host Factors

Patients with AML/MDS and those undergoing HCT are at highest risk for developing invasive IFIs.[12,14,27] Poor-risk disease and failure to reach complete remission are also factors likely to be associated with the development of IFI.[25,34] In addition to the primary cancer, patients with increased age,[35] concomitant diabetes,[24] iron overload,[36] or chronic lung disease may be at increased risk. Host genetics, driven primarily by polymorphisms to pattern recognition receptors, such as Toll-like receptors and Dectin-1, have been linked to primarily to IA.[37–40]

Exposures

Geographic areas are linked to endemic molds, such as the southwest (coccidiomycosis),[41] and the Ohio and Mississippi River valleys (histoplasmosis and blastomycosis).[42] Patients with frequent exposure to dust, dirt, or decaying vegetation, such as farmers or construction workers, and those who garden frequently are also potentially at increased risk.[43] Home or institutional water leaks and construction are also thought to increase risk.[44] Tobacco use and marijuana use may increase risk for fungal pneumonias.[45,46]

Treatment-related Complications

Neutropenia, either from the underlying malignancy or caused by treatment, is strongly associated with

Table 1
Epidemiologic risk factors associated with fungal pneumonia among patients with hematologic cancer

Associated Risk Factors	Risk
Host Factors	
Underlying Disease	
AML	↑↑↑
ALL	↑↑
Aplastic anemia[a]	↑↑
MDS	↑↑↑
Host Genetics[b]	
TLR-4, Dectin-1, IL-10, PTX-3, and other polymorphisms	↑↑
Other Host Factors	
Chronic lung disease	↑
Diabetes	↑
Iron overload	↑↑
Male gender	↑
Age >60 y	↑
Exposures	
Travel (endemic molds[a])	↑
Work-related exposure (eg, construction)	↑↑
Gardening/yard work	↑↑
Construction	↑
Tobacco/marijuana smoking	↑
Clinical Risk Factors	
Prolonged neutropenia (<500 µg/mL)	↑↑↑
Lymphopenia	↑↑
Hyperglycemia	↑
Therapy	
Hematopoietic cell transplant	↑↑↑
Type of transplant	
Allogeneic transplant	↑↑↑
Autologous transplant	↑
Donor status	
Unrelated donor	↑↑
Mismatched donor	↑↑
Conditioning	
Myeloablative conditioning	↑↑
GVHD	
Acute GVHD	↑↑↑
Chronic GVHD	↑
Immunosuppression	
Anti–T-cell therapy	↑↑
Myelosuppressive chemotherapy	↑↑↑
Steroids ≥1 mg/kg/d	↑↑↑
Other Infections	
CMV reactivation/disease	↑↑
Other pulmonary infections	↑

Abbreviations: CMV, cytomegalovirus; IL, interleukin; PTX3, pentraxin 3; TLR, toll-like receptors.
[a] Risk in patients with aplastic anemia depends on the level and duration of neutropenia.
[b] Selected polymorphisms noted; others have been reported.

development of IFIs. Risk is highest among patients expected to have fewer than 500 neutrophils/mm^3 for prolonged periods.[47,48] Some IFIs, such as cryptococcosis and fusariosis, are more associated with lymphopenia and T-cell dysfunction.[25,49] Among allogeneic HCT recipients, GVHD, the severity of GVHD, and need for glucocorticoids/immunosuppression are associated with IFIs.[6–8,13,14,17,50] Prolonged immunosuppression among patients with chronic GVHD also increases long-term risk.[51] Cytomegalovirus has been linked to posttransplant IFIs in multiple studies, particularly among patients who reactivate or develop invasive disease.[17,50] Malnutrition, hyperglycemia, and organ dysfunction likely increase overall risk.

CLINICAL PRESENTATION

Common symptoms of fungal pneumonia are fever, cough, chest pain, dyspnea, and hemoptysis,[52] but not all patients have pulmonary symptoms on presentation. Patients with tracheobronchitis may be more likely to present with wheezing and/or stridor.[53] Patients may have rhonchi, wheezing, or a normal lung examination.

Patients with fungal pneumonia may also present with other focal areas of involvement, such as skin nodules, oropharyngeal/palatal lesions, sinus, and/or central nervous system (CNS) involvement.

DIAGNOSIS OF FUNGAL PNEUMONIA
Radiologic Findings

Fungal pneumonia can present with consolidations, infiltrates, cavitations, or single or multiple nodules ($\geq$1 cm), on computed tomography (CT), which is considered the imaging modality of choice for assessing patients with suspected pulmonary infections.[54] Classically, the halo sign, which describes a nodule with surrounding ground-glass changes, is associated with fungal pneumonia (**Fig. 1**A, B), but can be seen with other pathogens. During neutrophil recovery, fungal pulmonary nodules may increase in both size and number despite appropriate therapy (see **Fig. 1**B). This increase is not thought to be caused by failure of therapy but by immune reconstitution, because neutrophils home to sites of infection and increase inflammation.[55] Cavitation can occur at presentation or during treatment. The reversed

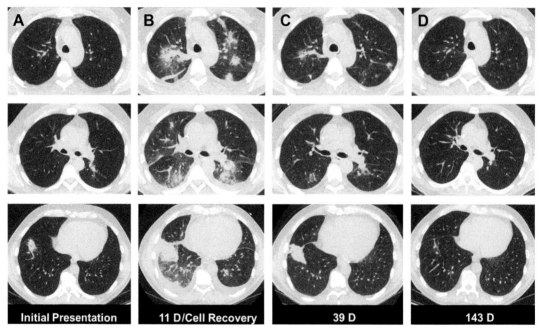

Fig. 1. Radiologic progression of aspergillus pneumonia in a patient with AML treated with voriconazole. (*A–D*) Chest CT images from the same study at the time frame noted at the bottom of each column. (*A*) At diagnosis when patient presented with fever, cough, and neutropenia. The patient was started on voriconazole therapy. Bronchoscopic evaluation was positive by galactomannan, culture, and polymerase chain reaction (PCR) for *Aspergillus fumigatus*. (*B*) Eleven days posttreatment at time point with neutrophil recovery. Patient had therapeutic levels of voriconazole and clinical symptoms had improved. Although CT appearance worsened (increased number and size of nodules), no changes were made to therapy. Halo signs are seen through bilateral lungs. (*C*) Thirty-nine days into treatment with voriconazole. (*D*) One-hundred and forty-three days into treatment with voriconazole, at which time therapy was stopped.

halo sign or bird's nest is a round nodule that has central ground-glass changes, surrounded by a crescent or ring of consolidation (**Fig. 2**). This sign is most frequently associated with Mucorales species infections.[56] Patients with fungal pneumonias may also present with lobar consolidations (**Fig. 3**) that mimic bacterial pneumonias. Because other nonfungal infections can present with pulmonary nodules, radiologic examination alone must be taken in context to avoid misdiagnosis. Several infectious and noninfectious diagnoses can lead to pulmonary nodules (**Box 2**, see **Fig. 2**).

LABORATORY TESTING
Microbiological Cultures

Isolation of fungal pathogens from sputum is considered part of the diagnostic criteria,[47] but most patients do not present with productive cough. Although a part of the work-up for some bacterial pneumonias, sputum is not a routine part of assessment for fungal disease at many centers because of poor sensitivity.[57] Fungal cultures from bronchoalveolar lavage (BAL) samples (**Fig. 4**) are more sensitive but still have a low overall yield (20%–50%).[58–60] Antifungal susceptibility testing from isolated molds can be useful when considering therapy options, but is only available in specialized laboratories.

Despite angioinvasion of filamentous molds, most are rarely found on blood cultures. Aspergillus spp detected from blood is often considered

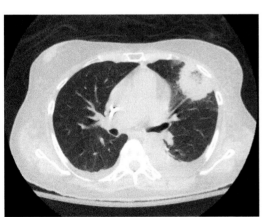

Fig. 2. A reversed halo sign (bird's nest) nodule seen on CT in patient with ALL. This patient was undergoing treatment of ALL, had a fever, and was found on CT scan to have this nodule. The patient was started empirically on liposomal amphotericin B because of the appearance and concern for mucormycosis. Bronchoscopic evaluation was negative for fungal pathogens, but positive on culture for Legionella micdadei. The patient had liposomal amphotericin B stopped and was treated with levofloxacin.

a contaminant because of the ubiquity of the organism in the environment.[61] Fusarium spp can be found in blood in 50% of cases with disseminated cases,[62] and Scedosporium prolificans can also more frequently present with positive blood cultures.[28] Dimorphic fungi such as cryptococcal yeast and Histoplasma capsulatum can also be identified from blood cultures.[63]

FUNGAL BIOMARKERS
Galactomannan

Galactomannan (GM), a heat-stable component of the cell wall of Aspergillus, is released during hyphal growth, and can be detected using an enzyme-linked immunosorbent assay (EIA).[64] Serum GM levels can be a helpful adjunct to the diagnosis of IA. Sensitivity varies in studies, by population at risk, predetermined cut points for positivity, and whether used for screening or diagnostic purposes.[65] Meta-analyses suggest that specificity of serum GM is around 70%, whereas specificity is closer to 85%.[66,67] Cross reaction between other species (eg, Fusarium and Penicillium spp), antibiotics,[68] serum proteins,[69] and gut bacteria can lead to false-positive results.[65] Serum levels may reflect overall outcome.[70]

BAL GM (see **Fig. 4**) has been shown in several studies to have a higher sensitivity and specificity for IA then serum GM.[60,65] However, sensitivity and specificity depend on the EIA cutoff for positivity (≥ 0.5 vs ≥ 1.0), and on the pretest probability of the patient population.[60,65] Studies have shown that BAL GM may be positive before serum testing, and thus may enhance early diagnosis in patients with less widespread disease.[71]

1,3-β-D-Glucan

Testing for the cell wall component 1,3-β-D-glucan has also been used in the diagnosis of IFI.[47] Similar to the GM assay, sensitivity is less than the specificity, ranging from 50% to 77% versus 85% to 99% respectively in 2 meta-analyses.[72,73] The test does not identify Cryptococcus and most Mucorales species, and is positive in patients with Pneumocystis jiroveci pneumonia and candidemia.[74] Sensitivity is affected by other factors, such as dialysis, intravenous immunoglobulin, and pseudomonas bacteremia.[65]

Other Serum Tests

Serum testing for endemic molds is an important component of diagnosis, particularly among patients not receiving antifungal prophylaxis and/or a history of associated exposure to endemic areas.[42,63,75] Serum cryptococcal antigen (CRAG)

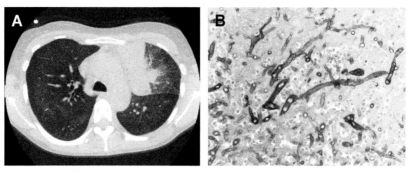

Fig. 3. Left upper lobe consolidation in a patient with AML and mucormycosis. (*A*) CT scan of patient with neutropenia, fever, and cough. Bronchoalveolar lavage was positive on PCR and culture for *Rhizopus* spp. The patient was treated with liposomal amphotericin B, and underwent surgical resection. (*B*) Silver stain of lung tissue for surgical resection showing ribbonlike hyphae consistent with Mucorales species.

can be useful as a diagnostic tool, but immunosuppressed patients with isolated pulmonary disease may have a negative assay.[76]

Evolving Diagnostic Tools

A number meta-analyses and clinical trials suggest that serum fungal polymerase chain reaction (PCR) tests may help with screening and diagnosis.[77–79] The use of PCR from BAL samples may be another important use, in which it may be equivalent to the GM assay in sensitivity for IA[72,73]; such assays may also allow detection of antifungal resistance mutations.[80] The routine use of PCR is less clear, as is its use for other fungal pathogens.[81,82] Current guidelines do not include PCR as a modality for the diagnosis of fungal pneumonias[47,48,74,83] because of the variety of assays and varied sensitivities. In a recent study, thermal desorption–gas chromatography/mass spectrometry identified a metabolic breath signature that was able to identify patients with IA[84]; however, these techniques require additional study and are not commercially available.

CYTOLOGY/PATHOLOGY/SURGICAL BIOPSY

Cytologic examination for hyphal elements from BAL has low overall sensitivity.[85] Because of the use of empiric antifungals and improvements in diagnostics, surgical biopsies are less commonly used for fungal diagnosis.[86] Lung biopsies via open surgical resection, video-assisted thoracoscopic surgery, or CT-guided biopsies have excellent sensitivity and specificity[87,88]; in contrast, transbronchial biopsies are both higher risk and lower yield.[89] *Aspergillus* spp are septate hyphae, with approximately 45° branching, whereas Mucorales species are often reported as nonseptate hyphae with wide-angle branching (see **Fig. 3**). *Fusarium* spp on biopsy are septate

with acute and right angles similar to other fungal species, but adventitial sporulation may be present; the presence of hyphae and yeastlike structures together on a biopsy are highly suggestive of fusariosis.[90] Biopsies can identify other infections or noninfectious causes, particularly among patients who continue to progress despite antifungal coverage.[86] Biopsies should undergo microbiological and histopathologic work-up, because these results may not always be concordant.[59,91] Skin and/or sinus biopsies in patients with focal findings are valuable when fungal pneumonia is suspected but microbiological confirmation cannot be obtained from a respiratory specimen (**Fig. 5**).

TREATMENT

Treatment of fungal pneumonia should be started before diagnosis if possible. Delays in therapy can lead to additional complications, dissemination, and poor outcomes. Empiric regimens may depend on local prevalence and patterns of antifungal prophylaxis, but are most often triazole regimens targeted toward IA and or Mucorales species.

Aspergillus Pneumonia

In national guidelines for the treatment of IA[48] the triazole voriconazole is recommended as first-line therapy for IA based on several randomized clinical trials that have shown safety, efficacy, and superiority to other antifungal agents.[92–94] Voriconazole has the advantage of more convenient dosing (oral and intravenous) and is thought to have less toxicity than deoxycholate or liposomal amphotericin B (LAMB), although head-to-head trials have compared voriconazole with deoxycholate amphotericin B only.[92] Voriconazole does have known side effects, such as

Box 2
Differential diagnosis of fungal pneumonia

Bacteria

- Pneumococcal pneumonia
- Gram-negative rod pneumonia (eg, Klebsiella or Pseudomonas pneumonia)
- *Nocardia* spp
- *Actinomycosis* spp
- *Legionella* spp
- Septic pulmonary emboli

Mycobacteria

- *Mycobacterium tuberculosis*
- Nontuberculous mycobacteria (eg, *Mycobacterium avium-intracellulare*)

Viral

- Cytomegalovirus pneumonia[a]
- Epstein-Barr virus–associated posttransplant lymphoproliferative disorder
- Respiratory viruses[a]
- Varicella zoster virus[a]

Inflammatory

- Acute respiratory distress syndrome
- Aspiration pneumonia
- Bronchiolitis obliterans
- Cryptogenic organizing pneumonia
- Diffuse alveolar hemorrhage
- Pulmonary alveolar proteinosis
- Sarcoidosis

Malignancy

- Lung cancer
- Leukemic infiltrates/granulocytic sarcoma
- Lymphoma
- Metastatic disease

Other

- Drug toxicity

[a] Viral pneumonias less frequently present with nodular disease, and when nodules are seen they are usually <1 cm in size.

CNS toxicity, hepatotoxicity, and QT prolongation, and has been associated with fluoride toxicity.[95] In addition, voriconazole has effects on cytochrome p450 enzymes, and therefore is associated with numerous drug-drug interactions.[96] Because pharmacokinetics can vary between patients, therapeutic drug monitoring (TDM) can ensure absorption and limit toxicity,[97] and is currently recommended.[48]

LAMB is considered an alternative to voriconazole, based in part on the AmBiLoad trial, which showed similar efficacy to voriconazole.[98] Deoxycholate amphotericin is associated with significantly more toxicity, particularly infusion reactions, nephrotoxicity, and electrolyte abnormalities, compared with LAMB, but these remain a major concern for all amphotericin-containing preparations. Isavuconazonium (Isavuconazole) is also considered second line, based on a randomized trial that showed that it was noninferior to voriconazole.[99] Although there are no randomized prospective trials of its use as primary therapy for IA, posaconazole is recommended as salvage therapy.[48] Combination therapy with triazoles and echinocandins is currently not recommended,[16,48] but can be considered in complicated patients or as salvage therapy. In those expected to have prolonged periods of neutropenia, granulocyte infusions can be considered as an adjunct to standard antifungal therapy, but this remains a point of debate.[100]

It is important to be aware that selected *Aspergillus* spp have intrinsic resistance to amphotericin B, including *Aspergillus tereus*,[101] whereas others are less sensitivity to azoles (eg, *A ustus*).[102] The emergence of triazole resistance has become an increasing concern, but has been reported primarily in Europe.[103,104] Resistance is focused on the Cyp51A gene, specifically an amino acid substitution at codon 98 (L98H) that can confer resistance to all the azoles.[103] New molecular tests for detection of resistance are now available.[80]

IA outcomes depend on the population at risk and underlying risk factors for IFI. HCT recipients have the lowest survival, with reports of 45% to 65% survival at 90 days,[10,14,105,106] and 33% at 1 year.[7] However, several of these studies include data before routine triazole use and most consider only all-cause mortality. Survival rates among other HMs are better, but mortalities remain high (25%–40%).[12,92,98,107]

Mucorales Species

There are a variety of species that make up the Mucorales family, but only small number that cause human clinical cases. *Rhizopus*, *Mucor*, *Rhizomucor*, *Lichtheimia*, and *Cunninghamella* spp are some of those most commonly reported.[27] LAMB is considered the primary antifungal agent of choice in patients with mucormycosis[74,108]; early treatment (≤3–5 days after presentation) is associated with increased survival.[27,109] Appropriate dosing of LAMB ranges from 5 to 10 mg/

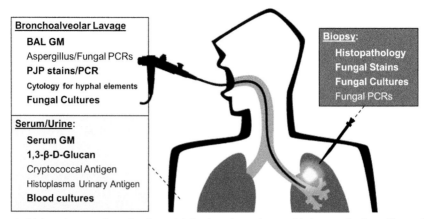

Fig. 4. Suggested laboratory work-up for fungal infections in patients with hematologic malignancies by site of testing. Patients at risk for fungal pneumonia should undergo evaluation to solidify this diagnosis. Tests that are considered standard portions of work-up are **bolded**. Decisions regarding work-up are highly dependent on local practices and patient presentation. In addition to tests noted earlier, providers should assess sinuses, perform a dermatologic examination, and evaluate any CNS symptoms by radiologic imaging. GM, galactomannan assay; PCR, polymerase chain reaction; PJP, *Pneumocystis jiroveci* pneumonia. (*Courtesy of* Kyoko Kurosawa, BS, Seattle, WA.)

kg, with the alternative of lipid-complex amphotericin B at 5 to 7.5 mg/kg; LAMB is preferred because of its superior side effect profile. Higher dosing can be considered in high-risk patients and those with CNS involvement, but is limited by renal toxicity.

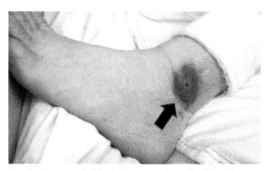

Fig. 5. Biopsy of skin lesions can be of critical importance in diagnosing invasive fungal infections. Fungal infections, particularly those that are disseminated, can present with skin manifestations. This lesion on the left ankle (*arrow*) is necrotic and surrounded by subcutaneous hemorrhage in a patient with AML, with prolonged neutropenia, and ongoing fevers. A biopsy of this lesion was positive for segmented, branching fungal hyphae; cultures from biopsies eventually grew *A fumigatus*. Although the patient had no active pulmonary symptoms, a CT scan of the chest completed during the work-up showed numerous pulmonary nodules consistent with fungal pneumonia. Clinicians caring for patients with hematologic malignancy at risk for fungal infections who present with painful, erythematous, or necrotic skin lesions should consider lesional biopsies (with culture and pathologic review) to help confirm the diagnosis.

Posaconazole can be considered for salvage or for step-down therapy after LAMB, particularly among patients who have had surgical intervention and those who have major side effects from LAMB.[110,111] When using posaconazole, the oral tablet formulation should be used whenever possible because of its enhanced bioavailability.[112] Isavuconazole has been shown in an open-label trial to be a comparable alternative to LAMB at 42 days posttreatment in a small study,[113] but prospective longer comparison trials are not available. Isavuconazole can be an alternative in patients who cannot tolerate LAMB, for salvage, or as a potential consolidation therapy after surgery/LAMB. Current guidelines do not recommend combination therapy,[114] but small studies and some experts suggest it should be considered in high-risk patients.[111,115]

A critical aspect of mucormycosis management is aggressive surgical debridement,[74,108] because combination LAMB with surgery may increase survival.[116] These data must be taken in context, because surgical patients may be more likely to have less aggressive disease and limited comorbid conditions, and therefore better outcomes.[111] Hyperbaric oxygen and granulocyte transfusions (in patients with prolonged neutropenia)[100] can be considered as adjunctive therapies. Despite aggressive therapy, overall survival remains low,[111] with attributable mortalities of more than 60%.[12,74,116]

Fusariosis

Fusarium solani species complex cause 60% of human infections, but multiple *Fusarium* spp are known to cause disease.[25] Optimal therapy for fusariosis remains unknown, and there are differing antifungal sensitivities between species.[90,117] If antifungal sensitivities are not available, guidelines recommend initial therapy with voriconazole or LAMB.[28] Because of the poor response to most single agents, combination therapy with triazole/LAMB, echinocandins, or terbinafine are often used.[25] Surgical debulking is recommended, but is often not possible because many patients present with dissemination.[28] Survival rates in fusariosis are approximately 30% in high-risk patients, but may be even lower in those with pulmonary involvement or dissemination.[28]

Cryptococcal Pneumonia

Cryptococcal infections are less frequent in patients with HM during therapy, because of routine fluconazole or other triazole prophylaxis. Current guidelines for cryptococcal infections are highly dependent on severity of disease and evidence of meningeal involvement.[118] Patients with proven cryptococcal pneumonia should undergo a lumbar puncture, and those with evidence of CNS disease, dissemination, severe acute respiratory distress syndrome, or high-level immunosuppression should be treated with LAMB and flucytosine, followed by fluconazole maintenance.[118] Because of the risk for dissemination, similar treatment regimens are recommended in patients with HM, but oral therapy with high-dose fluconazole can be considered with caution in select patients.[118] Data for the use of isavuconazole as a possible agent in *Cryptococcus* are emerging.[119] Survival is thought to range between 55% and 75%, but depends on host status, treatment response, and CNS involvement.[120]

Endemic Molds

The use of triazole prophylaxis among patients with HM limits the number of cases of endemic molds seen during therapy.[31] Specific guidelines for management are available,[121–123] and survival rates depend on pathogen, host factors, and level of dissemination.

Scedosporium, Scopularopsis, Paecilomyces, and Other Rare Filamentous Fungi

Recommendations for treatment of *Scedosporium* spp are limited by varied resistance among species; however, voriconazole is often the recommend first-line agent.[28] *Scedosporium prolificans* is considered resistant to all antifungals, but may respond to voriconazole/terbinafine combination therapy with surgical debridement.[124] *Scopularopsis* spp are often treated similarly to *Scedosporium* spp with voriconazole/terbinafine with or without an echinocandin combined with surgery.[28,125] Patients with *Paecilomyces variotii*, phaeohyphomycosis, and *Acremonium* spp should receive voriconazole as first line.[28,29] For these and other rare organisms, antifungal resistance testing is recommended, with the caveat that it may not reflect in-vitro efficacy. Overall survival for rare molds tends to be poor despite aggressive therapy.[28]

PREVENTION/PROPHYLAXIS
Screening and Preemptive Therapy

Serum GM has also been assessed as a screening tool for preemptive CT scanning and therapy in patients at high risk for fungal pneumonia.[79,126–128] A meta-analysis suggests that weekly or biweekly serum GM may detect IA early.[129] However, antifungal prophylaxis limits the sensitivity of serum GM testing.[130] Some organizations recommend biweekly serum GM screening in high-risk patients with HMs,[83] whereas others do not.[48] Studies suggest that serum PCR either alone or in combination with GM screening may provide future options for prevention.[65] Several studies suggest that the negative predictive value of the serum PCR may be its best value as a screening tool for IA.[77–79]

Antifungal Prophylaxis

Antifungal prophylaxis has become the standard for prevention of IFIs among high-risk HMs. Triazole antifungals are used at most centers, because they can be given orally, have good bioavailability, and have good efficacy in clinical trials. Although fluconazole has been shown to decrease IFIs, it has only proved to decrease the risk for candidiasis, and has no effect on other IFIs.[131] In high-risk patients, posaconazole has been shown to be effective at limiting IFIs in 2 large randomized controlled trials. The first showed a decrease in IFIs (1% vs 7%) and a survival advantage among patients with AML/MDS given posaconazole compared with fluconazole/itraconazole prophylaxis.[11] The second randomized trial compared posaconazole and fluconazole prophylaxis in HCT recipients with acute GVHD (grade II–IV), chronic extensive GVHD, or high-level immunosuppression.[132] Posaconazole led to fewer overall fungal complications (5% vs 9%, nonsignificant), but a smaller number of *Aspergillus* spp infections (2% vs 7%); overall mortality was no different between the two study groups.[132] In contrast, a randomized placebo controlled trial comparing voriconazole and fluconazole prophylaxis among HCT recipients did not show superiority.[128]

However, this study used a low dose of voriconazole (200 mg twice daily), did not use TDM, and had a lower number of IFIs, which may have limited results. To date, isavuconazole has not been studied as a prophylactic agent for IFI.

Many centers use posaconazole prophylaxis for high-risk patients (eg, neutropenia for prolonged periods or those with multiple risk factors) and fluconazole for low-risk patients (ie, nonneutropenic patients with limited risk factors). Postlicensure data have shown breakthrough cases of fungal infections among patients on posaconazole suspension, likely caused by poor absorption and bioavailability.[133] More concerning are reports that have shown shifts to more Mucorales species and poor outcomes with breakthrough infections.[134,135] No current data exist for oral posaconazole tablets as prophylaxis, but the enhanced bioavailability may help limit breakthroughs.[112] Although more limited antifungal spectrum, there are studies showing that echinocandins may provide an alternate for fungal prophylaxis in lower risk patients,[136] and likely they are better at limiting IFI complications post-HCT than fluconazole.[137,138] Many centers use echinocandin therapy as a bridge during periods when triazole therapy is limited by either drug-drug interactions or for patients who develop side effects from these agents. In patients who are undergoing HCT, prevention varies between centers, with some moving more toward routine prophylaxis with mold-active agents (eg, voriconazole or posaconazole), or the use of such agents limited to patients at higher risk for mold infections, including those receiving high-dose glucocorticoids for treatment of GVHD, numerous risk factors (eg, prolonged neutropenia), or with a prior history of fungal infections.

ENVIRONMENTAL/INFECTION CONTROL

Centers caring for patients with HMs and or HCT recipients should develop strategies for limiting environmental exposures to mold. Centralized construction practices and controls should be established within hospitals,[44,139] and units where HCT recipients are admitted should have appropriate high-efficiency particulate air filtration and air management as per national guidelines.[140] The value of air sampling remains controversial, because thresholds and minimal concentrations of fungal spores have yet to be determined.[44] Masking of patients during periods of construction when outside of protective units has been suggested to potentially help prevent mold infections,[141] but the value of routine masking has not been determined even in the highest risk populations.[140]

FUTURE DIRECTIONS

As therapy options for patients with HM continue to increase, and access to HCT expands, there is a need to continue progress in the diagnosis, treatment and prevention of major fungal pathogens. There is a need for additional antifungals and novel treatments for fungal infections, particularly for Mucorales and *Fusarium* spp. Future multicenter clinical trials with combination strategies, although challenging to enroll, are critical to address treatment choices for rare molds. Epidemiologic studies to further characterize the spread of azole-resistant *Aspergillus* spp are needed, as are new classes of antifungals to address this emerging resistance. Standardization of fungal PCR tests and expansion of new diagnostic modalities are needed improve diagnostic accuracy and enhance early detection. Future studies comparing novel antifungal (eg, isavuconazole) prophylaxis options, as well as treatment of breakthrough infections, are also needed. In addition, there is a need for large multicenter studies of masking and other infection control practices, to determine the best methods for limiting fungal infections among these high-risk patient populations.

REFERENCES

1. Gay F, Oliva S, Petrucci MT, et al. Chemotherapy plus lenalidomide versus autologous transplantation, followed by lenalidomide plus prednisone versus lenalidomide maintenance, in patients with multiple myeloma: a randomised, multicentre, phase 3 trial. Lancet Oncol 2015;16(16):1617–29.

2. Gooley TA, Chien JW, Pergam SA, et al. Reduced mortality after allogeneic hematopoietic-cell transplantation. N Engl J Med 2010;363(22):2091–101.

3. Kochenderfer JN, Dudley ME, Kassim SH, et al. Chemotherapy-refractory diffuse large B-cell lymphoma and indolent B-cell malignancies can be effectively treated with autologous T cells expressing an anti-CD19 chimeric antigen receptor. J Clin Oncol 2015;33(6):540–9.

4. Milano F, Gooley T, Wood B, et al. Cord-blood transplantation in patients with minimal residual disease. N Engl J Med 2016;375(10):944–53.

5. Barreto JN, Beach CL, Wolf RC, et al. The incidence of invasive fungal infections in neutropenic patients with acute leukemia and myelodysplastic syndromes receiving primary antifungal prophylaxis with voriconazole. Am J Hematol 2013;88(4):283–8.

6. Corzo-Leon DE, Satlin MJ, Soave R, et al. Epidemiology and outcomes of invasive fungal infections in

allogeneic haematopoietic stem cell transplant recipients in the era of antifungal prophylaxis: a single-centre study with focus on emerging pathogens. Mycoses 2015;58(6):325–36.

7. Kontoyiannis DP, Marr KA, Park BJ, et al. Prospective surveillance for invasive fungal infections in hematopoietic stem cell transplant recipients, 2001-2006: overview of the Transplant-Associated Infection Surveillance Network (TRANSNET) Database. Clin Infect Dis 2010;50(8):1091–100.

8. Garcia-Vidal C, Upton A, Kirby KA, et al. Epidemiology of invasive mold infections in allogeneic stem cell transplant recipients: biological risk factors for infection according to time after transplantation. Clin Infect Dis 2008;47(8):1041–50.

9. Sun Y, Meng F, Han M, et al. Epidemiology, management, and outcome of invasive fungal disease in patients undergoing hematopoietic stem cell transplantation in China: a multicenter prospective observational study. Biol Blood Marrow Transplant 2015;21(6):1117–26.

10. Upton A, Kirby KA, Carpenter P, et al. Invasive aspergillosis following hematopoietic cell transplantation: outcomes and prognostic factors associated with mortality. Clin Infect Dis 2007;44(4): 531–40.

11. Cornely OA, Maertens J, Winston DJ, et al. Posaconazole vs. fluconazole or itraconazole prophylaxis in patients with neutropenia. N Engl J Med 2007; 356(4):348–59.

12. Pagano L, Caira M, Candoni A, et al. The epidemiology of fungal infections in patients with hematologic malignancies: the SEIFEM-2004 study. Haematologica 2006;91(8):1068–75.

13. Pagano L, Caira M, Nosari A, et al. Fungal infections in recipients of hematopoietic stem cell transplants: results of the SEIFEM B-2004 study–Sorveglianza Epidemiologica Infezioni Fungine Nelle Emopatie Maligne. Clin Infect Dis 2007; 45(9):1161–70.

14. Neofytos D, Horn D, Anaissie E, et al. Epidemiology and outcome of invasive fungal infection in adult hematopoietic stem cell transplant recipients: analysis of Multicenter Prospective Antifungal Therapy (PATH) Alliance registry. Clin Infect Dis 2009; 48(3):265–73.

15. Mariette C, Tavernier E, Hocquet D, et al. Epidemiology of invasive fungal infections during induction therapy in adults with acute lymphoblastic leukemia: a GRAALL-2005 study. Leuk Lymphoma 2017;58(3):586–93.

16. Marr KA, Schlamm HT, Herbrecht R, et al. Combination antifungal therapy for invasive aspergillosis: a randomized trial. Ann Intern Med 2015; 162(2):81–9.

17. Montesinos P, Rodriguez-Veiga R, Boluda B, et al. Incidence and risk factors of post-engraftment

invasive fungal disease in adult allogeneic hematopoietic stem cell transplant recipients receiving oral azoles prophylaxis. Bone Marrow Transplant 2015;50(11):1465–72.

18. Biehl LM, Vehreschild JJ, Liss B, et al. A cohort study on breakthrough invasive fungal infections in high-risk patients receiving antifungal prophylaxis. J Antimicrob Chemother 2016;71(9): 2634–41.

19. Gil L, Styczynski J, Komarnicki M. Infectious complication in 314 patients after high-dose therapy and autologous hematopoietic stem cell transplantation: risk factors analysis and outcome. Infection 2007;35(6):421–7.

20. Rotstein C, Bow EJ, Laverdiere M, et al. Randomized placebo-controlled trial of fluconazole prophylaxis for neutropenic cancer patients: benefit based on purpose and intensity of cytotoxic therapy. The Canadian Fluconazole Prophylaxis Study Group. Clin Infect Dis 1999;28(2):331–40.

21. Gomes MZ, Mulanovich VE, Jiang Y, et al. Incidence density of invasive fungal infections during primary antifungal prophylaxis in newly diagnosed acute myeloid leukemia patients in a tertiary cancer center, 2009 to 2011. Antimicrob Agents Chemother 2014;58(2):865–73.

22. Torres HA, Bodey GP, Rolston KV, et al. Infections in patients with aplastic anemia: experience at a tertiary care cancer center. Cancer 2003;98(1): 86–93.

23. Quarello P, Saracco P, Giacchino M, et al. Epidemiology of infections in children with acquired aplastic anaemia: a retrospective multicenter study in Italy. Eur J Haematol 2012;88(6):526–34.

24. Slavin M, van Hal S, Sorrell TC, et al. Invasive infections due to filamentous fungi other than *Aspergillus*: epidemiology and determinants of mortality. Clin Microbiol Infect 2015;21(5):490. e1-10.

25. Campo M, Lewis RE, Kontoyiannis DP. Invasive fusariosis in patients with hematologic malignancies at a cancer center: 1998-2009. J Infect 2010; 60(5):331–7.

26. Marr KA, Carter RA, Boeckh M, et al. Invasive aspergillosis in allogeneic stem cell transplant recipients: changes in epidemiology and risk factors. Blood 2002;100(13):4358–66.

27. Kontoyiannis DP, Azie N, Franks B, et al. Prospective antifungal therapy (PATH) Alliance®: focus on mucormycosis. Mycoses 2014;57(4):240–6.

28. Tortorano AM, Richardson M, Roilides E, et al. ESCMID and ECMM joint guidelines on diagnosis and management of hyalohyphomycosis: *Fusarium* spp., *Scedosporium* spp. and others. Clin Microbiol Infect 2014;20(Suppl 3):27–46.

29. McCarty TP, Baddley JW, Walsh TJ, et al. Phaeohyphomycosis in transplant recipients: results from

the Transplant Associated Infection Surveillance Network (TRANSNET). Med Mycol 2015;53(5): 440–6.

30. Klingspor L, Saaedi B, Ljungman P, et al. Epidemiology and outcomes of patients with invasive mould infections: a retrospective observational study from a single centre (2005-2009). Mycoses 2015;58(8):470–7.

31. Kauffman CA, Freifeld AG, Andes DR, et al. Endemic fungal infections in solid organ and hematopoietic cell transplant recipients enrolled in the Transplant-Associated Infection Surveillance Network (TRANSNET). Transpl Infect Dis 2014; 16(2):213–24.

32. Cordonnier C, Cesaro S, Maschmeyer G, et al. *Pneumocystis jirovecii* pneumonia: still a concern in patients with haematological malignancies and stem cell transplant recipients. J Antimicrob Chemother 2016;71(9):2379–85.

33. Pappas PG, Kauffman CA, Andes DR, et al. Clinical practice guideline for the management of candidiasis: 2016 update by the Infectious Diseases Society of America. Clin Infect Dis 2016; 62(4):e1–50.

34. Pagano L, Busca A, Candoni A, et al. Risk stratification for invasive fungal infections in patients with hematological malignancies: SEIFEM recommendations. Blood Rev 2017. [Epub ahead of print].

35. Prentice HG, Kibbler CC, Prentice AG. Towards a targeted, risk-based, antifungal strategy in neutropenic patients. Br J Haematol 2000;110(2): 273–84.

36. Ozyilmaz E, Aydogdu M, Sucak G, et al. Risk factors for fungal pulmonary infections in hematopoietic stem cell transplantation recipients: the role of iron overload. Bone Marrow Transplant 2010; 45(10):1528–33.

37. Bochud PY, Chien JW, Marr KA, et al. Toll-like receptor 4 polymorphisms and aspergillosis in stem-cell transplantation. N Engl J Med 2008; 359(17):1766–77.

38. Sainz J, Lupianez CB, Segura-Catena J, et al. Dectin-1 and DC-SIGN polymorphisms associated with invasive pulmonary aspergillosis infection. PLoS One 2012;7(2):e32273.

39. Lambourne J, Agranoff D, Herbrecht R, et al. Association of mannose-binding lectin deficiency with acute invasive aspergillosis in immunocompromised patients. Clin Infect Dis 2009;49(10): 1486–91.

40. Cunha C, Aversa F, Lacerda JF, et al. Genetic PTX3 deficiency and aspergillosis in stem-cell transplantation. N Engl J Med 2014;370(5):421–32.

41. Thompson GR 3rd. Pulmonary coccidioidomycosis. Semin Respir Crit Care Med 2011;32(6): 754–63.

42. Kauffman CA. Endemic mycoses: blastomycosis, histoplasmosis, and sporotrichosis. Infect Dis Clin North Am 2006;20(3):645–62, vii.

43. Partridge-Hinckley K, Liddell GM, Almyroudis NG, et al. Infection control measures to prevent invasive mould diseases in hematopoietic stem cell transplant recipients. Mycopathologia 2009;168(6): 329–37.

44. Kanamori H, Rutala WA, Sickbert-Bennett EE, et al. Review of fungal outbreaks and infection prevention in healthcare settings during construction and renovation. Clin Infect Dis 2015;61(3): 433–44.

45. Ruchlemer R, Amit-Kohn M, Raveh D, et al. Inhaled medicinal cannabis and the immunocompromised patient. Support Care Cancer 2015;23(3):819–22.

46. Verweij PE, Kerremans JJ, Voss A, et al. Fungal contamination of tobacco and marijuana. JAMA 2000;284(22):2875.

47. De Pauw B, Walsh TJ, Donnelly JP, et al. Revised definitions of invasive fungal disease from the European Organization for Research and Treatment of Cancer/Invasive Fungal Infections Cooperative Group and the National Institute of Allergy and Infectious Diseases Mycoses Study Group (EORTC/MSG) Consensus Group. Clin Infect Dis 2008;46(12):1813–21.

48. Patterson TF, Thompson GR 3rd, Denning DW, et al. Practice guidelines for the diagnosis and management of aspergillosis: 2016 update by the Infectious Diseases Society of America. Clin Infect Dis 2016;63(4):e1–60.

49. Kontoyiannis DP, Peitsch WK, Reddy BT, et al. Cryptococcosis in patients with cancer. Clin Infect Dis 2001;32(11):E145–50.

50. Fukuda T, Boeckh M, Carter RA, et al. Risks and outcomes of invasive fungal infections in recipients of allogeneic hematopoietic stem cell transplants after nonmyeloablative conditioning. Blood 2003; 102(3):827–33.

51. Marr KA, Carter RA, Crippa F, et al. Epidemiology and outcome of mould infections in hematopoietic stem cell transplant recipients. Clin Infect Dis 2002;34(7):909–17.

52. Pagano L, Girmenia C, Mele L, et al. Infections caused by filamentous fungi in patients with hematologic malignancies. A report of 391 cases by GIMEMA Infection Program. Haematologica 2001; 86(8):862–70.

53. Fernandez-Ruiz M, Silva JT, San-Juan R, et al. *Aspergillus* tracheobronchitis: report of 8 cases and review of the literature. Medicine (Baltimore) 2012;91(5):261–73.

54. Marom EM, Kontoyiannis DP. Imaging studies for diagnosing invasive fungal pneumonia in immunocompromised patients. Curr Opin Infect Dis 2011; 24(4):309–14.

55. Miceli MH, Maertens J, Buve K, et al. Immune reconstitution inflammatory syndrome in cancer patients with pulmonary aspergillosis recovering from neutropenia: Proof of principle, description, and clinical and research implications. Cancer 2007;110(1):112–20.

56. Georgiadou SP, Sipsas NV, Marom EM, et al. The diagnostic value of halo and reversed halo signs for invasive mold infections in compromised hosts. Clin Infect Dis 2011;52(9):1144–55.

57. Horvath JA, Dummer S. The use of respiratory-tract cultures in the diagnosis of invasive pulmonary aspergillosis. Am J Med 1996;100(2):171–8.

58. Fisher CE, Stevens AM, Leisenring W, et al. Independent contribution of bronchoalveolar lavage and serum galactomannan in the diagnosis of invasive pulmonary aspergillosis. Transpl Infect Dis 2014;16(3):505–10.

59. Tarrand JJ, Lichterfeld M, Warraich I, et al. Diagnosis of invasive septate mold infections. A correlation of microbiological culture and histologic or cytologic examination. Am J Clin Pathol 2003; 119(6):854–8.

60. Maertens J, Maertens V, Theunissen K, et al. Bronchoalveolar lavage fluid galactomannan for the diagnosis of invasive pulmonary aspergillosis in patients with hematologic diseases. Clin Infect Dis 2009;49(11):1688–93.

61. Simoneau E, Kelly M, Labbe AC, et al. What is the clinical significance of positive blood cultures with *Aspergillus* sp in hematopoietic stem cell transplant recipients? A 23 year experience. Bone Marrow Transplant 2005;35(3):303–6.

62. Muhammed M, Coleman JJ, Carneiro HA, et al. The challenge of managing fusariosis. Virulence 2011; 2(2):91–6.

63. Kauffman CA. Histoplasmosis: a clinical and laboratory update. Clin Microbiol Rev 2007;20(1): 115–32.

64. Lehrnbecher T, Robinson PD, Fisher BT, et al. Galactomannan, beta-D-glucan, and polymerase chain reaction-based assays for the diagnosis of invasive fungal disease in pediatric cancer and hematopoietic stem cell transplantation: a systematic review and meta-analysis. Clin Infect Dis 2016; 63(10):1340–8.

65. Ambasta A, Carson J, Church DL. The use of biomarkers and molecular methods for the earlier diagnosis of invasive aspergillosis in immunocompromised patients. Med Mycol 2015;53(6): 531–57.

66. Leeflang MM, Debets-Ossenkopp YJ, Wang J, et al. Galactomannan detection for invasive aspergillosis in immunocompromised patients. Cochrane Database Syst Rev 2015;(12):CD007394.

67. Pfeiffer CD, Fine JP, Safdar N. Diagnosis of invasive aspergillosis using a galactomannan assay: a meta-analysis. Clin Infect Dis 2006; 42(10):1417–27.

68. Boonsarngsuk V, Niyompattama A, Teosirimongkol C, et al. False-positive serum and bronchoalveolar lavage *Aspergillus* galactomannan assays caused by different antibiotics. Scand J Infect Dis 2010; 42(6–7):461–8.

69. Ko JH, Peck KR, Lee JY, et al. Multiple myeloma as a major cause of false-positive galactomannan tests in adult patients with cancer. J Infect 2016; 72(2):233–9.

70. Fisher CE, Stevens AM, Leisenring W, et al. The serum galactomannan index predicts mortality in hematopoietic stem cell transplant recipients with invasive aspergillosis. Clin Infect Dis 2013;57(7): 1001–4.

71. Becker MJ, Lugtenburg EJ, Cornelissen JJ, et al. Galactomannan detection in computerized tomography-based broncho-alveolar lavage fluid and serum in haematological patients at risk for invasive pulmonary aspergillosis. Br J Haematol 2003;121(3):448–57.

72. Torelli R, Sanguinetti M, Moody A, et al. Diagnosis of invasive aspergillosis by a commercial real-time PCR assay for Aspergillus DNA in bronchoalveolar lavage fluid samples from high-risk patients compared to a galactomannan enzyme immunoassay. J Clin Microbiol 2011;49(12):4273–8.

73. Heng SC, Chen SC, Morrissey CO, et al. Clinical utility of *Aspergillus* galactomannan and PCR in bronchoalveolar lavage fluid for the diagnosis of invasive pulmonary aspergillosis in patients with haematological malignancies. Diagn Microbiol Infect Dis 2014;79(3):322–7.

74. Skiada A, Lanternier F, Groll AH, et al. Diagnosis and treatment of mucormycosis in patients with hematological malignancies: guidelines from the 3rd European Conference on Infections in Leukemia (ECIL 3). Haematologica 2013;98(4):492–504.

75. Crum NF, Lederman ER, Stafford CM, et al. Coccidioidomycosis: a descriptive survey of a re-emerging disease. Clinical characteristics and current controversies. Medicine (Baltimore) 2004; 83(3):149–75.

76. Baddley JW, Perfect JR, Oster RA, et al. Pulmonary cryptococcosis in patients without HIV infection: factors associated with disseminated disease. Eur J Clin Microbiol Infect Dis 2008;27(10):937–43.

77. Cruciani M, Mengoli C, Loeffler J, et al. Polymerase chain reaction blood tests for the diagnosis of invasive aspergillosis in immunocompromised people. Cochrane Database Syst Rev 2015;(10): CD009551.

78. Mengoli C, Cruciani M, Barnes RA, et al. Use of PCR for diagnosis of invasive aspergillosis: systematic review and meta-analysis. Lancet Infect Dis 2009;9(2):89–96.

79. Barnes RA, Stocking K, Bowden S, et al. Prevention and diagnosis of invasive fungal disease in high-risk patients within an integrative care pathway. J Infect 2013;67(3):206–14.

80. Chong GM, van der Beek MT, von dem Borne PA, et al. PCR-based detection of *Aspergillus fumigatus* Cyp51A mutations on bronchoalveolar lavage: a multicentre validation of the AsperGenius assay® in 201 patients with haematological disease suspected for invasive aspergillosis. J Antimicrob Chemother 2016;71(12):3528–35.

81. Lengerova M, Racil Z, Hrncirova K, et al. Rapid detection and identification of mucormycetes in bronchoalveolar lavage samples from immunocompromised patients with pulmonary infiltrates by use of high-resolution melt analysis. J Clin Microbiol 2014;52(8):2824–8.

82. Millon L, Herbrecht R, Grenouillet F, et al. Early diagnosis and monitoring of mucormycosis by detection of circulating DNA in serum: retrospective analysis of 44 cases collected through the French Surveillance Network of Invasive Fungal Infections (RESSIF). Clin Microbiol Infect 2016;22(9):810.e1-8.

83. Marchetti O, Lamoth F, Mikulska M, et al. ECIL recommandations for the use of biological markers for the diagnosis of invasive fungal diseases in leukemic patients and hematopoietic SCT recipients. Bone Marrow Transplant 2012;47(6):846–54.

84. Koo S, Thomas HR, Daniels SD, et al. A breath fungal secondary metabolite signature to diagnose invasive aspergillosis. Clin Infect Dis 2014;59(12):1733–40.

85. Hope WW, Walsh TJ, Denning DW. Laboratory diagnosis of invasive aspergillosis. Lancet Infect Dis 2005;5(10):609–22.

86. Cheng GS, Stednick Z, Madtes DK, et al. Decline in the use of surgical biopsy for diagnosis of pulmonary disease in hematopoietic cell transplantation recipients in an era of improved diagnostics and empirical therapy. Biol Blood Marrow Transplant 2016;22(12):2243–9.

87. de Bazelaire C, Coffin A, Cohen-Zarade S, et al. CT-guided biopsies in lung infections in patients with haematological malignancies. Diagn Interv Imaging 2013;94(2):202–15.

88. Theodore S, Liava'a M, Antippa P, et al. Surgical management of invasive pulmonary fungal infection in hematology patients. Ann Thorac Surg 2009;87(5):1532–8.

89. Hofmeister CC, Czerlanis C, Forsythe S, et al. Retrospective utility of bronchoscopy after hematopoietic stem cell transplant. Bone Marrow Transplant 2006;38(10):693–8.

90. Nucci M, Anaissie E. Fusarium infections in immunocompromised patients. Clin Microbiol Rev 2007;20(4):695–704.

91. Sangoi AR, Rogers WM, Longacre TA, et al. Challenges and pitfalls of morphologic identification of fungal infections in histologic and cytologic specimens: a ten-year retrospective review at a single institution. Am J Clin Pathol 2009;131(3):364–75.

92. Herbrecht R, Denning DW, Patterson TF, et al. Voriconazole versus amphotericin B for primary therapy of invasive aspergillosis. N Engl J Med 2002;347(6):408–15.

93. Herbrecht R, Patterson TF, Slavin MA, et al. Application of the 2008 definitions for invasive fungal diseases to the trial comparing voriconazole versus amphotericin B for therapy of invasive aspergillosis: a collaborative study of the Mycoses Study Group (MSG 05) and the European Organization for Research and Treatment of Cancer Infectious Diseases Group. Clin Infect Dis 2015;60(5):713–20.

94. Denning DW, Ribaud P, Milpied N, et al. Efficacy and safety of voriconazole in the treatment of acute invasive aspergillosis. Clin Infect Dis 2002;34(5):563–71.

95. Barajas MR, McCullough KB, Merten JA, et al. Correlation of pain and fluoride concentration in allogeneic hematopoietic stem cell transplant recipients on voriconazole. Biol Blood Marrow Transplant 2016;22(3):579–83.

96. Niwa T, Imagawa Y, Yamazaki H. Drug interactions between nine antifungal agents and drugs metabolized by human cytochromes P450. Curr Drug Metab 2014;15(7):651–79.

97. Mikus G, Scholz IM, Weiss J. Pharmacogenomics of the triazole antifungal agent voriconazole. Pharmacogenomics 2011;12(6):861–72.

98. Cornely OA, Maertens J, Bresnik M, et al. Liposomal amphotericin B as initial therapy for invasive mold infection: a randomized trial comparing a high-loading dose regimen with standard dosing (AmBiLoad trial). Clin Infect Dis 2007;44(10):1289–97.

99. Maertens JA, Raad II, Marr KA, et al. Isavuconazole versus voriconazole for primary treatment of invasive mould disease caused by *Aspergillus* and other filamentous fungi (SECURE): a phase 3, randomised-controlled, non-inferiority trial. Lancet 2016;387(10020):760–9.

100. Price TH, Boeckh M, Harrison RW, et al. Efficacy of transfusion with granulocytes from G-CSF/dexamethasone-treated donors in neutropenic patients with infection. Blood 2015;126(18):2153–61.

101. Baddley JW, Marr KA, Andes DR, et al. Patterns of susceptibility of *Aspergillus* isolates recovered from patients enrolled in the Transplant-Associated Infection Surveillance Network. J Clin Microbiol 2009;47(10):3271–5.

102. Panackal AA, Imhof A, Hanley EW, et al. *Aspergillus ustus* infections among transplant recipients. Emerg Infect Dis 2006;12(3):403–8.

103. Verweij PE, Zhang J, Debets AJ, et al. In-host adaptation and acquired triazole resistance in *Aspergillus fumigatus*: a dilemma for clinical management. Lancet Infect Dis 2016;16(11): e251–60.

104. Verweij PE, Mellado E, Melchers WJ. Multiple-triazole-resistant aspergillosis. N Engl J Med 2007; 356(14):1481–3.

105. Steinbach WJ, Marr KA, Anaissie EJ, et al. Clinical epidemiology of 960 patients with invasive aspergillosis from the PATH Alliance registry. J Infect 2012;65(5):453–64.

106. Baddley JW, Andes DR, Marr KA, et al. Factors associated with mortality in transplant patients with invasive aspergillosis. Clin Infect Dis 2010; 50(12):1559–67.

107. Slobbe L, Polinder S, Doorduijn JK, et al. Outcome and medical costs of patients with invasive aspergillosis and acute myelogenous leukemia-myelodysplastic syndrome treated with intensive chemotherapy: an observational study. Clin Infect Dis 2008;47(12):1507–12.

108. Cornely OA, Cuenca-Estrella M, Meis JF, et al. European Society of Clinical Microbiology and Infectious Diseases (ESCMID) Fungal Infection Study Group (EFISG) and European Confederation of Medical Mycology (ECMM) 2013 joint guidelines on diagnosis and management of rare and emerging fungal diseases. Clin Microbiol Infect 2014;20(Suppl 3):1–4.

109. Chamilos G, Lewis RE, Kontoyiannis DP. Delaying amphotericin B-based frontline therapy significantly increases mortality among patients with hematologic malignancy who have zygomycosis. Clin Infect Dis 2008;47(4):503–9.

110. Greenberg RN, Mullane K, van Burik JA, et al. Posaconazole as salvage therapy for zygomycosis. Antimicrob Agents Chemother 2006;50(1):126–33.

111. Kontoyiannis DP, Lewis RE. How I treat mucormycosis. Blood 2011;118(5):1216–24.

112. Wiederhold NP. Pharmacokinetics and safety of posaconazole delayed-release tablets for invasive fungal infections. Clin Pharmacol 2016; 8:1–8.

113. Marty FM, Ostrosky-Zeichner L, Cornely OA, et al. Isavuconazole treatment for mucormycosis: a single-arm open-label trial and case-control analysis. Lancet Infect Dis 2016;16(7):828–37.

114. Kyvernitakis A, Torres HA, Jiang Y, et al. Initial use of combination treatment does not impact survival of 106 patients with haematologic malignancies and mucormycosis: a propensity score analysis. Clin Microbiol Infect 2016;22(9): 811.e1-8.

115. Spellberg B, Ibrahim A, Roilides E, et al. Combination therapy for mucormycosis: why, what, and how? Clin Infect Dis 2012;54(Suppl 1):S73–8.

116. Roden MM, Zaoutis TE, Buchanan WL, et al. Epidemiology and outcome of zygomycosis: a review of 929 reported cases. Clin Infect Dis 2005;41(5): 634–53.

117. Guarro J. Fusariosis, a complex infection caused by a high diversity of fungal species refractory to treatment. Eur J Clin Microbiol Infect Dis 2013; 32(12):1491–500.

118. Perfect JR, Dismukes WE, Dromer F, et al. Clinical practice guidelines for the management of cryptococcal disease: 2010 update by the Infectious Diseases Society of America. Clin Infect Dis 2010; 50(3):291–322.

119. Thompson GR 3rd, Rendon A, Ribeiro Dos Santos R, et al. Isavuconazole treatment of cryptococcosis and dimorphic mycoses. Clin Infect Dis 2016;63(3):356–62.

120. Schmalzle SA, Buchwald UK, Gilliam BL, et al. *Cryptococcus neoformans* infection in malignancy. Mycoses 2016;59(9):542–52.

121. Galgiani JN, Ampel NM, Blair JE, et al. 2016 Infectious Diseases Society of America (IDSA) clinical practice guideline for the treatment of coccidioidomycosis. Clin Infect Dis 2016;63(6):e112–46.

122. Chapman SW, Dismukes WE, Proia LA, et al. Clinical practice guidelines for the management of blastomycosis: 2008 update by the Infectious Diseases Society of America. Clin Infect Dis 2008; 46(12):1801–12.

123. Wheat LJ, Freifeld AG, Kleiman MB, et al. Clinical practice guidelines for the management of patients with histoplasmosis: 2007 update by the Infectious Diseases Society of America. Clin Infect Dis 2007; 45(7):807–25.

124. Tong SY, Peleg AY, Yoong J, et al. Breakthrough *Scedosporium prolificans* infection while receiving voriconazole prophylaxis in an allogeneic stem cell transplant recipient. Transpl Infect Dis 2007; 9(3):241–3.

125. Yao L, Wan Z, Li R, et al. In vitro triple combination of antifungal drugs against clinical *Scopulariopsis* and *Microascus* species. Antimicrob Agents Chemother 2015;59(8):5040–3.

126. Cordonnier C, Pautas C, Maury S, et al. Empirical versus preemptive antifungal therapy for high-risk, febrile, neutropenic patients: a randomized, controlled trial. Clin Infect Dis 2009;48(8): 1042–51.

127. Maertens J, Theunissen K, Verhoef G, et al. Galactomannan and computed tomography-based preemptive antifungal therapy in neutropenic patients at high risk for invasive fungal infection: a prospective feasibility study. Clin Infect Dis 2005;41(9): 1242–50.

128. Wingard JR, Carter SL, Walsh TJ, et al. Randomized, double-blind trial of fluconazole versus voriconazole for prevention of invasive fungal infection after allogeneic hematopoietic cell transplantation. Blood 2010;116(24):5111–8.

129. Arvanitis M, Anagnostou T, Mylonakis E. Galactomannan and polymerase chain reaction-based screening for invasive aspergillosis among high-risk hematology patients: a diagnostic meta-analysis. Clin Infect Dis 2015;61(8):1263–72.

130. Marr KA, Laverdiere M, Gugel A, et al. Antifungal therapy decreases sensitivity of the *Aspergillus* galactomannan enzyme immunoassay. Clin Infect Dis 2005;40(12):1762–9.

131. Winston DJ, Chandrasekar PH, Lazarus HM, et al. Fluconazole prophylaxis of fungal infections in patients with acute leukemia. Results of a randomized placebo-controlled, double-blind, multicenter trial. Ann Intern Med 1993;118(7):495–503.

132. Ullmann AJ, Lipton JH, Vesole DH, et al. Posaconazole or fluconazole for prophylaxis in severe graft-versus-host disease. N Engl J Med 2007;356(4):335–47.

133. Winston DJ, Bartoni K, Territo MC, et al. Efficacy, safety, and breakthrough infections associated with standard long-term posaconazole antifungal prophylaxis in allogeneic stem cell transplantation recipients. Biol Blood Marrow Transplant 2011;17(4):507–15.

134. Auberger J, Lass-Florl C, Aigner M, et al. Invasive fungal breakthrough infections, fungal colonization and emergence of resistant strains in high-risk patients receiving antifungal prophylaxis with posaconazole: real-life data from a single-centre institutional retrospective observational study. J Antimicrob Chemother 2012;67(9):2268–73.

135. Lerolle N, Raffoux E, Socie G, et al. Breakthrough invasive fungal disease in patients receiving posaconazole primary prophylaxis: a 4-year study. Clin Microbiol Infect 2014;20(11):O952–9.

136. Hiramatsu Y, Maeda Y, Fujii N, et al. Use of micafungin versus fluconazole for antifungal prophylaxis in neutropenic patients receiving hematopoietic stem cell transplantation. Int J Hematol 2008;88(5):588–95.

137. van Burik JA, Ratanatharathorn V, Stepan DE, et al. Micafungin versus fluconazole for prophylaxis against invasive fungal infections during neutropenia in patients undergoing hematopoietic stem cell transplantation. Clin Infect Dis 2004;39(10):1407–16.

138. Ziakas PD, Kourbeti IS, Mylonakis E. Systemic antifungal prophylaxis after hematopoietic stem cell transplantation: a meta-analysis. Clin Ther 2014;36(2):292–306.e1.

139. Centers for Disease Control and Prevention. Guidelines for environmental infection control in healthcare facilities: recommendations of CDC and the Healthcare Infection Control Practices Advisory Committee (HICPAC). MMWR Recomm Rep 2003;52(No. RR-10):1–48.

140. Tomblyn M, Chiller T, Einsele H, et al. Guidelines for preventing infectious complications among hematopoietic cell transplantation recipients: a global perspective. Biol Blood Marrow Transplant 2009;15(10):1143–238.

141. Raad I, Hanna H, Osting C, et al. Masking of neutropenic patients on transport from hospital rooms is associated with a decrease in nosocomial aspergillosis during construction. Infect Control Hosp Epidemiol 2002;23(1):41–3.

Viral Pneumonia in Patients with Hematopoietic Cell Transplantation and Hematologic Malignancies

 CrossMark

Margaret L. Green, MD, MPH[a,b,*]

KEYWORDS

- Pneumonia • Hematopoietic cell transplantation • Hematologic malignancy
- Community respiratory virus infection • Cytomegalovirus

KEY POINTS

- Viral pneumonia is a common pulmonary complication in patients with HCT/HM and is associated with high morbidity and mortality.
- Because of nonspecific imaging findings, and high rates of coinfection with other viral, bacterial, and fungal pathogens, microbiologic diagnosis generally requires bronchoalveolar lavage with samples sent for culture, direct fluorescent antibody and nucleic acid testing as available.
- CMV remains the most common cause of viral pneumonia in HCT/HM, but adoption of preemptive therapy strategies and changes in transplant techniques over the last few decades have resulted in significant improvement in the incidence and mortality associated with CMV pneumonia.
- Community respiratory virus (CRV) infections, such as influenza, parainfluenza, and respiratory syncytial virus, are common. Fewer patients develop lower tract disease; however, once established, mortality rates are high.
- Infection prevention practices in the community and health care setting are critical in limiting the acquisition and spread of CRVs in this highly susceptible patient population.

INTRODUCTION

Patients undergoing hematopoietic cell transplantation (HCT) or treatment of hematologic malignancy (HM) have profound impairment of cell-mediated and humoral immunity. As such they are at risk of lower respiratory tract infection from reactivation of latent infections, such as cytomegalovirus (CMV), and progression of community-acquired upper respiratory tract infections, such as respiratory syncytial virus (RSV) influenza A and B. The clinical presentation of these infections is varied, and diagnosis is often complicated by high rates of coinfection with bacterial, fungal, and other viral pathogens (**Table 1**).[1–4] This article reviews the epidemiology of the major viral pathogens for pneumonia in patients with HCT/HM with discussion of evidence-based prevention strategies and treatments.

Disclosure: Dr M.L. Green has received research funding from Merck and Astellas Global Pharma. No other relationships to disclose.

[a] University of Washington, 1959 NE Pacific Street, Box 359930, Seattle, WA 98195, USA; [b] Fred Hutchinson Cancer Research Center, 1100 Fairview Avenue North, Seattle, WA 98109, USA
* Fred Hutchinson Cancer Research Center, 1100 Fairview Avenue North, Seattle, WA 98109.
E-mail address: mlgreen@fredhutch.org

Clin Chest Med 38 (2017) 295–305
http://dx.doi.org/10.1016/j.ccm.2016.12.009
0272-5231/17/© 2016 Elsevier Inc. All rights reserved.

Table 1
Incidence of infection, incidence of pneumonia, associated mortality rates, and treatments of most common causes of viral pneumonia in patients with HCT or HM

Virus	Incidence of Infection	Progression to Pneumonia	Mortality	Treatment
Cytomegalovirus	50%–90% seroprevalence	1%–8% after allogeneic HCT with pre-emptive therapy 1%–5% other populations with no surveillance	60%–80%	Ganciclovir or foscarnet
Influenza A and B (FluA and FluB)	33% of symptomatic patients	14%–30%	15%–28%	Oseltamivir or other neuraminidase inhibitors
Respiratory syncytial virus	14%–30% of symptomatic patients	40%–75%	28%–55%	No direct-acting therapy; inhaled ribavirin most studied
Parainfluenza virus	1%–10% of all patients	30%	17%–46%	None currently licensed; DAS-181 in phase III trials
Adenovirus	8%–17% after allogeneic HCT, 6% after autologous	~8%	N/A	Cidofovir

DIAGNOSIS OF VIRAL PNEUMONIA
Clinical Presentation

Presenting signs and symptoms of viral pneumonia are variable. Most patients have fever and cough, with hypoxia and increased work of breathing of varying degrees depending on the extent of the infection. Upper respiratory tract infection symptoms, such as nasal congestion, rhinorrhea, sinusitis, myalgias, and fatigue, may be present for infections caused by community respiratory viruses (CRVs).

Imaging

Computed tomography (CT) is helpful in distinguishing between infectious and noninfectious causes of lung disease in this patient population and also between viral and fungal or bacterial infections.[5,6] Viral pneumonias are similar in appearance on CT often demonstrating small centrilobular nodules, patchy bilateral areas of ground glass opacities and consolidation, bronchial wall thickening, and tree-in-bud opacities (**Fig. 1**). If there is significant bronchiolitis, air trapping can also be evident.[5–10]

Diagnostic Sampling

Fiberoptic bronchoscopy with bronchoalveolar lavage is the predominant sampling method to confirm a diagnosis of viral pneumonia in the HCT/HM population. Although sampling of the upper respiratory tract with nasopharyngeal aspirate/wash may provide an early identification of the involved virus or viruses, sampling of the lower tract is usually recommended to confirm the diagnosis and to exclude other copathogens. Because of the risk of hemorrhage in these patients who often have thrombocytopenia, endobronchial biopsy is usually avoided. Surgical lung biopsy, which was once the principle method by which lung abnormalities were evaluated after HCT, is now rarely performed.[11]

Virologic Diagnosis

Standard viral cultures are of waning utility in the diagnosis of viral pneumonias because it can take up to 2 weeks to become positive and several more recently identified respiratory viruses, such as human metapneumovirus, coronaviruses, and bocavirus, are notoriously difficult to isolate in culture. For most viral pathogens, molecular methods of viral detection, such as direct or indirect fluorescent antibody tests or nucleic acid tests, can be used to give reliable results with a rapid turnaround time. Multiplex polymerase chain reaction (PCR) panels have the advantage of being able to test for multiple viruses at the same time and are more sensitive than fluorescent antibody tests.[12–17]

A

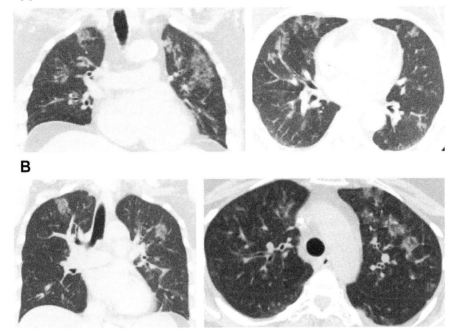

B

Fig. 1. (*A*) Transverse and coronal views of CT imaging for a patient with HCT with adenovirus and rhinovirus pneumonia, demonstrating patchy bilateral infiltrates with ground glass opacities and tree-in-bud pattern. (*B*) Transverse and coronal view of CT imaging for a patient with HCT with pneumonia caused by parainfluenza virus type 3. Note scattered nodular infiltrates with ground glass opacities.

The diagnosis of CMV pneumonia, however, continues to rely on the use of standard viral or shell vial culture, histopathology, or immunohistochemical testing.[18] The assumption has been that the CMV PCR tests would be too sensitive and have a low positive predictive value for CMV pneumonitis.[19–22] However, because of the operational advantages of PCR testing with much faster turnaround time, efforts are underway to estimate a quantitative CMV viral load threshold that would be more predictive of CMV pneumonitis rather than asymptomatic shedding.

CYTOMEGALOVIRUS
Epidemiology

CMV is the most common cause of viral pneumonia after allogeneic HCT. Early reports indicated an incidence of 20% to 70% with an associated mortality of 85% to 90%.[23–25] The development of ganciclovir resulted in significant improvements in the mortality associated with CMV pneumonia but with mortality rates still 60% to 80% focus shifted to prevention of disease.[26–29] The use of ganciclovir for prophylaxis decreased the incidence of pneumonitis and other CMV end-organ disease, but was associated with increased rates of neutropenia and late-occurring

disease (ie, after Day 100 posttransplant).[25,30–33] In the current era of preemptive therapy, where patients are monitored for CMV replication with either pp65 antigen or CMV DNA PCR in the blood or plasma and antiviral treatment is initiated before the development of CMV pneumonia, the incidence of CMV pneumonia is now only 1% to 3% in the early posttransplant period (100 days posttransplant).[34–36] An additional 1% to 8% of patients develop CMV pneumonia within the first year after transplant.[36–38]

Risk factors for development of CMV pneumonia after allogeneic HCT are CMV seropositivity, recipient of a cord blood graft, HLA-mismatched donors, myeloablative conditioning regimens, acute and chronic graft-versushost disease (GVHD), and use of T-cell-depleted stem cells.[34,36,39–43]

CMV pneumonia is much less common in patients who have received an autologous transplant, or in patients receiving treatment of HM with incidence of 1% to 5% reported in the absence of surveillance and preemptive therapy.[44–48]

Treatment

Ganciclovir (5 mg/kg intravenous [IV] every 12 hours) remains the first-line treatment for CMV pneumonitis.[49] Based on the results of three non-randomized studies,[50–52] CMV immunoglobulin was often recommended as adjunctive treatment. However, more recent analyses have called into question the additional benefit of this therapy.[29,47,53,54] Duration of treatment is generally induction therapy for 21 to 28 days, followed by 21 to 28 days of maintenance therapy (ganciclovir, 5 mg/kg IV every 24 hours). Foscarnet (90 mg/kg IV every 12 hours) may be used in the setting of neutropenia because it is associated with less bone marrow suppression than ganciclovir, but commonly causes significant nephrotoxicity.

Antiviral resistance mutations have been identified in the viral encoded UL97 kinase, required only by ganciclovir, and the viral DNA polymerase, the target of ganciclovir, foscarnet, and cidofovir.[55] Fortunately, antiviral resistance is a rare occurrence in patients with HCT/HM occurring in 0% to 4% of patients with CMV reactivation.[56–58] Foscarnet, cidofovir, and brincidofovir (an oral nucleotide analogue and prodrug of cidofovir) could be used for treatment of resistant CMV caused by UL97 mutations. Maribavir and letermovir, two agents currently undergoing clinical trials, have distinct mechanisms of action that may make them useful for treatment of resistant CMV disease; however, little is known of their genetic barrier to resistance.[59–62]

Other Herpesviruses

Reactivation of latent varicella zoster virus and herpes simplex virus in immunocompromised patients can result in disseminated disease with pneumonia and was a significant clinical problem for patients with HCT/HM.[63,64] Long-term prophylaxis with acyclovir or valacyclovir has been the standard of care for more than a decade.[65–68] Cases still rarely occur in patients who have discontinued acyclovir prophylaxis, but generally respond well to high-dose parenteral acyclovir.[69–71]

COMMUNITY RESPIRATORY VIRUSES

CRVs are a common cause of infection in patients with HCT/HM; however, the risk of pneumonia varies by virus type and patient risk factors. Several of the viruses, such as influenza and RSV, have significant seasonal variation of incidence, whereas others, such as parainfluenza virus (PIV) and adenovirus, tend to cause disease year round. Outbreaks on oncology and HCT hospital wards and ambulatory clinics have been described for many of these viruses,[72–76] emphasizing the importance of infection-prevention policies and procedures that can prevent the

transmission of viruses among highly susceptible patients. This is particularly challenging with this patient population because of prolonged viral shedding, which often lasts weeks or months.[77–79]

Influenza

Influenza is diagnosed in approximately 1% of patients with HCT/HM during treatment, and in 33% of patients presenting with respiratory virus symptoms.[80–82] Progression to pneumonia occurs in 14% to 30% of patients and is associated with mortality rates of 15% to 28%.[80–83] During the 2009 H1N1 influenza pandemic, rates of pneumonia were much higher (>50%), but mortality was similar.[84] Risk factors for development of pneumonia include lymphopenia (<100 cells/μL), neutropenia (<500 cells/μL), steroid use at time of diagnosis, and absence of antiviral treatment.[80,81,83,84]

Neuraminidase inhibitors, primarily oseltamivir, are currently the standard of care for influenza treatment and postexposure prophylaxis. Oseltamivir resistance has been described but remains uncommon.[85–88] In the setting of documented or suspected oseltamivir resistance, or in patients who have impaired enteric absorption, inhaled zanamivir or the newly licensed parenteral peramivir have been used.[89–91]

Seasonal vaccination with the trivalent inactivated vaccine is recommended for all health care workers caring for patients with HCT/HM, family members, and household contacts. Additionally, it is recommended that patients undergoing treatment of leukemia and lymphoma are vaccinated because it may reduce the risk of hospitalization for respiratory illness.[92–95] Ideally, vaccine should be administered at least 2 weeks before any cytotoxic therapy. For HCT recipients, vaccination of patients less than 6 months after transplant is ineffective and is generally not recommended.[66,95,96] Chemoprophylaxis after exposure is recommended for patients with HCT within 1 year of transplant or for patients with HM during chemotherapy.[66,97]

Respiratory Syncytial Virus

Infection with RSV is more common than influenza, occurring in 7% to 10% of patients undergoing allogeneic HCT.[98,99] Among patients with HCT/HM presenting with viral respiratory symptoms, RSV is diagnosed in 14% to 30%.[81,99] Involvement of the lower respiratory tract occurs in 40% to 75% of infected patients.[81,98,99] Risk factors for progression to pneumonia include patient age, allogeneic HCT, mismatched or unrelated donor, GVHD, myeloablative conditioning regimens, infection less than 30 days post-transplant, prolonged lymphopenia, and lack of ribavirin-based therapy.[81,98–101] RSV pneumonia is associated with mortality rates of 28% to 55%.[100,102,103] Treatment with inhaled ribavirin has been shown in several retrospective studies to be associated with decreased rates of progression and a 67% to 83% reduction in the risk of mortality after RSV infection.[100,102] Based on these data, many centers use inhaled ribavirin (2 g for 2 hours every 8 hours for 10 days) in select, high-risk patient populations.[66,104] However, because of recent increases in the cost of this formulation, the use of systemic (oral or parenteral) ribavirin is increasing despite a paucity of evidence to support this practice.[102,105,106] There are a few noteworthy agents with novel mechanisms of action that are currently in trial: GS5806, an oral RSV entry inhibitor; and ALS8176, a nucleoside RSV polymerase inhibitor.[107,108] Finally, pneumonia caused by RSV has been associated with a significant airflow decline by 1 year posttransplant, an important long-term sequela of this common infection.[109]

Parainfluenza Virus

Unlike influenza and RSV, PIV infections occur without much seasonal variation. The incidence of PIV infection in patients with HCT/HM is 1% to 10%, and 30% of infected patients develop pneumonia; most cases are caused by PIV type 3.[110–113] Death occurs in 17% to 46% of patients who develop pneumonia.[110,112,113] Risk factors for development of pneumonia include high-dose corticosteroid use, lymphopenia, neutropenia, infection occurring early posttransplantation, the presence of copathogens, and a higher Acute Physiology and Chronic Health Evaluation II score.[110,113,114] There are currently no licensed treatments for PIV pneumonia. Ribavirin has been used with little noted improvement in mortality or clinical response.[110,114] DAS181, an investigational sialidase fusion protein that works by removing sialic acid–containing receptors from respiratory epithelial cells, preventing PIV from binding, has been successfully used in several cases of adult and pediatric PIV pneumonia in HCT/HM and is currently in phase III clinical trials.[115,116]

Adenovirus

Human adenovirus (HAdV) infections can cause significant disseminated disease in patients with HCT/HM, including severe pneumonia. The most severe disease occurs after HCT, especially in children, and in patients with HM treated with alemtuzumab.[117–119] Adenovirus infection occurs in 8% to 17% of patients undergoing allogeneic HCT, with most cases occurring in children.[120,121] A total of 10% of patients develop HAdV end-organ disease; the lungs are involved in 75% of these cases.[120,121] Infection is less common after autologous HCT, occurring in only 6% of patients, and end-organ disease including pneumonia is rare. In addition to T-cell depletion, risk factors for HAdV disease are lymphopenia, receipt of cord blood grafts, GVHD requiring increased or prolonged immunosuppression, and absence of HAdV-specific T-cell responses.[122] Patients with adenoviral pneumonia often have involvement at other sites, such as the gut and liver, and mortality rates with disseminated disease are high. First-line treatment of HAdV disease including pneumonitis is cidofovir (5 mg/kg once weekly, or 1 mg/kg three times weekly) and reduction in immunosuppression whenever possible.[66,122–124]

Other Community Respiratory Viruses

Other common CRVs, such as human metapneumovirus, novel coronaviruses (eg, SARS-CoV, MERS-CoV), and even human rhinovirus, cause lower respiratory tract infection in patients with HCT/HM.[125–128] Although each of these viruses have their own specific biology and epidemiology, the risk factors for pneumonia that have been identified for other CRVs, such as lymphopenia and infection occurring early after HCT, are shared. Because there are yet no direct-acting treatments for these viruses, efforts to prevent infection in these highly immunosuppressed patients remains paramount. Current guidelines recommend preventing contact from symptomatic health care workers and family members, daily screening of health care workers and visitors to inpatient units for symptoms, active surveillance for CRV disease, and isolation of symptomatic patients with recognition that viral shedding is prolonged in this patient population.[129,130]

SUMMARY

The profound and prolonged immunosuppression experienced by patients undergoing HCT and intensive chemotherapy for HM results in rates of viral pneumonia that far surpass the incidence in the general population. Patients with viral pneumonia generally present with fever; hypoxia; and often bilateral, patchy nodular infiltrates with or without surrounding ground glass opacities on high-resolution CT imaging. Because the imaging findings do not help distinguish among different viral etiologies, and these patients commonly have other viral, bacterial, and fungal coinfections, a microbiologic diagnosis typically requires fiberoptic bronchoscopy with bronchoalveolar lavage.

Although CMV remains the most common cause of viral pneumonia in this population, efforts to treat CMV replication early in its course and changes in transplant practices have resulted in improvements in the incidence and associated mortality of CMV pneumonia. Taken together, CRV infections also occur commonly in this patient population. However, the rates of progression to pneumonia vary depending on the virus with influenza, RSV, and PIV causing lower tract disease more commonly than adenovirus, human metapneumovirus, and rhinovirus, and patient risk factors relating to the degree of immunosuppression (ie, lymphopenia, early posttransplant, steroid use). Once established, however, pneumonia caused by these infections is associated with high mortality rates in part because of the lack of direct-acting antiviral agents for most of these viruses. Infection prevention practices that limit the acquisition of CRVs by patients with HCT/HM and decrease the risk of spread within the clinics and inpatient settings are of particular importance.

REFERENCES

1. Ison MG, Hayden FG, Kaiser L, et al. Rhinovirus infections in hematopoietic stem cell transplant recipients with pneumonia. Clin Infect Dis 2003; 36(9):1139–43.

2. Shannon VR, Andersson BS, Lei X, et al. Utility of early versus late fiberoptic bronchoscopy in the evaluation of new pulmonary infiltrates following hematopoietic stem cell transplantation. Bone Marrow Transplant 2009;45(4):647–55.

3. Oren I, Hardak E, Zuckerman T, et al. Does molecular analysis increase the efficacy of bronchoalveolar lavage in the diagnosis and management of respiratory infections in hemato-oncological patients? Int J Infect Dis 2016;50:48–53.

4. Hardak E, Avivi I, Berkun L, et al. Polymicrobial pulmonary infection in patients with hematological malignancies: prevalence, co-pathogens, course and outcome. Infection 2016;44(4):491–7.

5. Miller WTJ, Mickus TJ, Barbosa EJ, et al. CT of viral lower respiratory tract infections in adults: comparison among viral organisms and between viral and bacterial infections. AJR Am J Roentgenol 2011; 197(5):1088–95.

6. Kanne JP, Godwin JD, Franquet T. Viral pneumonia after hematopoietic stem cell transplantation: high-resolution CT findings. J Thorac Imaging 2007; 22(3):292–9.

7. Franquet T, Rodriguez S, Martino R, et al. Thin-section CT findings in hematopoietic stem cell transplantation recipients with respiratory virus

pneumonia. AJR Am J Roentgenol 2006;187(4): 1085–90.

8. Herbst T, Van Deerlin VM, Miller WTJ. The CT appearance of lower respiratory infection due to parainfluenza virus in adults. AJR Am J Roentgenol 2013;201(3):550–4.

9. Shiley KT, Van Deerlin VM, Miller WTJ. Chest CT features of community-acquired respiratory viral infections in adult inpatients with lower respiratory tract infections. J Thorac Imaging 2010;25(1):68–75.

10. Kim M-C, Kim MY, Lee HJ, et al. CT findings in viral lower respiratory tract infections caused by parainfluenza virus, influenza virus and respiratory syncytial virus. Medicine 2016;95(26):e4003.

11. Cheng G-S, Stednick Z, Madtes DK, et al. Decline in the use of surgical biopsy for diagnosis of pulmonary disease in hematopoietic cell transplantation recipients in an era of improved diagnostics and empirical therapy. Biol Blood Marrow Transplant 2016;22:2243–9.

12. Osiowy C. Direct detection of respiratory syncytial virus, parainfluenza virus, and adenovirus in clinical respiratory specimens by a multiplex reverse transcription-PCR assay. J Clin Microbiol 1998; 36(11):3149–54.

13. Coiras MT, Aguilar JC, Garcia ML, et al. Simultaneous detection of fourteen respiratory viruses in clinical specimens by two multiplex reverse transcription nested-PCR assays. J Med Virol 2004; 72(3):484–95.

14. Templeton KE, Scheltinga SA, Beersma MFC, et al. Rapid and sensitive method using multiplex real-time PCR for diagnosis of infections by influenza a and influenza B viruses, respiratory syncytial virus, and parainfluenza viruses 1, 2, 3, and 4. J Clin Microbiol 2004;42(4):1564–9.

15. Fan J, Henrickson KJ, Savatski LL. Rapid simultaneous diagnosis of infections with respiratory syncytial viruses A and B, influenza viruses A and B, and human parainfluenza virus types 1, 2, and 3 by multiplex quantitative reverse transcription-polymerase chain reaction-enzyme hybridization assay (Hexaplex). Clin Infect Dis 1998;26(6): 1397–402.

16. Choudhary ML, Anand SP, Heydari M, et al. Development of a multiplex one step RT-PCR that detects eighteen respiratory viruses in clinical specimens and comparison with real time RT-PCR. J Virol Methods 2013;189(1):15–9.

17. van Elden L, van Kraaij M. Polymerase chain reaction is more sensitive than viral culture and antigen testing for the detection of respiratory viruses in adults with hematological cancer and pneumonia. Clin Infect Dis 2002;34(2):177–83.

18. Ljungman P, Griffiths P, Paya C. Definitions of cytomegalovirus infection and disease in transplant recipients. Clin Infect Dis 2002;34(8):1094–7.

19. Fajac A, Stephan F, Ibrahim A, et al. Value of cytomegalovirus detection by PCR in bronchoalveolar lavage routinely performed in asymptomatic bone marrow recipients. Bone Marrow Transplant 1997; 20(7):581–5.

20. Cathomas G, Morris P, Pekle K, et al. Rapid diagnosis of cytomegalovirus pneumonia in marrow transplant recipients by bronchoalveolar lavage using the polymerase chain reaction, virus culture, and the direct immunostaining of alveolar cells. Blood 1993;81(7):1909–14.

21. Eriksson BM, Brytting M, Zweygberg-Wirgart B, et al. Diagnosis of cytomegalovirus in bronchoalveolar lavage by polymerase chain reaction, in comparison with virus isolation and detection of viral antigen. Scand J Infect Dis 1993;25(4): 421–7.

22. Tan SK, Burgener EB, Waggoner JJ, et al. Molecular and culture-based bronchoalveolar lavage fluid testing for the diagnosis of cytomegalovirus pneumonitis. Open Forum Infect Dis 2016;3(1):ofv212.

23. Krowka MJ, Rosenow EC. Pulmonary complications of bone marrow transplantation. Chest 1985; 87(2):237–46.

24. Meyers JD, Flournoy N, Thomas ED. Risk factors for cytomegalovirus infection after human marrow transplantation. J Infect Dis 1986;153(3):478–88.

25. Schmidt GM, Horak DA, Niland JC, et al. A randomized, controlled trial of prophylactic ganciclovir for cytomegalovirus pulmonary infection in recipients of allogeneic bone marrow transplants; the City of Hope-Stanford-Syntex CMV Study Group. N Engl J Med 1991;324(15):1005–11.

26. Winston DJ, Ho WG, Bartoni K, et al. Ganciclovir therapy for cytomegalovirus infections in recipients of bone marrow transplants and other immunosuppressed patients. Rev Infect Dis 1988;10(Suppl 3): S547–53.

27. Crumpacker C, Marlowe S, Zhang JL, et al. Treatment of cytomegalovirus pneumonia. Rev Infect Dis 1988;10(Suppl 3):S538–46.

28. Erice A, Jordan MC, Chace BA, et al. Ganciclovir treatment of cytomegalovirus disease in transplant recipients and other immunocompromised hosts. JAMA 1987;257(22):3082–7.

29. Erard V, Guthrie KA, Seo S, et al. Reduced mortality of cytomegalovirus pneumonia after hematopoietic cell transplantation due to antiviral therapy and changes in transplantation practices. Clin Infect Dis 2015;61(1):31–9.

30. Goodrich JM, Mori M, Gleaves CA, et al. Early treatment with ganciclovir to prevent cytomegalovirus disease after allogeneic bone marrow transplantation. N Engl J Med 1991;325(23):1601–7.

31. Winston DJ, Ho WG, Bartoni K, et al. Ganciclovir prophylaxis of cytomegalovirus infection and disease in allogeneic bone marrow transplant recipients. Results of a placebo-controlled, double-blind trial. Ann Intern Med 1993;118(3):179–84.

32. Boeckh M, Gooley TA, Myerson D, et al. Cytomegalovirus pp65 antigenemia-guided early treatment with ganciclovir versus ganciclovir at engraftment after allogeneic marrow transplantation: a randomized double-blind study. Blood 1996;88(10):4063.

33. Nguyen Q, Champlin R, Giralt S, et al. Late cytomegalovirus pneumonia in adult allogeneic blood and marrow transplant recipients. Clin Infect Dis 1999;28(3):618–23.

34. Ljungman P, Perez-Bercoff L, Jonsson J, et al. Risk factors for the development of cytomegalovirus disease after allogeneic stem cell transplantation. Haematologica 2006;91(1):78–83.

35. Marty FM, Ljungman P, Papanicolaou GA, et al. Maribavir prophylaxis for prevention of cytomegalovirus disease in recipients of allogeneic stem-cell transplants: a phase 3, double-blind, placebo-controlled, randomised trial. Lancet Infect Dis 2011;11(4):284–92.

36. Green ML, Leisenring W, Stachel D, et al. Efficacy of a viral load-based, risk-adapted, preemptive treatment strategy for prevention of cytomegalovirus disease after hematopoietic cell transplantation. Biol Blood Marrow Transplant 2012;18(11): 1687–99.

37. Boeckh M, Leisenring W, Riddell SR, et al. Late cytomegalovirus disease and mortality in recipients of allogeneic hematopoietic stem cell transplants: importance of viral load and T-cell immunity. Blood 2003;101(2):407–14.

38. Boeckh M, Nichols WG, Chemaly RF, et al. Valganciclovir for the prevention of complications of late cytomegalovirus infection after allogeneic hematopoietic cell transplantation. Ann Intern Med 2015; 162(1):1.

39. Miller W, Flynn P, McCullough J, et al. Cytomegalovirus infection after bone marrow transplantation: an association with acute graft-v-host disease. Blood 1986;67(4):1162.

40. Dahi PB, Perales MA, Devlin SM, et al. Incidence, nature and mortality of cytomegalovirus infection after double-unit cord blood transplant. Leuk Lymphoma 2015;56(6):1799–805.

41. Milano F, Pergam SA, Xie H, et al. Intensive strategy to prevent CMV disease in seropositive umbilical cord blood transplant recipients. Blood 2011; 118(20):5689–96.

42. Hertenstein B, Hampl W, Bunjes D, et al. In vivo/ ex vivo T cell depletion for GVHD prophylaxis influences onset and course of active cytomegalovirus infection and disease after BMT. Bone Marrow Transplant 1995;15(3):387–93.

43. van Burik J-AH, Carter SL, Freifeld AG, et al. Higher risk of cytomegalovirus and aspergillus infections in recipients of T cell-depleted unrelated bone

marrow: analysis of infectious complications in patients treated with T cell depletion versus immunosuppressive therapy to prevent graft-versus-host disease. Biol Blood Marrow Transplant 2007; 13(12):1487–98.

44. Chemaly RF, Torres HA, Hachem RY, et al. Cytomegalovirus pneumonia in patients with lymphoma. Cancer 2005;104(6):1213–20.

45. Nguyen Q, Estey E, Raad I, et al. Cytomegalovirus pneumonia in adults with leukemia: an emerging problem. Clin Infect Dis 2001;32(4):539–45.

46. Konoplev S, Champlin RE, Giralt S. Cytomegalovirus pneumonia in adult autologous blood and marrow transplant recipients. Transplantation 2001;27(8):877–81.

47. Ljungman P, Biron P, Bosi A, et al. Cytomegalovirus interstitial pneumonia in autologous bone marrow transplant recipients. Infectious disease working party of the European Group for bone marrow transplantation. Bone Marrow Transplant 1994; 13(2):209–12.

48. Jain R, Trehan A, Mishra B, et al. Cytomegalovirus disease in children with acute lymphoblastic leukemia. Pediatr Hematol Oncol 2016;33(4):239–47.

49. Boeckh M, Ljungman P. How we treat cytomegalovirus in hematopoietic cell transplant recipients. Blood 2009;113(23):5711–9.

50. Emanuel D, Cunningham I, Jules-Elysee K, et al. Cytomegalovirus pneumonia after bone marrow transplantation successfully treated with the combination of ganciclovir and high-dose intravenous immune globulin. Ann Intern Med 1988;109(10):777–82.

51. Reed EC, Bowden RA, Dandliker PS, et al. Treatment of cytomegalovirus pneumonia with ganciclovir and intravenous cytomegalovirus immunoglobulin in patients with bone marrow transplants. Ann Intern Med 1988;109(10):783–8.

52. Schmidt GM, Kovacs A, Zaia JA, et al. Ganciclovir/immunoglobulin combination therapy for the treatment of human cytomegalovirus-associated interstitial pneumonia in bone marrow allograft recipients. Transplantation 1988;46(6):905–7.

53. Machado CM, Dulley FL, Boas LS, et al. CMV pneumonia in allogeneic BMT recipients undergoing early treatment of pre-emptive ganciclovir therapy. Bone Marrow Transplant 2000;26(4):413–7.

54. Ljungman P, Engelhard D, Link H, et al. Treatment of interstitial pneumonitis due to cytomegalovirus with ganciclovir and intravenous immune globulin: experience of European Bone Marrow Transplant Group. Clin Infect Dis 1992;14(4):831–5.

55. Lurain NS, Chou S. Antiviral drug resistance of human cytomegalovirus. Clin Microbiol Rev 2010; 23(4):689–712.

56. Avery RK, Arav-Boger R, Marr KA, et al. Outcomes in transplant recipients treated with foscarnet for ganciclovir-resistant or refractory cytomegalovirus infection. Transplantation 2016;100(10):e74–80.

57. Choi SH, Hwang J-Y, Park K-S, et al. The impact of drug-resistant cytomegalovirus in pediatric allogeneic hematopoietic cell transplant recipients: a prospective monitoring of UL97 and UL54 gene mutations. Transpl Infect Dis 2014;16(6):919–29.

58. Eckle T, Prix L, Jahn G, et al. Drug-resistant human cytomegalovirus infection in children after allogeneic stem cell transplantation may have different clinical outcomes. Blood 2000;96(9):3286–9.

59. Avery RK, Marty FM, Strasfeld L, et al. Oral maribavir for treatment of refractory or resistant cytomegalovirus infections in transplant recipients. Transpl Infect Dis 2010;12(6):489–96.

60. Schubert A, Ehlert K, Schuler-Luettmann S, et al. Fast selection of maribavir resistant cytomegalovirus in a bone marrow transplant recipient. BMC Infect Dis 2013;13:330.

61. Chou S. Approach to drug-resistant cytomegalovirus in transplant recipients. Curr Opin Infect Dis 2015;28(4):293–9.

62. Kaul DR, Stoelben S, Cober E, et al. First report of successful treatment of multidrug-resistant cytomegalovirus disease with the novel anti-CMV compound AIC246. Am J Transplant 2011;11(5):1079–84.

63. Locksley RM, Flournoy N, Sullivan KM, et al. Infection with varicella-zoster virus after marrow transplantation. J Infect Dis 1985;152(6):1172–81.

64. Koc Y, Miller KB, Schenkein DP, et al. Varicella zoster virus infections following allogeneic bone marrow transplantation: frequency, risk factors, and clinical outcome. Biol Blood Marrow Transplant 2000;6(1):44–9.

65. Baden LR, Bensinger W, Angarone M. Prevention and treatment of cancer-related infections. J Natl Compr Canc Netw 2012;10(11):1412–45.

66. Tomblyn M, Chiller T, Einsele H, et al. Guidelines for preventing infectious complications among hematopoietic cell transplantation recipients: a global perspective. Biol Blood Marrow Transplant 2009; 15(10):1143–238.

67. Boeckh M, Kim HW, Flowers MED, et al. Long-term acyclovir for prevention of varicella zoster virus disease after allogeneic hematopoietic cell transplantation–a randomized double-blind placebo-controlled study. Blood 2006;107(5):1800–5.

68. Erard V, Guthrie KA, Varley C, et al. One-year acyclovir prophylaxis for preventing varicella-zoster virus disease after hematopoietic cell transplantation: no evidence of rebound varicella-zoster virus disease after drug discontinuation. Blood 2007;110(8):3071–7.

69. Perren TJ, Powles RL, Easton D, et al. Prevention of herpes zoster in patients by long-term oral

acyclovir after allogeneic bone marrow transplantation. Am J Med 1988;85(2A):99–101.

70. Kim DH, Kumar D, Messner HA, et al. Clinical efficacy of prophylactic strategy of long-term low-dose acyclovir for varicella-zoster virus infection after allogeneic peripheral blood stem cell transplantation. Clin Transplant 2008;22(6):770–9.

71. Kim DH, Messner H, Minden M, et al. Factors influencing varicella zoster virus infection after allogeneic peripheral blood stem cell transplantation: low-dose acyclovir prophylaxis and pre-transplant diagnosis of lymphoproliferative disorders. Transpl Infect Dis 2008;10(2):90–8.

72. Weinstock DM, Eagan J, Malak SA, et al. Control of influenza A on a bone marrow transplant unit. Infect Control Hosp Epidemiol 2000;21(11):730–2.

73. Mattner F, Sykora K-W, Meissner B, et al. An adenovirus type F41 outbreak in a pediatric bone marrow transplant unit. Pediatr Infect Dis J 2008; 27(5):419–24.

74. Abdallah A, Rowland KE, Schepetiuk SK, et al. An outbreak of respiratory syncytial virus infection in a bone marrow transplant unit: effect on engraftment and outcome of pneumonia without specific antiviral treatment. Bone Marrow Transplant 2003; 32(2):195–203.

75. Hodson A, Kasliwal M, Streetly M, et al. A parainfluenza-3 outbreak in a SCT unit: sepsis with multi-organ failure and multiple co-pathogens are associated with increased mortality. Bone Marrow Transplant 2011;46(12):1545–50.

76. Chu HY, Englund JA, Podczervinski S, et al. Nosocomial transmission of respiratory syncytial virus in an outpatient cancer center. Biol Blood Marrow Transplant 2014;20(6):844–51.

77. Campbell AP, Guthrie KA, Englund JA, et al. Clinical outcomes associated with respiratory virus detection before allogeneic hematopoietic stem cell transplant. Clin Infect Dis 2015;61(2): 192–202.

78. de Lima CRA, Mirandolli TB, Carneiro LC, et al. Prolonged respiratory viral shedding in transplant patients. Transpl Infect Dis 2014;16(1):165–9.

79. Lehners N, Tabatabai J, Prifert C, et al. Long-term shedding of influenza virus, parainfluenza virus, respiratory syncytial virus and nosocomial epidemiology in patients with hematological disorders. PLoS One 2016;11(2):e0148258.

80. Nichols WG, Guthrie KA, Corey L, et al. Influenza infections after hematopoietic stem cell transplantation: risk factors, mortality, and the effect of antiviral therapy. Clin Infect Dis 2004;39(9): 1300–6.

81. Chemaly RF, Ghosh S, Bodey GP, et al. Respiratory viral infections in adults with hematologic malignancies and human stem cell transplantation recipients. Medicine 2006;85(5):278–87.

82. Yousuf HM, Englund J, Couch R, et al. Influenza among hospitalized adults with leukemia. Clin Infect Dis 1997;24(6):1095–9.

83. Ljungman P. Respiratory virus infections in stem cell transplant patients: the European experience. Biol Blood Marrow Transplant 2001;7(Suppl): 5S–7S.

84. Choi S-M, Boudreault AA, Xie H, et al. Differences in clinical outcomes after 2009 influenza A/H1N1 and seasonal influenza among hematopoietic cell transplant recipients. Blood 2011;117(19): 5050–6.

85. Tramontana AR, George B, Hurt AC, et al. Oseltamivir resistance in adult oncology and hematology patients infected with pandemic (H1N1) 2009 virus, Australia. Emerg Infect Dis 2010;16(7):1068–75.

86. Couturier BA, Bender JM, Schwarz MA, et al. Oseltamivir-resistant influenza A 2009 H1N1 virus in immunocompromised patients. Influenza Other Respir Viruses 2010;4(4):199–204.

87. Pollara CP, Piccinelli G, Rossi G, et al. Nosocomial outbreak of the pandemic influenza A (H1N1) 2009 in critical hematologic patients during seasonal influenza 2010-2011: detection of oseltamivir resistant variant viruses. BMC Infect Dis 2013; 13:127.

88. Renaud C, Kuypers J, Englund JA. Emerging oseltamivir resistance in seasonal and pandemic influenza A/H1N1. J Clin Virol 2011;52(2):70–8.

89. Yu Y, Garg S, Yu PA, et al. Peramivir use for treatment of hospitalized patients with influenza A(H1N1)pdm09 under emergency use authorization, October 2009-June 2010. Clin Infect Dis 2012;55(1):8–15.

90. Hernandez JE, Adiga R, Armstrong R, et al. Clinical experience in adults and children treated with intravenous peramivir for 2009 influenza A (H1N1) under an Emergency IND program in the United States. Clin Infect Dis 2011;52(6):695–706.

91. Muthuri SG, Venkatesan S, Myles PR, et al. Effectiveness of neuraminidase inhibitors in reducing mortality in patients admitted to hospital with influenza A H1N1pdm09 virus infection: a meta-analysis of individual participant data. Lancet Respir Med 2014;2(5):395–404.

92. Shahgholi E, Ehsani MA, Salamati P, et al. Immunogenicity of trivalent influenza vaccine in children with acute lymphoblastic leukemia during maintenance therapy. Pediatr Blood Cancer 2010;54(5): 716–20.

93. Cheuk DKL, Chiang AKS, Lee TL, et al. Vaccines for prophylaxis of viral infections in patients with hematological malignancies. Cochrane Database Syst Rev 2011;3:CD006505.

94. Baden LR, Swaminathan S, Angarone M, et al. Prevention and treatment of cancer-related infections, version 2.2016, NCCN clinical practice guidelines

in oncology. J Natl Compr Canc Netw 2016;14(7): 882–913.

95. Rubin LG, Levin MJ, Ljungman P, et al. 2013 IDSA clinical practice guideline for vaccination of the immunocompromised host. Clin Infect Dis 2014; 58(3):e44–100.

96. Engelhard D, Nagler A, Hardan I, et al. Antibody response to a two-dose regimen of influenza vaccine in allogeneic T cell-depleted and autologous BMT recipients. Bone Marrow Transplant 1993;11(1):1–5.

97. Engelhard D, Mohty B, La Camara de R, et al. European guidelines for prevention and management of influenza in hematopoietic stem cell transplantation and leukaemia patients: summary of ECIL-4 (2011), on behalf of ECIL, a joint venture of EBMT, EORTC, ICHS, and ELN. Transpl Infect Dis 2013;15(3):219–32.

98. Nichols WG, Gooley T, Boeckh M. Community-acquired respiratory syncytial virus and parainfluenza virus infections after hematopoietic stem cell transplantation: the Fred Hutchinson Cancer Research Center experience. Biol Blood Marrow Transplant 2001;7(Suppl):11S–5S.

99. Martino R, Porras RP, Rabella N, et al. Prospective study of the incidence, clinical features, and outcome of symptomatic upper and lower respiratory tract infections by respiratory viruses in adult recipients of hematopoietic stem cell transplants for hematologic malignancies. Biol Blood Marrow Transplant 2005;11(10):781–96.

100. Shah DP, Ghantoji SS, Shah JN, et al. Impact of aerosolized ribavirin on mortality in 280 allogeneic haematopoietic stem cell transplant recipients with respiratory syncytial virus infections. J Antimicrob Chemother 2013;68(8):1872–80.

101. Shah DP, Ghantoji SS, Ariza-Heredia EJ, et al. Immunodeficiency scoring index to predict poor outcomes in hematopoietic cell transplant recipients with RSV infections. Blood 2014;123:1–7.

102. Waghmare A, Campbell AP, Xie H, et al. Respiratory syncytial virus lower respiratory disease in hematopoietic cell transplant recipients: viral RNA detection in blood, antiviral treatment, and clinical outcomes. Clin Infect Dis 2013;57(12):1731–41.

103. Khanna N, Widmer AF, Decker M, et al. Respiratory syncytial virus infection in patients with hematological diseases: single-center study and review of the literature. Clin Infect Dis 2008;46(3):402–12.

104. Hirsch HH, Martino R, Ward KN, et al. Fourth European Conference on Infections in Leukaemia (ECIL-4): guidelines for diagnosis and treatment of human respiratory syncytial virus, parainfluenza virus, metapneumovirus, rhinovirus, and coronavirus. Clin Infect Dis 2012;56(2):258–66.

105. Chemaly RF, Aitken SL, Wolfe CR, et al. Aerosolized ribavirin: the most expensive drug for pneumonia. Transpl Infect Dis 2016;18(4):634–6.

106. Beaird OE, Freifeld A, Ison MG, et al. Current practices for treatment of respiratory syncytial virus and other non-influenza respiratory viruses in high-risk patient populations: a survey of institutions in the Midwestern Respiratory Virus Collaborative. Transpl Infect Dis 2016;18(2):210–5.

107. DeVincenzo JP, McClure MW, Symons JA, et al. Activity of Oral ALS-008176 in a respiratory syncytial virus challenge study. N Engl J Med 2015; 373(21):2048–58.

108. DeVincenzo JP, Whitley RJ, Mackman RL, et al. Oral GS-5806 activity in a respiratory syncytial virus challenge study. N Engl J Med 2014;371(8): 711–22.

109. Erard V, Chien JW, Kim HW, et al. Airflow decline after myeloablative allogeneic hematopoietic cell transplantation: the role of community respiratory viruses. J Infect Dis 2006;193(12):1619–25.

110. Chemaly RF, Hanmod SS, Rathod DB, et al. The characteristics and outcomes of parainfluenza virus infections in 200 patients with leukemia or recipients of hematopoietic stem cell transplantation. Blood 2012;119(12):2738–45.

111. Srinivasan A, Wang C, Yang J, et al. Parainfluenza virus infections in children with hematologic malignancies. Pediatr Infect Dis J 2011;30(10):855–9.

112. Wendt CH, Weisdorf DJ, Jordan MC, et al. Parainfluenza virus respiratory infection after bone marrow transplantation. N Engl J Med 1992; 326(14):921–6.

113. Schiffer JT, Kirby K, Sandmaier B, et al. Timing and severity of community acquired respiratory virus infections after myeloablative versus nonmyeloablative hematopoietic stem cell transplantation. Haematologica 2009;94(8):1101–8.

114. Nichols WG, Corey L, Gooley T, et al. Parainfluenza virus infections after hematopoietic stem cell transplantation: risk factors, response to antiviral therapy, and effect on transplant outcome. Blood 2001;98(3):573–8.

115. Waghmare A, Wagner T, Andrews R, et al. Successful treatment of parainfluenza virus respiratory tract infection with DAS181 in 4 immunocompromised children. J Pediatr Infect Dis Soc 2015; 4(2):114–8.

116. Chen Y-B, Driscoll JP, McAfee SL, et al. Treatment of parainfluenza 3 infection with DAS181 in a patient after allogeneic stem cell transplantation. Clin Infect Dis 2011;53(7):e77–80.

117. de Mezerville MHN, Tellier R, Richardson S, et al. Adenoviral infections in pediatric transplant recipients. Pediatr Infect Dis J 2006;25(9):815–8.

118. Roch N, Salameire D, Gressin R, et al. Fatal adenoviral and enteroviral infections and an Epstein-Barr virus positive large B-cell lymphoma after alemtuzumab treatment in a patient with refractory Sézary syndrome. Scand J Infect Dis 2009;40(4):343–6.

119. Karlsson C, Lundin J, Kimby E, et al. Phase II study of subcutaneous alemtuzumab without dose escalation in patients with advanced-stage, relapsed chronic lymphocytic leukaemia. Br J Haematol 2009;144(1):78–85.

120. Bruno B, Gooley T, Hackman RC, et al. Adenovirus infection in hematopoietic stem cell transplantation: effect of ganciclovir and impact on survival. Biol Blood Marrow Transplant 2003;9(5):341–52.

121. Baldwin A, Kingman H, Darville M, et al. Outcome and clinical course of 100 patients with adenovirus infection following bone marrow transplantation. Bone Marrow Transplant 2000;26(12):1333–8.

122. Matthes-Martin S, Feuchtinger T, Shaw PJ, et al. European guidelines for diagnosis and treatment of adenovirus infection in leukemia and stem cell transplantation: summary of ECIL-4 (2011). Transpl Infect Dis 2012;14(6):555–63.

123. Yusuf U, Hale GA, Carr J, et al. Cidofovir for the treatment of adenoviral infection in pediatric hematopoietic stem cell transplant patients. Transplantation 2006;81(10):1398–404.

124. Legrand F, Berrebi D, Houhou N, et al. Early diagnosis of adenovirus infection and treatment with cidofovir after bone marrow transplantation in children. Bone Marrow Transplant 2001;27(6): 621–6.

125. Oliveira RR, Machado AF, Tateno AF, et al. Frequency of human metapneumovirus infection in hematopoietic SCT recipients during 3 consecutive years. Bone Marrow Transplant 2008;42(4):265–9.

126. Rattray RM, Press RD. The clinical impact of coronavirus infection in patients with hematologic malignancies and hematopoietic stem cell transplant recipients. J Clin Virol 2015;68:1–5.

127. Renaud C, Xie H, Seo S, et al. Mortality rates of human metapneumovirus and respiratory syncytial virus lower respiratory tract infections in hematopoietic cell transplantation recipients. Biol Blood Marrow Transplant 2013;19(8):1220–6.

128. Seo S, Gooley TA, Kuypers JM, et al. Human metapneumovirus infections following hematopoietic cell transplantation: factors associated with disease progression. Clin Infect Dis 2016;63(2): 178–85.

129. Dykewicz CA, National Center for Infectious Diseases, Centers for Disease Control and Prevention, Infectious Diseases Society of America, American Society for Blood and Marrow Transplantation. Guidelines for preventing opportunistic infections among hematopoietic stem cell transplant recipients: focus on community respiratory virus infections. Biol Blood Marrow Transplant 2001; 7(Suppl):19S–22S.

130. Sullivan KM, Dykewicz CA, Longworth DL, et al. Preventing opportunistic infections after hematopoietic stem cell transplantation: the Centers for Disease Control and Prevention, Infectious Diseases Society of America, and American Society for Blood and Marrow Transplantation Practice Guidelines and beyond. Hematol Am Soc Hematol Educ Program 2001;392–421.

Evaluation of Pulmonary Disease in Patients with Malignancy

Pulmonary Function and Pretransplant Evaluation of the Hematopoietic Cell Transplant Candidate

Guang-Shing Cheng, MD[a,b],*

KEYWORDS

- Pretransplant evaluation • Hematopoietic cell transplantation • Pulmonary function tests
- Pulmonary complications • Risk assessment • FEV$_1$ • DLCO

KEY POINTS

- Pretransplant pulmonary function tests establish lung function baseline and help detect pulmonary disease in hematopoietic cell transplant candidates.
- Pretransplant impairments in lung function are associated with an increase in posttransplant pulmonary complications and mortality.
- The use of formal risk assessment tools can aid in prognostication and clinical decision making before hematopoietic cell transplantation.

INTRODUCTION

Of all the organ-specific complications that can occur after allogeneic and autologous hematopoietic cell transplantation (HCT), pulmonary complications remain among the most significant in terms of incidence and impact on outcome of HCT recipients. Historically, pulmonary complications, infectious and noninfectious, affected up to 50% of HCT recipients and continues to be a primary cause of mortality in the early posttransplant period.[1] Early acute complications such as idiopathic pneumonia syndrome are less common in a contemporaneous era of transplantation; however, there remains significant use of the intensive care unit for respiratory failure in this population with an incidence of acute respiratory failure of up to 15% to 25% in allogeneic HCT recipients.[2] Patients who survive beyond 1 year and are cured of their original condition continue to experience pulmonary complications, which contribute to early mortality compared with the general population as well as other cancer patients.[3,4] The goal of this article is to update the practicing chest physician on current practices in HCT, discuss the impact of pulmonary dysfunction on the outcome of HCT recipients as well as the relevance of pretransplant pulmonary function evaluation, and provide recommendations for clinical practice.

RECENT DEVELOPMENTS IN HEMATOPOIETIC CELL TRANSPLANTATION

HCT has evolved from a salvage therapy for terminal malignancies to a widely accepted, life-saving procedure for a number of hematologic malignancies and nonmalignant conditions. As of December 2012, 1 million transplants have been

Disclosure Statement: The author has nothing to disclose.
[a] Clinical Research Division, Fred Hutchinson Cancer Research Center, 1100 Fairview Avenue North, D5-360, Seattle, WA 98109-1024, USA; [b] Division of Pulmonary and Critical Care Medicine, University of Washington School of Medicine, 1959 NE Pacific, Campus Box 356522, Seattle, WA 98195-6522, USA
* Fred Hutchinson Cancer Research Center, 1100 Fairview Avenue North, D5-360, Seattle, WA 98109-1024.
E-mail address: gcheng2@fredhutch.org

Clin Chest Med 38 (2017) 307–316
http://dx.doi.org/10.1016/j.ccm.2016.12.014
0272-5231/17/© 2017 Elsevier Inc. All rights reserved.

chestmed.theclinics.com

performed,[5] and more than 50,000 transplants are performed annually worldwide.[6] The rate of allogeneic transplants continues to increase. Since the first infusion of isolated marrow cells into terminally ill cancer patients in 1957, the technology and indications for HCT have expanded dramatically, in part owing to improved HLA typing, allowing for unrelated donors, the use of peripheral blood stem cells, cord blood cells, and now the use of haploidentical donors.

Historically, HCT was limited to younger patients owing to the significant toxicities associated with myeloablative conditioning regimens, which involve supralethal doses of total body irradiation (TBI) and high doses of chemotherapeutic agents. TBI is a well-documented cause of interstitial pneumonitis and severe pulmonary toxicity.[7,8] Although intensification of conditioning regimens reduced relapse of disease, the degree of nonrelapse mortality was unacceptably high for older patients or those with significant comorbidities. Observations that patients who developed graft-versus-host disease had lower rates of relapse led to the recognition of the graft-versus-tumor effect, in which the immune effects of the donor cells eliminate the malignancy. As a consequence, the intensity of the conditioning regimens could be reduced, allowing the use of HCT in older, previously ineligible patients. The use of reduced intensity conditioning, which used smaller doses of chemoradiation to achieve marrow ablation, and nonmyeloablative conditioning regimens has contributed to the expansion of HCT for patients with lower risk disease and with medical comorbidities.[9,10]

Although survival after HCT has improved in recent years with reduction in regimen-related toxicities as well as improvements in infectious prophylaxis, prophylaxis for graft-versus-host disease, and supportive care, HCT remains a treatment modality with significant risks for morbidity and mortality.[11] Given the significant medical, personal, social, and financial resources required to undertake HCT, meticulous evaluation of potential candidates is of utmost importance. Because acute respiratory failure from infectious and noninfectious causes contributes significantly to early nonrelapse mortality, lung function continues to carry significant weight in the assessment of eligibility and selection of a suitable transplant regimen.

ROLE OF PULMONARY FUNCTION TESTING BEFORE HEMATOPOIETIC CELL TRANSPLANTATION

As with preoperative evaluation in nontransplant settings, the pretransplant evaluation is done to ensure that a patient has sufficient physiologic fitness to survive the significant physiologic stresses associated with conditioning and engraftment and includes evaluation of cardiac, renal, hepatic, as well as pulmonary function. Although the majority of patients who present for transplantation have normal lung function, pulmonary function tests (PFTs) will identify patients who have serious pulmonary comorbidities that would limit candidacy for transplant. Overall, the prevalence of abnormalities in PFTs is greater for nonmyeloablative regimens compared with myeloablative regimens owing to the more permissive eligibility requirements.[12]

Given the expanded options for less toxic conditioning regimens in contemporary practice, very few patients will be denied transplant based on lung function alone. Most HCT centers routinely perform PFTs before transplant to establish a baseline by which to reference post-HCT lung function in the event of respiratory insufficiency. Lung function abnormalities before transplantation may be a result of toxic chemoradiation therapy, the sequelae of suppurative lung infections brought on by neutropenia, or preexisting medical lung disease such as smoking-related chronic obstructive pulmonary disease. At the minimum, PFTs are performed just before transplant, at day 80 to 100 after transplant, and then at 1 year.[13] It is recommended that patients who are at higher risk for developing late noninfectious complications, such as those with chronic graft-versus-host disease, undergo PFT screening more frequently.[14] The diagnosis of bronchiolitis obliterans syndrome, a late noninfectious pulmonary complication, is contingent on recognizing new spirometric decline compared with an established pretransplant baseline.[15]

In addition to establishing baseline lung function, pretransplant PFTs can aid in the prognostication and identification of individuals at greater risk for posttransplant complications and mortality. However, the practical usefulness of lung function parameters for prognostication remains a matter of debate, because these predictive tools are based on data from single centers in which transplant protocols, including the extensive use of TBI in myeloablative regimens, may not reflect current practices. There continues to be controversy about which parameters and the degree to which these impairments contribute to pulmonary complications and nonrelapse mortality, and specifically respiratory-related mortality, although there is general agreement that pulmonary dysfunction contributes to worse outcomes.

Spirometric Parameters

The impairment of forced expiratory volume in 1 second (FEV_1) is the lung function parameter associated most robustly with outcome; however, the evidence is limited to a few modest and large single-center retrospective cohort studies. The definition of early pulmonary complications varies, but includes the spectrum of acute lung injury syndromes and any cause of respiratory failure requiring mechanical ventilation. Early complications are generally accepted as occurring before day 100.[16] Studies from the 1980s and 1990s showed that a reduced FEV_1 was associated with early complications; however, the association with mortality remained controversial, perhaps owing to the relatively small numbers of patients and fatal respiratory events.[17–19] Notably, Crawford and Fisher[19] analyzed 1297 predominantly allogeneic HCT recipients (82%) during an early era of transplantation (1986–1990) and showed that gas exchange abnormalities, and not spirometric parameters or lung volumes, were associated with increased mortality.

In a larger, more contemporary cohort of 2852 allogeneic HCT recipients from the same center, Parimon and colleagues[20] showed that progressively more abnormal pretransplant FEV_1 was associated independently with stepwise increased risk of early respiratory failure, with an HR of 2.7 to 2.9 (95% confidence interval [CI], 1.7–4.2), and that a pretransplant FEV_1 of less than 70% predicted was associated with a 1.7- to 2.2-fold increase in mortality. Notably, diffusing capacity of carbon monoxide (DLCO) was also associated significantly with both outcomes and was independent of the degree of FEV_1 impairment. Based on these findings, the authors developed a pretransplant Lung Function Score (LFS) based on the combination of these 2 parameters (**Table 1**). For the first time, the posttransplant risk of respiratory failure and all-cause mortality could be quantified and stratified using pretransplant PFTs.[20] This measure was subsequently incorporated into the Pre-Transplant Assessment of Mortality (PAM), which will be discussed elsewhere in this article. The risk of mortality with an FEV_1 of less than 60% predicted has been shown to be reduced in patients undergoing nonmyeloablative versus myeloablative regimens, providing justification to consider nonmyeloablative regimens in patients with reduced lung function.[12]

Although rarely considered, indices of small airways dysfunction may add prognostic value to the pretransplant PFTs. Small airways dysfunction may precede a clinical decline in FEV_1, and therefore may be more sensitive in detecting patients at risk, particularly in the pediatric population. Analyses in children regarding the association of FEV_1 with early respiratory complications and overall survival are mixed, likely owing to the small cohorts, the inherent challenges of accurate measurements in this population, and the varying definitions of pulmonary complications, which remains predominantly infectious in children.[21,22] In a cohort of 410 children, pretransplant reduction of forced expiratory flow between 25% and 75% of forced vital capacity (FVC) was more common than FEV_1 decline, was lower in children with a pulmonary complication, and was predictive of a pulmonary complication, whereas FEV_1 was not.[22] The overall incidence of reduced pretransplant than FEV_1 abnormalities was low in this cohort, which may have impacted the discriminatory sensitivity of this parameter. A Japanese group applied an index of small airways obstruction to an predominantly adult population, 50% of vital capacity to 25% of vital capacity, to the pretransplant LFS, which had an improved discriminatory function for a group with the greatest risk for mortality.[20,23] Notably, the revised LFS was correlated

Table 1		
The pretransplant Lung Function Score for recipients of allogeneic hematopoietic cell transplantation		
Pretransplant LFS	**Pretransplant LFS Category**	**Description**
2	I	Normal
3–4	II	Mildly decreased
5–6	III	Moderately decreased
7–8	IV	Severely decreased

LFS is based on the sum of the score assigned to a forced expiratory volume in 1 second and percent diffusing capacity of carbon monoxide predicted, as follows: >80% = 1, 70% to 80% = 2, 60% to 70% = 3, <60% = 4.

Abbreviation: LFS, Lung Function Score.

Adapted from Parimon T, Madtes DK, Au DH, et al. Pretransplant lung function, respiratory failure, and mortality after stem cell transplantation. Am J Respir Crit Care Med 2005;172(3):388; with permission of the American Thoracic Society.

with age and degree of cigarette smoking, which was prevalent in 51% of this cohort. These observations are intriguing but require further investigation in larger cohorts.

Preexisting airflow obstruction, as defined by a reduced FEV$_1$/FVC, has not been associated with early complications and mortality in early studies, likely because the FEV$_1$ and FVC in pretransplant studies are highly correlated, and patients with clinically significant obstructive lung disease would have been ineligible for myeloablative transplant.[17,19,20] It is reasonable to extrapolate that patients with pretransplant obstructive lung disease and a reduction in FEV$_1$ would be at greater risk for poorer outcomes given the data on FEV$_1$. Reduced pretransplant FEV$_1$/FVC, however, has been associated with airflow obstruction at 1 year posttransplantation, which is a feature of bronchiolitis obliterans syndrome.[24,25]

Lung Volumes

Transplant candidates may have a restrictive pattern on PFTs for a variety of reasons: toxicity from prior chemotherapy and radiation therapy, neuromuscular weakness, or bulky and advanced intrathoracic disease.[13] Very few studies have focused on reduced total lung capacity (TLC) as a risk factor for outcomes, although TLC is usually included in studies investigating PFTs in general. Reduced pretransplant TLC is noted in fewer than 10% of patients presenting for HCT and has been associated with increased risk of early pulmonary complications in a number of studies involving both autologous and allogeneic recipients.[17,20,26,27] Crawford and Fisher's early study suggested a role for reduced TLC in predicting mortality (relative risk, 1.20; 95% CI, 1.09–1.32), but this did not add predictive value to the model when measurements of gas exchange (diffusing capacity and PA-aO$_2$) were included.[19] Reduced TLC correlated with FVC (r = 0.80) and FEV$_1$ (r = 0.61); therefore, this factor was not included in the development of the LFS.[20]

In a more recent study involving the largest series of 2595 allogeneic recipients specifically investigating the impact of restrictive lung disease, the majority of patients with a pretransplant TLC of less than 80% did not have any evidence of chest wall abnormality or parenchymal disease on radiographic imaging. There was a 2-fold greater risk of early respiratory failure and nonrelapse mortality that remained significant even if the most stringent definitions of restrictive lung disease were applied to subjects without evidence of parenchymal or chest wall disease, suggesting that pretransplant neuromuscular weakness may have contributed

to the patient's outcome.[26] These findings were corroborated in reduced-intensity conditioning allogeneic transplant recipients, in which a pretransplant TLC of less than 80% predicted was the only lung function parameter that was significantly associated with both pulmonary complications and nonrelapse mortality. One explanation for this finding is that reduced TLC from neuromuscular weakness reflects a heavily pretreated status, which increases the risk of poor outcomes. Of note, these subjects had a median of 6 prior lines of therapy compared with the entire cohort.[27]

Gas Exchange Abnormalities

Diffusing capacity refers to the lungs' ability in allowing oxygen to move from the air to the blood and is a function of the thickness of the alveolar membrane, the surface area available for gas exchange.[28] Most commonly assessed by the single breath (DLCO), sometimes referred to as the transfer factor, this measurement may also reflect the capillary blood volume, cardiac output, and heterogeneity in ventilation and diffusing capacity in anatomic regions of the lung and other conditions.[29] Because of the high prevalence of anemia in the transplant population, the DLCO calculation is always corrected for hemoglobin, rather than volume.[13] The measurement is also subject to various small correction factors for the specific equipment and technicalities. Therefore, there is potentially substantial variation in the predicted values between laboratories. Given these caveats, the interpretation of a reduced DLCO is frequently unclear, but nonetheless may reflect a global process that suggests the physiologic fitness of an individual—hence, DLCO has been given significant weight in the pretransplant assessment.

Many of the studies mentioned in this discussion of spirometry and lung volumes have also assessed the contribution of DLCO to respiratory failure and mortality. In Crawford and Fisher's influential early analysis, a DLCO of less than 80% had the greatest risk of mortality in a multivariate model (relative risk, 1.43; 95% CI, 1.26–1.64) followed by an alveolar-arterial partial pressure of oxygen difference (PA-aO$_2$) of greater than 20 mm Hg (relative risk, 1.28; 95% CI, 104–1.55) when adjusted for age, diagnosis, malignancy status, HLA matching, and after pulmonary function parameters were entered in a stepwise fashion.[19] The probability of receiving mechanical ventilation was greater if there were abnormalities in these parameters, but the risk of death was similar whether patients were ventilated or not, suggesting that death associated with reduced DLCO is not solely owing to respiratory failure. A follow-up study of this cohort found that a reduced DLCO of less than 70% predicted was an independent risk factor for the development of severe hepatic venoocclusive disease, with an odds ratio of 2.4 (95% CI, 1.0–5.4), suggesting that a reduced DLCO may reflect systemic endothelial cell damage present in the lungs and other organs such as the liver.[30] As noted, Parimon and colleagues[20] showed that a progressively worse DLCO was independently associated with stepwise increase in the likelihood for early respiratory failure, with a DLCO of 70% to 80% predicted conferring an HR of 1.7 (95% CI, 1.3–2.2) and a DLCO of less than 60% predicted conferring an HR of 3.4 (95% CI, 2.1–5.4). The DLCO added increased predictive value to the LFS for both early respiratory failure and mortality when considered with the FEV_1 (**Table 2**).[20]

Based on these studies, a DLCO threshold of 60% in the absence of other comorbid conditions was recommended as a cutoff for transplant for myeloablative regimens as recently as 2009. However, based on multiple studies suggesting that outcomes depend on a number of patient-related comorbidities and factors but are not limited to DLCO, the 60% threshold was evaluated in a retrospective analysis of 56 autologous recipients and 165 allogeneic recipients who received HCT with a DLCO of less than 60%. When the cohort was stratified by level of DLCO impairment (50%–60%, 40%–50%, <40%), there were no differences in the risk of respiratory failure or nonrelapse mortality. This finding was similar when allogeneic recipients were stratified by myeloablative or nonmyeloablative conditioning, suggesting that pretransplantation DLCO should not be the sole criteria for determining transplant eligibility. Interestingly, the majority of patients at day 80 experienced an improvement in DLCO.[31] It should be noted that the small numbers of patients with a DLCO of less than 40% included in this study likely reflects the fact that they were excluded from HCT.

A widened pretransplant $PA-aO_2$ is also associated with worse outcomes, but it is likely correlated to the degree of DLCO impairment.[20] Given the low incidence of a $PA-aO_2$ of greater than 20, there is little added usefulness in obtaining an arterial blood gas for routine pretransplant PFTs, although it can be helpful to assess oxygenation when there is a borderline DLCO.

LUNG FUNCTION AND TOOLS FOR RISK ASSESSMENT

Taken together, these observations of pretransplant lung function parameters confirm the clinical notion that reduced lung function contributes to worse outcomes. Myeloablative regimens have eligibility requirements of DLCO of greater than 50% to 60% predicted, which has more recently been modified to 50% at most centers.[32] whereas nonmyeloablative regimens have a DLCO requirement of greater than 40% predicted, with some regimens allowing patients as low as 30% predicted. The FEV_1 cutoffs are variable or unspecified, but in general an FEV_1 of less than 40% predicted is a contraindication for accepted protocols.

The most robust parameters—FEV_1 and DLCO, reflecting different aspects of lung function—have been incorporated into risk assessment tools to help prognosticate a patient's risk of dying from the transplant itself. Impairments in lung function reflect pretransplant comorbidities, which have a significant impact on survival and quality of life.[33] These risk stratification schemes have been developed for allogeneic HCT owing to the higher risk of organ damage and nonrelapse mortality compared with autologous HCT.[34] The 2 most clinically relevant schemes for pulmonologists are described.

Table 2
Pretransplant Lung Function Score and its association with early respiratory failure in a single center cohort of 2811 allogeneic HCT recipients

Pretransplant LFS Category	No Respiratory Failure (n = 2424), n (%)	Respiratory Failure (n = 387), n (%)	HR (95% CI)	P Value
I	1789 (74)	232 (60)	Referent	—
II	489 (20)	98 (25)	1.4 (1.3–1.6)	<.001
III	112 (5)	43 (11)	2.2 (1.8–2.6)	<.001
IV	34 (1)	14 (4)	3.1 (2.3–4.2)	<.001

Abbreviations: CI, confidence interval; HCT, hematopoietic cell transplantation; HR, hazard ratio; LFS, Lung Function Score.

Reprinted from Parimon T, Madtes DK, Au DH, et al. Pretransplant lung function, respiratory failure, and mortality after stem cell transplantation. Am J Respir Crit Care Med 2005;172(3):388; with permission of the American Thoracic Society.

The Pretransplant Assessment of Mortality Score

In a follow-up to the LFS, Parimon and colleagues[35] developed the Pretransplant Assessment of Mortality (PAM) from a patient sample of 2802 patients who underwent allogeneic HCT between 1990 and 2002. The authors' goal was to construct a simple tool that could reliably predict all-cause mortality within the first 2 years after transplantation.[35] Clinically significant factors in a multivariate Cox regression model included age, donor type, disease risk, conditioning regimen, serum creatinine, serum alanine aminotransferase level, FEV_1, and DLCO (**Table 3**). Each factor was assigned a score based on its weight in the multivariate model, which were summed to provide a score, which was broken down into quartiles by the hazard ratio for death. This scoring system was internally validated, which also accounted for the increasing use of nonmyeloablative conditioning regimens after 1997.

Because of the evolving nature of HCT practice, these assessment tools require periodic recalibration to reflect the population at risk. The original PAM score was based on a cohort with a high prevalence of myeloablative transplants with TBI. However, as more nonmyeloablative regimens became available to older patients, the original PAM variables needed to be reconsidered. In addition, additional risk stratification of the disease indication, specifically for acute myeloid leukemia and myelodysplastic syndromes, have been refined further.[36,37] In a reassessment of PAM in a contemporary cohort of 1549 patients, higher PAM scores were still associated with increasing 2-year mortality, but the association was weaker.[38] The authors chose a parsimonious approach in incorporating select factors that reflected the strongest associations for mortality into their model. Interestingly, DLCO fell out as a significant predictor of nonrelapse mortality (see **Table 3**). A possible explanation is that the range of DLCO measurements narrowed as patients in the recent cohort were highly selected based on other eligibility criteria, thus eliminating the ability to discriminate significant risk strata.

Hematopoietic Cell Transplantation-Specific Comorbidity Index

While the goal of the PAM was to provide a global assessment of mortality risk by combining patient risk factors with transplant characteristics, the hematopoietic cell transplantation-specific comorbidity index (HCT-CI) was developed to assess primarily the impact of a patient's pretransplant medical status. Sorror and colleagues[39] used a

Table 3 Clinical variables used in PAM and revised PAM scores	
PAM (2005)	**Revised PAM (2015)**
Patient age (y) • <60 • >60	Patient age (y) • <65 • ≥65
Donor type[a] • Matched related • Mismatched related • Unrelated	Donor type[b] • Matched related • Mismatched related • Unrelated, 10/10 • Unrelated, ≤9/10 • Cord blood
Disease risk[c] • Low • Intermediate • High	Disease risk[d] • Low • Intermediate • High • Very high
Conditioning regimen • Nonmyelablative • Non-TBI • TBI ≤12 Gy • TBI >12 Gy	FEV_1% predicted • Continuous variable
FEV_1% predicted • >80% • 70%–80% • <70%	Patient/donor CMV status • −/− • −/+ • +/− • +/+
DLCO % predicted • >80% • 70%–80% • <70%	
Serum alanine aminotransferase level • ≤ or >49 U/L	
Serum creatinine level • ≤ or >1.2 mg/dL	

Abbreviations: CMV, cytomegalovirus; DLCO, diffusing capacity of carbon monoxide; FEV_1, forced expiratory volume in 1 second; PAM, pretransplant assessment of mortality; TBI, total body irradiation.
[a] Matching determined according to HLA-A, HLA-B, and HLA-DR compatibility.
[b] Matching based on HLA-B, HLA-B, HLA-DR, and HLA-DQ compatibility.
[c] Disease risk determined based on outcomes observed at study center.
[d] Disease risk determined by risk index developed by Armand and colleagues[36] and myelodysplastic syndrome risk categories defined by Deeg and colleagues.[37]

cohort of 1055 subjects to score the impact of different comorbidities on 2-year nonrelapse mortality. The approach modified a well-accepted generalized risk assessment tool, the Charlson Comorbidity Index, to a population being considered for allogeneic HCT. The HCT-CI took into account transplant-specific organ complications as well as the different comorbidities encountered in HCT recipients owing to eligibility criteria.[40] Seventeen separate comorbidities (**Box 1**), including

---

Box 1
Comorbidities considered in the hematopoietic cell transplantation-specific comorbidity index

Arrhythmia

Cardiac dysfunction

- CAD, CHF, EF $\leq 50\%$

Cardiac valvular disease

Inflammatory bowel disease

Diabetes requiring medications

Cerebrovascular disease

Psychiatric disturbance

Hepatic dysfunction, mild

- Chronic hepatitis
- Bilirubin up to 1.5 × ULN
- AST/ALT up to 2.5 × ULN

Hepatic dysfunction, severe

- Cirrhosis
- Bilirubin greater than 1.5 × ULN
- AST/ALT greater than 2.5 × ULN

Obesity

- Body mass index >35 kg/m^2

Rheumatologic condition

Infection requiring ongoing treatment

Peptic ulcer disease requiring treatment

Renal dysfunction, moderate/severe

- Serum creatinine >2 mg/dL

Pulmonary dysfunction, moderate

- DLCO and/or FEV$_1$ 66% to 80% of predicted
- Dyspnea with slight activity

Pulmonary dysfunction, severe

- DLCO and/or FEV$_1$ 66% to 80% of predicted
- Dyspnea with slight activity

Prior solid malignancy excluding nonmelanoma skin cancer

Abbreviations: ALT, alanine aminotransferase; AST, aspartate aminotransferase; CAD, coronary artery disease; CHF, congestive heart failure; DLCO, diffusing capacity of carbon monoxide; EF, ejection fraction; FEV$_1$, forced expiratory volume in 1 second; ULN, upper limit of normal.

---

moderate pulmonary impairment (defined as DLCO and/or FEV$_1$ 66%–80% predicted, or dyspnea on slight activity) and severe pulmonary impairment (DLCO and/or FEV$_1$ $\leq 65\%$ or dyspnea at rest or requiring oxygen) were given a weighted score, which was summed to a composite score for 3 separate risk groups, which were low (0), intermediate (1–2), and high (≥ 3). This showed good discrimination of nonrelapse mortality, and has since been validated in other institutions on contemporary cohorts in both allogeneic and autologous HCT.[41,42] The HCT-CI is now widely accepted as a research tool to identify coexisting medical problems that should be measured in clinical trials and applied in retrospective studies. As a bedside tool for clinical decision making, a high score may have implications for the type of conditioning protocol used for the patient. As with the PAM score, the HCT-CI may not necessarily supersede clinical judgment, but can serve as a disclosure of anticipated risk.

ROLE OF OTHER RISK FACTORS IN PULMONARY COMPLICATIONS

The contribution of cigarette smoking to morbidity and mortality after HCT is controversial. Cigarette smoking is frequently included in retrospective risk factor analyses for pulmonary complications, but a robust contribution to morbidity and mortality has not been shown definitely.[17,18,43,44] This may be owing to the difficulty of quantifying smoking exposure a self-reported measure. Increased risk of respiratory complications in cigarette smokers was shown in a retrospective study of 845 allogeneic transplant recipients. An association with respiratory failure may have been mediated in part by lung function abnormalities or to the cardiovascular effects of cigarette smoking.[44] A recent report suggested that tobacco smoking is associated with pulmonary infections after HCT in a dose-dependent fashion. The cumulative incidence of pulmonary complications was 26% in never smokers, 36% in low-dose smokers, and 46% in high-dose smokers.[45]

Harris and colleagues[46] reported recently an association of gut microbiota with pulmonary infiltrates after allogeneic HCT. Pulmonary complications were prevalent in 70% of a cohort of 94 patients who were enrolled previously in a prospective study for the sequencing of 16S ribosomal RNA of the fecal microbiome patients undergoing allogeneic transplantation. Pulmonary infiltrates were associated with a high HCT-CI index, use of fluoroquinolones, low baseline fecal microbiota diversity, as well as posttransplant dominance of gammaproteobacteria, a phylum that includes nosocomial gram-negative pathogens of the lung such as *Klebsiella* and *Escherichia* spp. In addition, dominance of the gamma-proteobacteria in the gut as well as the development of pulmonary complications were independent risk factors for mortality. These intriguing findings suggest a role for the gut–lung axis in the pathogenesis of pulmonary disease after HCT and potential biomarker candidates for pretransplant risk assessment; further research is needed to elaborate on these findings.[46]

RECOMMENDATIONS FOR PULMONARY EVALUATION BEFORE HEMATOPOIETIC STEM CELL TRANSPLANTATION

The most common reasons for a pulmonologist to be consulted before proceeding with HCT are for the evaluation of abnormalities in either PFTs or chest imaging. Because active infection is a contraindication for proceeding with conditioning and transplantation, patients with chest imaging abnormalities should be evaluated for infectious etiologies. Usually, the consultation is directed specifically toward the question of whether a patient can proceed with transplant in light of a PFT abnormality. A series of stepwise considerations are recommended as follows.

Is There a Reversible Etiology of the Underlying Abnormality?

Reduced FEV_1 and DLCO are the most common abnormal pretransplant parameters. FEV_1 abnormalities may reflect preexisting airways disease, such as asthma or chronic obstructive pulmonary disease, or ventilatory dysfunction from neuromuscular weakness. An isolated DLCO abnormality may reflect a variety of etiologies, but in many instances the patient is asymptomatic and there will be no apparent explanation after a workup that includes a transthoracic echocardiogram to exclude pulmonary hypertension and chest tomography to exclude occult interstitial lung disease. An arterial blood gas measurement may be required to ensure adequate oxygenation; if there is evidence of hypoxemia, further evaluation with exercise oximetry is warranted.

Can Transplantation Be Reasonably Delayed if Further Workup and Treatment Are Warranted?

Modifiable etiologies of lung dysfunction such as asthma and infection should be treated before transplantation to reduce the transplant-related risk. An isolated, asymptomatic reduction in DLCO without resting hypoxemia in which the basic workup (arterial blood gas, echocardiogram, chest imaging) has not revealed a distinct etiology is generally not a reason to delay transplantation. Decisions on whether or not to move forward with transplantation in a patient with significant lung dysfunction necessarily need to be closely discussed with the transplant physician, as the oncologic issues may ultimately outweigh the risk of pulmonary morbidity. It is rare that a patient will be denied a transplant solely owing to PFT abnormalities, but reduced lung function may alter the specific protocol for conditioning, which has additional clinical implications, because the efficacy in achieving remission or resolution of the underlying disease depends on the disease status as well as the regimen selected.

If Transplantation Cannot Be Delayed, What Is the Risk of Going into Transplant with Such an Abnormality? Does the Pretransplant Risk Outweigh the Potential Benefit of Transplantation?

In cases when the urgency of the transplant precludes additional diagnostics or treatment for lung dysfunction, the primary question is whether the patient is still an appropriate candidate for a specific conditioning regimen vis-à-vis additional risk for mortality from pulmonary dysfunction. Here, the PAM score can be helpful in counseling patients as well as the transplant team with regard to their overall risk for mortality. A simple online calculator for the revised PAM score is available at pamscore.org. Although the PAM score can be calculated in the office with only 5 readily available factors, the score does not take into account the patient's functional status or other lung function parameters. The HCT-CI more comprehensively considers the patient's functional status with the PFT parameters; however, the calculation of HCT-CI can be time consuming because it requires data that may not be readily available to the consulting pulmonologist at the point of service. An online calculator for the HCT-CI can be found at hctci.org. An estimate of the risk of mortality as per the PAM or HCT-CI serves as a disclosure of the risk of proceeding with the potentially lifesaving and life-threatening procedure of HCT. Clearly, if the risk of dying from the procedure exceeds the benefit of cure, then HCT should not be performed. Ultimately, the decision to proceed with a transplant comes down to a carefully weighed assessment of the risks and benefits for a specific patient performed by the entire team, which includes the consulting pulmonologist.

SUMMARY

The lungs are a significant site of injurious side effects from allogeneic HCT. The routine assessment of lung function is essential for determining eligibility and pretransplant risk reduction for this lifesaving but potentially morbid procedure. As indications for HCT expand and become available to a wider range of individuals with comorbidities, it will be important to update the validity of lung function parameters in the risk assessment of posttransplant pulmonary complications and mortality.

REFERENCES

1. Soubani AO, Miller KB, Hassoun PM. Pulmonary complications of bone marrow transplantation. Chest 1996;109(4):1066–77.

2. Yadav H, Nolan ME, Bohman JK, et al. Epidemiology of acute respiratory distress syndrome following hematopoietic stem cell transplantation. Crit Care Med 2016;44(6):1082–90.

3. Chow EJ, Cushing-Haugen KL, Cheng GS, et al. Morbidity and mortality differences between hematopoietic cell transplantation survivors and other cancer survivors. J Clin Oncol 2017;35(3):306–13.

4. Atsuta Y, Hirakawa A, Nakasone H, et al. Late mortality and causes of death among long-term survivors after allogeneic stem cell transplantation. Biol Blood Marrow Transplant 2016;22(9):1702–9.

5. Niederweiser D, Pasquini M, Aljurf M, et al. Global Hematopoietic Stem Cell Transplantation (HSCT) at one million: an achievement of pioneers and foreseeable challenges for the next decade. A report from the Worldwide Network for Blood and Marrow Transplantation (WBMT). Blood 2012;122(21):2133.

6. Pasquini M, Zhu X. Current uses and outcomes of hematopoietic stem cell transplantation: CIBMTR Summary Slides. 2015. Available at: http://www.cibmtr.org. Accessed January 29, 2017.

7. Kelsey CR, Horwitz ME, Chino JP, et al. Severe pulmonary toxicity after myeloablative conditioning using total body irradiation: an assessment of risk factors. Int J Radiat Oncol Biol Phys 2011;81(3):812–8.

8. Abugideiri M, Nanda RH, Butker C, et al. Factors influencing pulmonary toxicity in children undergoing allogeneic hematopoietic stem cell transplantation in the setting of total body irradiation-based myeloablative conditioning. Int J Radiat Oncol Biol Phys 2016;94(2):349–59.

9. Deeg HJ, Sandmaier BM. Who is fit for allogeneic transplantation? Blood 2010;116(23):4762–70.

10. Gyurkocza B, Sandmaier BM. Conditioning regimens for hematopoietic cell transplantation: one size does not fit all. Blood 2014;124(3):344–53.

11. Gooley TA, Chien JW, Pergam SA, et al. Reduced mortality after allogeneic hematopoietic-cell transplantation. N Engl J Med 2010;363(22):2091–101.

12. Chien JW, Maris MB, Sandmaier BM, et al. Comparison of lung function after myeloablative and 2 Gy of total body irradiation-based regimens for hematopoietic stem cell transplantation. Biol Blood Marrow Transplant 2005;11(4):288–96.

13. Chien JW, Madtes DK, Clark JG. Pulmonary function testing prior to hematopoietic stem cell transplantation. Bone Marrow Transplant 2005;35(5):429–35.

14. Carpenter PA, Kitko CL, Elad S, et al. National Institutes of Health Consensus Development Project on criteria for clinical trials in chronic graft-versus-host disease: V. The 2014 Ancillary Therapy and Supportive Care Working Group Report. Biol Blood Marrow Transplant 2015;21(7):1167–87.

15. Jagasia MH, Greinix HT, Arora M, et al. National Institutes of Health Consensus Development Project on criteria for clinical trials in chronic graft-versus-host disease: I. The 2014 Diagnosis and Staging Working Group Report. Biol Blood Marrow Transplant 2015;21(3):389–401.e1.

16. Cheng GS, Madtes DK. Acute pulmonary complications of bone marrow and stem cell transplantation. In: Lee SJ, Donahoe MP, editors. Hematologic abnormalities and acute lung syndromes. Basel (Switzerland): Springer International; 2016. p. 147–74.

17. Ghalie R, Szidon JP, Thompson L, et al. Evaluation of pulmonary complications after bone marrow transplantation: the role of pretransplant pulmonary function tests. Bone Marrow Transplant 1992;10(4):359–65.

18. Ho VT, Weller E, Lee SJ, et al. Prognostic factors for early severe pulmonary complications after hematopoietic stem cell transplantation. Biol Blood Marrow Transplant 2001;7(4):223–9.

19. Crawford SW, Fisher L. Predictive value of pulmonary function tests before marrow transplantation. Chest 1992;101(5):1257–64.

20. Parimon T, Madtes DK, Au DH, et al. Pretransplant lung function, respiratory failure, and mortality after stem cell transplantation. Am J Respir Crit Care Med 2005;172(3):384–90.

21. Kaya Z, Weiner DJ, Yilmaz D, et al. Lung function, pulmonary complications, and mortality after allogeneic blood and marrow transplantation in children. Biol Blood Marrow Transplant 2009;15(7):817–26.

22. Srinivasan A, Srinivasan S, Sunthankar S, et al. Pre-hematopoietic stem cell transplant lung function and pulmonary complications in children. Ann Am Thorac Soc 2014;11(10):1576–85.

23. Nakamae M, Yamashita M, Koh H, et al. Lung function score including a parameter of small airway disease as a highly predictive indicator of survival after allogeneic hematopoietic cell transplantation. Transpl Int 2016;29(6):707–14.

24. Chien JW, Martin PJ, Gooley TA, et al. Airflow obstruction after myeloablative allogeneic hematopoietic stem cell transplantation. Am J Respir Crit Care Med 2003;168(2):208–14.

25. Chien JW, Martin PJ, Flowers ME, et al. Implications of early airflow decline after myeloablative allogeneic stem cell transplantation. Bone Marrow Transplant 2004;33(7):759–64.

26. Ramirez-Sarmiento A, Orozco-Levi M, Walter EC, et al. Influence of pretransplantation restrictive lung disease on allogeneic hematopoietic cell transplantation outcomes. Biol Blood Marrow Transplant 2010; 16(2):199–206.

27. Pinana JL, Martino R, Barba P, et al. Pulmonary function testing prior to reduced intensity conditioning allogeneic stem cell transplantation in an unselected patient cohort predicts posttransplantation pulmonary complications and outcome. Am J Hematol 2012;87(1):9–14.

28. Powell FL, Wagner PE, West JB. Ventilation, blood flow, and gas exchange. Murray and Nadel's textbook of respiratory medicine. 6th edition. Philadelphia: Elsevier Saunders; 2015. p. 44–75.

29. West JB. Respiratory physiology: the essentials. 8th edition. Philadelphia: Lippincott Williams and Wilkins; 2008.

30. Matute-Bello G, McDonald GD, Hinds MS, et al. Association of pulmonary function testing abnormalities and severe veno-occlusive disease of the liver after marrow transplantation. Bone Marrow Transplant 1998;21(11):1125–30.

31. Chien JW, Sullivan KM. Carbon monoxide diffusion capacity: how low can you go for hematopoietic cell transplantation eligibility? Biol Blood Marrow Transplant 2009;15(4):447–53.

32. Hamadani M, Craig M, Awan FT, et al. How we approach patient evaluation for hematopoietic stem cell transplantation. Bone Marrow Transplant 2010;45(8):1259–68.

33. Sorror M. Impacts of pretransplant comorbidities on allogeneic hematopoietic cell transplantation (HCT) outcomes. Biol Blood Marrow Transplant 2009;15(1 Suppl):149–53.

34. Elsawy M, Sorror ML. Up-to-date tools for risk assessment before allogeneic hematopoietic cell transplantation. Bone Marrow Transplant 2016; 51(10):1283–300.

35. Parimon T, Au DH, Martin PJ, et al. A risk score for mortality after allogeneic hematopoietic cell transplantation. Ann Intern Med 2006;144(6):407–14.

36. Armand P, Gibson CJ, Cutler C, et al. A disease risk index for patients undergoing allogeneic stem cell transplantation. Blood 2012;120(4):905–13.

37. Deeg HJ, Scott BL, Fang M, et al. Five-group cytogenetic risk classification, monosomal karyotype, and outcome after hematopoietic cell transplantation for MDS or acute leukemia evolving from MDS. Blood 2012;120(7):1398–408.

38. Au BK, Gooley TA, Armand P, et al. Reevaluation of the pretransplant assessment of mortality score after allogeneic hematopoietic transplantation. Biol Blood Marrow Transplant 2015;21(5):848–54.

39. Sorror ML, Maris MB, Storb R, et al. Hematopoietic cell transplantation (HCT)-specific comorbidity index: a new tool for risk assessment before allogeneic HCT. Blood 2005;106(8):2912–9.

40. Charlson ME, Pompei P, Ales KL, et al. A new method of classifying prognostic comorbidity in longitudinal studies: development and validation. J Chronic Dis 1987;40(5):373–83.

41. Sorror ML, Logan BR, Zhu X, et al. Prospective validation of the predictive power of the hematopoietic cell transplantation comorbidity index: a center for International Blood and Marrow Transplant Research Study. Biol Blood Marrow Transplant 2015;21(8): 1479–87.

42. ElSawy M, Storer BE, Pulsipher MA, et al. Multicentre validation of the prognostic value of the haematopoietic cell transplantation- specific comorbidity index among recipient of allogeneic haematopoietic cell transplantation. Br J Haematol 2015; 170(4):574–83.

43. Savani BN, Montero A, Wu C, et al. Prediction and prevention of transplant-related mortality from pulmonary causes after total body irradiation and allogeneic stem cell transplantation. Biol Blood Marrow Transplant 2005;11(3):223–30.

44. Tran BT, Halperin A, Chien JW. Cigarette smoking and outcomes after allogeneic hematopoietic stem cell transplantation. Biol Blood Marrow Transplant 2011;17(7):1004–11.

45. Hanajiri R, Kakihana K, Kobayashi T, et al. Tobacco smoking is associated with infectious pulmonary complications after allogeneic hematopoietic stem cell transplantation. Bone Marrow Transplant 2015; 50(8):1141–3.

46. Harris B, Morjaria SM, Littmann ER, et al. Gut microbiota predict pulmonary infiltrates after allogeneic hematopoietic cell transplantation. Am J Respir Crit Care Med 2016;194(4):450–63.

Diagnostic Evaluation of Pulmonary Abnormalities in Patients with Hematologic Malignancies and Hematopoietic Cell Transplantation

Bianca Harris, MD, MSc[a],*, Alexander I. Geyer, MD[a,b]

KEYWORDS

- Pulmonary complications • Lung infiltrates • Hematopoietic cell transplant
- Hematologic malignancy • Diagnosis • Pneumonia • Bronchoscopy

KEY POINTS

- Patients with hematologic malignancies and recipients of hematopoietic cell transplantation are highly susceptible to pulmonary complications.
- Early diagnosis of pulmonary complications is challenging. Delayed diagnosis limits opportunity for targeted treatment, and may contribute to poor outcomes, including mortality.
- An integrated clinicoradiologic approach to diagnosing pulmonary complications provides some insight into their nature, and guides the risk/benefit assessment in pursuing lung sampling.
- Diagnostic bronchoscopy should be considered promptly in these immunocompromised populations, especially in the presence of high-risk features, such as neutropenia and posttransplant status.

INTRODUCTION

Pulmonary complications (PC) of hematologic malignancies (HM) and their treatments, including hematopoietic cell transplantation (HCT), are common causes of morbidity and mortality.[1,2] Despite advances in management,[3] these patients remain highly susceptible to lung injury involving one or more anatomic compartments of the lower respiratory tract (LRT), especially the lung parenchyma. Vulnerability to parenchymal PCs is multifactorial, determined largely by the type, magnitude, and duration of impaired immune defense.[4] This risk is compounded further by treatment-related toxicities, complex comorbidities, and recurrent nosocomial exposures.

Patients at greatest risk for infectious PCs include those with prolonged neutropenia[5] and recipients of HCT.[6] Infectious and noninfectious parenchymal PCs occur in up to 70% of allogeneic HCT patients[1] (25% after autologous HCT[7]), frequently in the acute setting,[8] and represent the most common cause for admission to the intensive care unit.[9] PCs significantly increase mortality, both during treatment (eg, during induction therapy for acute leukemias[10]) and in later periods, after HCT.[1,11] This predisposition requires clinical vigilance in the formulation of a differential diagnosis, in performing prompt diagnostic investigations, and in the initiation of treatment.

Disclosure Statement: The authors have nothing to disclose.
[a] Pulmonary Service, Department of Medicine, Memorial Sloan Kettering Cancer Center, 1275 York Avenue, New York, NY 10065, USA; [b] Weill Cornell Medical College, 1300 York Avenue, New York, NY 10065, USA
* Corresponding author.
E-mail address: harrisb@mskcc.org

Clin Chest Med 38 (2017) 317–331
http://dx.doi.org/10.1016/j.ccm.2016.12.008
0272-5231/17/© 2016 Elsevier Inc. All rights reserved.

In practice, a specific cause of pulmonary disease is frequently undiagnosed ante mortem in this population.[12-14] An elusive understanding of disease mechanisms, notably inflammatory HCT-related PCs, may contribute to this disparity. However, the lack of a diagnosis also reflects delayed, if not altogether deferred, diagnostic sampling of the LRT in the setting of excessive patient risk and/or provider preference. It has been suggested that diagnostic uncertainty regarding PCs may impact mortality after HCT.[15,16] Difficulty obtaining a timely diagnosis naturally interferes with the clinician's ability to target treatment, leading to prolonged empirical management of many PCs. With the institution of these broad therapies come exposures to unnecessary toxicities, ripe conditions for the emergence of antibiotic resistance, and possibly the acceleration of poor outcomes.

Given the incidence of acute and often fatal PCs in this highly immunocompromised population, a comprehensive approach to the diagnostic evaluation of PCs in HM and HCT patients is essential. The integration of information regarding high-risk host features, abnormal chest imaging patterns, and noninvasive test results informs decisions to pursue lung sampling via minimally invasive techniques, such as fiberoptic bronchoscopy (FOB), or other modalities. The goal of this paper is to provide an overview of the considerations and practices in the diagnostic approach to the adult HM and HCT patient with respiratory signs and symptoms, with a focus on investigating PCs involving the lung parenchyma.

DIAGNOSTIC APPROACH
Context

An initial survey of the clinical landscape is essential to ascertain PC risk and to determine subsequent diagnostic steps. Timing of presentation, host characteristics, immune deficits, treatment-related factors, and past exposures may each impact the risk/benefit equation for LRT sampling in an HM or HCT patient with new pulmonary infiltrates on chest imaging. The identification of high-risk features (eg, prolonged neutropenia or known mold exposure) may also raise suspicion of a specific disease entity (eg, invasive fungal infection), early enough to expedite lung sampling while initiating presumptive therapy.

Immune defects

Understanding the timing of respiratory symptom onset relative to immunosuppressive treatments[17] can help to narrow the differential diagnosis of PCs. Defects in innate, cell-mediated, and humoral immunity, as well as splenic defects, each predispose to infection by specific organisms[18] (Table 1).

Table 1
Immune defects and associated pathogens in hematologic malignancies and HCT

Immune Impairment	Potential Causes	Spectrum of Respiratory Infections
Neutrophil number/function	Leukemia Lymphoma Myelodysplastic syndrome Cytoreductive therapies Corticosteroids Hematopoietic stem cell transplant	Gram-negative bacilli Gram-positive cocci Invasive molds (eg, *Aspergillus* spp, *Mucorales*, *Fusarium*, *Scedosporium*)

T lymphocytes	Lymphoma
	Corticosteroids
	T-cell depletion
	Drugs
	  Calcineurin inhibitors
	  Mammalian target of rapamycin inhibitors
		Intracellular bacteria (eg, *Nocardia*, mycobacteria, legionella)
		Viruses (eg, respiratory viruses, latent Herpesviridae)
		Fungi (eg, *Pneumocystis jirovecii*, *Cryptococcus* spp, *Histoplasma capsulatum*, *Coccidioides* spp, *Aspergillus* spp, *Micorales*, *Fusarium*, *Scedosporium*)
		Parasites (eg, *Strongyloides* spp, *Toxoplasma* spp)

B lymphocytes and humoral immunity	Leukemia Multiple myeloma Anti–B-cell antibodies Splenectomy Plasmapheresis Drugs	Encapsulated bacterial (eg, *Pneumococcus*, *H influenza*) *Mycoplasma* spp

Neutropenia is the most common individual risk factor for cancer-related pneumonia, and a greater than 20% risk of febrile neutropenia (FN) can be expected with specific chemotherapy regimens for many types of HM.[19] The underlying HM may also exacerbate treatment-related deficits in cell function,[20] albeit less predictably.

Recipients of HCTs have additional treatment-related risk factors for PCs, including intensity of the conditioning regimen, stem cell source, prolonged cytopenias, and intensified immunosuppression for graft-versus-host disease.[1,6] Pretransplant conditioning confers a shared susceptibility to PCs both before and after engraftment[6] (**Fig. 1**). Preengraftment PCs are usually infectious and occur within 30 days of HCT. These commonly include Gram-negative bacterial pneumonias in the setting of neutropenia and/or mucositis. Early postengraftment PCs, which occur

between days 30 and 100, typically include infectious processes associated with impaired cellular immunity. Late- postengraftment PCs tend to develop after day 100, typically after immune reconstitution. Atypical processes may occur outside of these expected windows based on additional host risk factors (eg, opportunistic infection late after engraftment in the setting of delayed antibody response[21]). PCs occurring before engraftment, which are predominantly infectious, are associated with significantly lower mortality compared with those that develop later.[1]

It is more difficult to predict the timing of noninfectious PCs after HCT. A spectrum of acute lung injury syndromes may parallel endothelial damage that can occur at other organ sites (eg, the liver) early after HCT.[2,22] Preengraftment syndrome and diffuse alveolar hemorrhage develop soon after allogeneic or autologous HCT, whereas

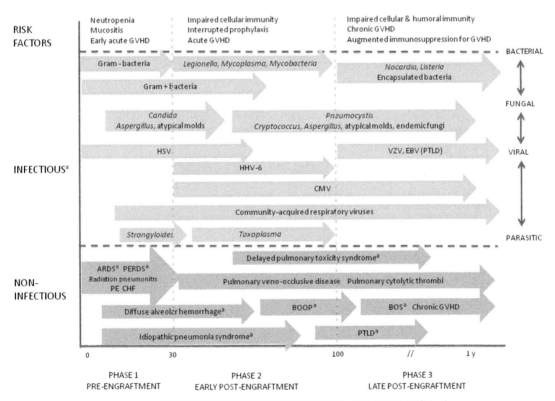

Fig. 1. Infectious and noninfectious pulmonary complications of hematopoietic cell transplantation. ARDS, acute respiratory distress syndrome; BOOP, bronchiolitis obliterans organizing pneumonia; BOS, bronchiolitis obliterans syndrome; CHF, congestive heart failure; CMV, cytomegalovirus; EBV, Epstein–Barr virus; GVHD, graft-versus-host disease; HHV-6, human herpes virus-6; HSV, herpes simplex virus; PE, pulmonary embolism; PERDS, periengraftment respiratory distress syndrome; PTLD, posttransplant lymphoproliferative disorder; VZV, varicella zoster virus. [a] Consider diagnostic bronchoscopy to (1) establish or rule out an infectious etiology, and/or (2) diagnose a noninfectious etiology for the pulmonary complication. (*Reproduced from* Harris B, Lowy FD, Stover DE, et al. Diagnostic bronchoscopy in solid-organ and hematopoietic stem cell transplantation. Ann Am Thorac Soc 2013;10(1):41; with permission.)

idiopathic pneumonia syndrome occurs somewhat later, albeit during the first 100 days after allogenic HCT. Although these processes are variably steroid responsive, both diffuse alveolar hemorrhage and idiopathic pneumonia syndrome are associated with high mortality,[23,24] and mortality after preengraftment syndrome tends to be significantly less.[25] Of note, acute respiratory distress syndrome in HCT subjects is most often associated with an infectious etiology, and carries a very high mortality in the setting of invasive fungal disease.[26] Thus, early recognition and appropriate intervention for both infectious and noninfectious transplant-related PCs is imperative to successful outcomes.

Risk factors

The medical histories of HM and HCT patients are among the most complex, representing unique disease chronologies, treatment courses/responses, and comorbidities. A history of tobacco smoking[10,27] and conditions such as chronic obstructive pulmonary disease predispose LRT colonization by bacterial pathogens,[28] thereby increasing the risk of infectious PCs. The development of mucositis, a common complication of myeloablative chemotherapies, may impair airway clearance and nutritional intake, thereby increasing the risk of pneumonia and bacteremic events.[29] Noninfectious causes of PCs may be suggested by a history of pneumotoxic chemotherapy (eg, bleomycin, alkylating agents, radiation therapy, non–cancer-related medications (eg, amiodarone), and transfusion of blood products. A history of pulmonary disease or cardiac dysfunction may increase risk of drug-related lung toxicities influence the acuity of their presentation.

Pretransplant pulmonary function should be considered in the assessment of PC risk after HCT, in particular. Reduced lung function, as measured by pulmonary function testing, has been associated with severe PCs occurring early after HCT.[30] Abnormalities in the diffusing lung capacity for carbon monoxide and the forced expiratory volume in 1 second also contribute to the HCT-Co-morbidity Index, a validated prognostic indicator of posttransplant mortality.[31,32] Ongoing investigations of microbial biomarkers in allogeneic HCT recipients suggest that changes in gut flora, which commonly occur within days of initiating pretransplant conditioning and antimicrobial prophylaxis,[33] may increase the likelihood of developing PCs.[1] This may occur either via direct translocation of infectious agents, or indirectly via stimulation of an aberrant pulmonary inflammatory response. Importantly, gut microbiota changes and PCs may be significant and independent predictors of transplant-related mortality.[1,33,34] This finding highlights a need for continued development of tools for identifying at-risk populations.

Exposures

Although many common respiratory tract infections arise from the patient's own microbial flora, others are contracted through exposure to sick individuals or environmental sources. Eliciting such exposures is important in surveying the landscape for potential infections, both de novo (eg, multidrug-resistant organisms in the hospital setting) and with reactivation of latent infections. Patients should be questioned about travel or residence in areas with exposures to *Mycobacterium tuberculosis* and endemic fungal organisms, including *Histoplasma capsulatum*, *Coccidioides immitis*, *Blastomyces dermatitidis*, and others. Inquiry regarding exposures to house pets, birds, farm animals, aerosolized water sources, and disturbed soil dust can provide clues to infections caused by diverse organisms, such as Nocardia species (spp), Legionella *spp*, *Toxoplasma gondii*, and *Cryptococcus neoformans*. Immunologic evidence of the patient's (and donor's, in the case of allogeneic HCT) history of latent infection with cytomegalovirus, Epstein–Barr virus, *T gondii*, or *M tuberculosis* need to be reviewed carefully. These exposures should be kept in mind in considering additional noninvasive or invasive diagnostic investigations to pursue beyond routine testing.

Presentation

PCs can broadly be categorized as infectious, inflammatory, malignant, or "other" (**Fig. 2**). Processes within each group share a common identity based on their predominant pathophysiology, although with some overlap, as in Epstein–Barr virus–related posttransplant lymphoproliferative disorder. The presence of abnormal vital signs (eg, fever, hypoxemia) and respiratory symptoms (eg, dyspnea, cough) does not readily distinguish between PC processes, whose presentations may vary further by underlying HM.[35] For example, hemoptysis may suggest alveolar hemorrhage; however, its absence is common in diffuse alveolar hemorrhage. Hypoxemia with an elevated alveolar-arterial gradient may suggest *Pneumocystis jirovecii* pneumonia as the etiology of patchy ground glass opacities on chest imaging, but further investigation for an alternate explanation, such as pulmonary embolism, may be required if radiographic findings seem out of proportion to the gas exchange abnormality. The acuity of presentation may provide

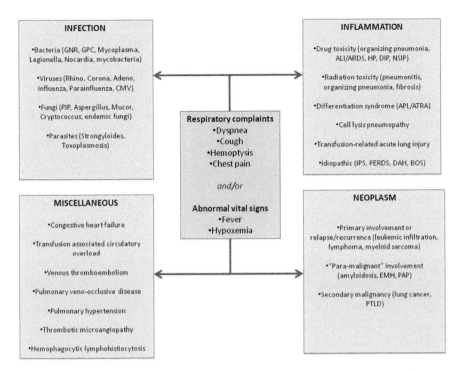

Fig. 2. Spectrum of pulmonary complications in patients with hematologic malignancies and in hematopoietic cell transplant recipients. ALI, acute lung injury; APL, acute promyelocytic leukemia; ARDS, acute respiratory distress syndrome; ATRA, all-trans retinoic acid; BOS, bronchiolitis obliterans syndrome; CMV, cytomegalovirus; DAH, diffuse alveolar hemorrhage; DIP, desquamative interstitial pneumonia; EMH, extramedullary hematopoiesis; GNR, gram-negative rods; GPC, gram-positive cocci; HP, hypersensitivity pneumonitis; IPS, idiopathic pneumonia syndrome; NSIP, nonspecific interstitial pneumonia; PAP, pulmonary alveolar proteinosis; PERDS, periengraftment respiratory distress syndrome; PJP, *Pneumocystis jiroveci* pneumonia; PTLD, posttransplant lymphoproliferative disease.

additional insight into the differential diagnosis in the appropriate context; for example, acute hypoxemia and new crackles in the setting of a blood product transfusion may suggest suggestive of transfusion-related acute lung injury or transfusion-associated circulation overload. However, further investigation into the PC cause is indicated more often than not.

Chest Imaging

Modality

Chest imaging is generally obtained for diagnosis of HMs with pulmonary manifestations, and for working up a suspicious sign or unexplained fever during management. The latter indication is common after HCT[35] and in the setting of neutropenia, where 15% of patients with FN present with lung infiltrates.[36] The distribution and morphology of infiltrates can help to refine the PC differential diagnosis, although a diminished inflammatory response may alter or delay the appearance of typical findings. There are significant limitations to the sensitivity of chest radiographs

for diagnosing PCs in HM and HCT patients, even when combined with clinical data.[37,38] In 1 study of febrile immunocompromised patients, one-half of those with a negative chest radiograph had parenchymal abnormalities detected on computed tomography (CT) imaging of the chest.[37] Thus, a reliance on CT imaging of the chest as the initial diagnostic imaging modality is commonplace in the management of the compromised host with respiratory complaints.[39] Chest CT is also performed routinely for disease surveillance during treatment of certain HMs (eg, lymphoma) and may be useful for comparison when diagnostic chest radiographs suggest a new PC. The special role of high-resolution CT has been considered useful in HM and HCT subgroups; however, their interpretation is not considered "unambiguous."[39–41] PET scanning may be useful for the evaluation of a solitary pulmonary nodule,[42] and MRI may be required when a subject cannot receive iodinated contrast for a CT study, although a noncontrast CT is generally sufficient for the evaluation of parenchymal infiltrates.

Abnormal parenchymal patterns

Table 2 shows differential diagnoses to consider in the HM or HCT patient presenting with common parenchymal patterns on chest CT, including airspace consolidation, ground glass opacities, nodules, and reticular changes. Radiographic findings may be typical of certain clinical scenarios, for example, symmetric ground glass opacities with sharp margins in prior radiation fields suggest radiation pneumonitis, and diffuse reticular markings during a leukemic blast crisis may support pulmonary leukostasis. The differential may be justifiably narrowed quickly enough to warrant empiric treatment without more thorough investigation in select cases. However, radiographic abnormalities frequently overlap or are ill-defined, and their management may present conflict. For example, bacterial and fungal pneumonias often present as focal or multifocal airspace consolidation, as does noninfectious organizing pneumonia. Given that organizing pneumonia would require steroids for treatment, and that steroids would likely exacerbate an infectious process, further investigation is paramount. Along with the integration of information regarding underlying patient risk factors, clinical presentation, and abnormal imaging, results of noninvasive testing help to determine the next steps in management.

Table 2
Abnormal parenchymal findings in hematologic malignancies and hematopoietic cell transplantation patients warranting consideration of lung sampling for diagnosis

Radiographic Abnormalities[a]	Onset	Distribution/Sign
Airspace consolidation	Acute: Infection (bacteria) Subacute/chronic: Infection (fungi, *Nocardia* or *Actinomyces spp*, mycobacteria), drug toxicity, COP/BOOP, malignancy	Focal: Infection (bacteria), malignancy Multi-focal/diffuse: Infection (bacteria, fungi/mold), COP/BOOP, drug toxicity, malignancy Air-bronchogram: Infection (bacteria)
Ground-glass attenuation	Acute: Infection (early PJP, CMV, HHV-6, CARV, atypical bacteria), alveolar hemorrhage, IPS,[b] acute radiation pneumonitis, eosinophilic pneumonia, pulmonary edema, ARDS, TRALI Subacute/chronic: Infection (CMV, atypicals), drug/radiation toxicity, malignancy, PAP, PVOD[b]	Multi-focal/diffuse: Infection (PJP, CMV, CARV, HHV-6), drug/radiation toxicity, DAH, IPS,[b] PERDS,[b] COP/BOOP, ARDS, TRALI Mosaic attenuation & air trapping: BOS[b]/chronic GVHD
Nodules & mass lesions	Acute: Infection (necrotizing bacteria, eg, *Pseudomonas*, *Staphylococcus aureus*, *Klebsiella spp*; *Aspergillus spp*) Subacute/chronic: Infection (fungi, *Nocardia*, mycobacteria), malignancy	Halo-sign: *Aspergillus* infection Reversed Halo-sign: COP Tree-in-bud: Infection (atypical bacteria, mycobacteria, fungi), mucoid impaction Diffuse centrilobular nodules: viral bronchiolitis, late BOS[b]
Interstitial infiltrates	Acute: Infection (late PJP, viruses, atypical bacteria), pulmonary edema, ARDS, TRALI Subacute/chronic: Infection (mycobacteria), drug/radiation toxicity, malignancy (leukemic infiltration), PAP, PVOD[b]	Multi-focal/diffuse: Infection (PJP, viruses, atypical bacteria), pulmonary edema, ARDS, TRALI, malignancy (leukemic infiltration), PAP Crazy-paving: PAP, pulmonary edema, DAH

Abbreviations: ARDS, acute respiratory distress syndrome; BOOP, bronchiolitis obliterans organizing pneumonia; BOS, bronchiolitis obliterans syndrome; CARV, community-acquired respiratory virus; CMV, cytomegalovirus; COP, cryptogenic organizing pneumonia; DAH, diffuse alveolar hemorrhage; GVHD, graft-versus-host disease; HHV-6, human herpes virus 6; IPS, idiopathic pneumonia syndrome; PAP, pulmonary alveolar proteinosis; PERDS, periengraftment respiratory distress syndrome; PJP, *Pneumocystis jirovecii* pneumonia; PVOD, pulmonary veno-occlusive disease; TRALI, transfusion-related acute lung injury.
[a] In some cases, findings may be apparent on chest radiography, but chest computed tomography scans, especially when performed at high resolution, allow for earlier detection. Common radiologic patterns include airspace consolidation, ground-glass attenuation, interstitial infiltrates, and nodular/mass lesions.
[b] Unique to hematopoietic cell transplant recipients.

Noninvasive Testing

Infectious workup

Together with chest imaging, the results of noninvasive diagnostic testing narrow the differential diagnosis for an infectious PC (**Fig. 3**). Routine microbiological and serologic investigations of serum, urine, and respiratory specimens (nasopharyngeal swabs, sputum, tracheal aspirates) are usually obtained at the time of clinical presentation. Additional assays are requested based on risk features of the patient, for example, endemic fungal exposures; and chest CT patterns, for example, nodule infiltrates, which may heighten suspicion for atypical processes. In recent years, culture-based methods of pathogen isolation from respiratory secretions or blood have been supplemented or supplanted by molecular testing techniques, such as polymerase chain reaction,

for diagnosis of infectious PCs (**Table 3**). At our institution, polymerase chain reaction for the identification of *P jirovecii*, *M tuberculosis*, and community-acquired respiratory viruses is performed routinely on respiratory samples of appropriate HM and HCT patients. Antigen testing in serum (eg, Aspergillus galactomannan, beta-D glucan, cryptococcal and histoplasma antigens), and in urine (eg, *Streptococcus pneumoniae* and *Legionella pneumophila* antigens), are obtained in appropriate patients. In some cases, the negative predictive value may be most valuable, as with beta-D glucan, where only moderate diagnostic value is mitigated by its high negative predictive value in critically ill HM patients.[43] As with any test results, preexisting clinical suspicion is essential for their interpretation, to avoid overdiagnosis or underdiagnosis, and to ensure appropriate treatment decisions.

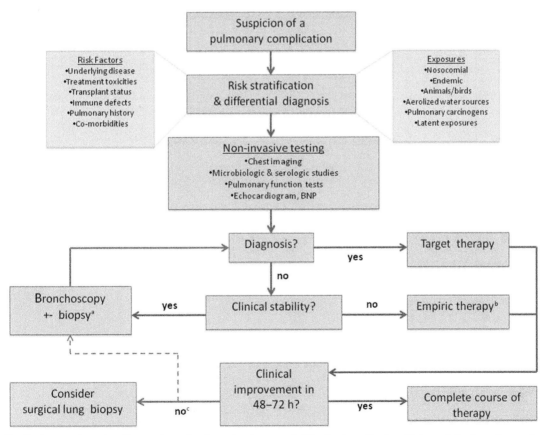

Fig. 3. Approach to the diagnostic evaluation of pulmonary infiltrates in patients with hematologic malignancies and in hematopoietic cell transplant recipients. [a] Transbronchial lung biopsy is generally reserved for suspicion of invasive viral, fungal or mycobacterial disease. [b] The unstable transplant patient who becomes clinically stable may benefit from early diagnostic bronchoscopy within 48 to 72 hours of initiating therapy (*dashed line*). [c] Diagnostic bronchoscopy should be considered before surgical lung biopsy in cases refractory to empiric therapy (*dotted line*). BNP, B-natriuretic peptide. (*Adapted from* Harris B, Lowy FD, Stover DE, et al. Diagnostic bronchoscopy in solid-organ and hematopoietic stem cell transplantation. Ann Am Thorac Soc 2013;10(1):44; with permission.)

Table 3
Diagnostic evaluation of bronchoscopic specimens for specific infectious pulmonary complications of hematologic malignancies and HCT

Infectious Etiology	Microbiology (BAL, PSB, TBLB)	Pathology (BAL, EBB, TBLB)	Additional Studies (BAL, Other)	Comments
Bacteria • Common pathogens • Mycobacteria • Nocardia	• Stain (Gram, acid-fast) and culture[a] • PCR[b]	• Cytology (BAL)[c]	• Legionella DFA (BAL) • Urine antigens, serology[d]	• Nosocomial and community-acquired Gram-positive and Gram-negative bacteria • 10^5 CFU (BAL) and 10^3 CFU (PSB) suggests pneumonia • Patterns of antimicrobial resistance for example, MRSA, VRE, ESBL
Fungi • Candida spp. • Pneumocystis • Aspergillus • Atypical molds • Endemic fungi	• Stain (KOH, Giemsa, Silver, Calcofluor white) and culture[a] • PCR[b]	Cytology (BAL)[c] Tissue invasion (TBLB) Airway infection (EBB) II	Pneumocystis IFA/DFA/PCR (BAL) A Galactomannan (BAL, serum) Urine and serum antigens, serology[d]	• Atypical molds: Mucorales, Fusarium, Scedosporium species • Endemic fungi: C neoformans, H capsulatum, C immitis, B dermatitidis
Viruses Herpesviruses, respiratory viruses	Stain (Papanicolaou) and culture[a] PCR[b]	Cytology (BAL)[c] Tissue invasion (TBLB)[e]	CMV DFA (BAL) Serum antigen and viral load[d] Nasal swab PCR[b]	• Herpesviruses: CMV, EBV, HSV, VZV, HHV-6, • CARVs: adenovirus, coronaviruses, enterovirus, human metapneumovirus, influenza, parainfluenza, respiratory syncytial virus, rhinovirus
Parasites Toxoplasma, Strongyloides	PCR	Immunostain (BAL) Larvae (BAL)	Serology, peripheral cell count, stool studies[d]	• BAL microscopy and serology for evaluation of protozoal lung diseases, such as pulmonary malaria or leishmaniasis, and other parasitic processes may be considered in the context of specific travel exposures.

Abbreviations: BAL, bronchoalveolar lavage; CARV, community-acquired respiratory virus; CFU, colony forming unit; CMV, cytomegalovirus; DFA, direct fluorescent antibody; EBB, endobronchial biopsy; EBV, Epstein–Barr virus; ESBL, extended spectrum beta lactam; HCT, hematopoietic cell transplantation; HHV-6, human herpes virus-6; HSV, herpes simplex virus; IFA, indirect fluorescent antibody; KOH, potassium hydroxide stain; MRSA, methicillin-resistant *S aureus*; PCR, polymerase chain reaction; PSB, protected specimen brushing; spp, species; TBLB, transbronchial lung biopsy; VRE, vancomycin-resistant Enterococcus; VZV, varicella zoster virus.

[a] Direct stains are lacking for atypical organisms such as *M pneumoniae* and *C pneumonia*, and special media is required for culture of *L pneumophila*. Culture is unavailable for *P jirovecii*, and most fungi are difficult to cultivate in the clinical laboratory. Viral staining and culture is predominantly done for CMV. Culture is uncommonly performed for the identification of *T gondii* or *S stercoralis*.

[b] Multiplex PCR is available for a comprehensive panel of respiratory viruses and atypical bacteria, including *L pneumonia, C pneumoniae, M pneumoniae,* and *B pertussis.* PCR for *M tuberculosis* is routinely performed on samples with a positive acid-fast stain or in smear-negative specimens from a high-risk patient.

[c] Cytology with special stains is generally performed for the identification of organisms that are difficult to cultivate in the laboratory, including acid-fast bacteria, fungi (including *Pneumocystis*) and CMV.

[d] Other tests that may assist in microbiologic diagnosis include complement fixation and cold agglutinins for *Mycoplasma* in serum and urine antigen testing for *S pneumonia* and *L pneumophila* serotype 1. Non-BAL antigen testing may also be done for *C neoformans* (serum), *H capsulatum* (serum, urine), and *B dermatitidis* (serum, urine), as well as HSV, RSV, influenza A and B, and adenovirus 40/41 (all serum). Viral load provides information pertaining to CMV activity. Nasopharyngeal swab for PCR of CARV may be useful before bronchoscopy. Serology, peripheral cell count (eg, eosinophilia) and stool studies may be useful adjunctive tests for parasitic causes of infection, notably *Strongyloides.*

[e] Tissue invasion is commonly caused by fungi (*Aspergillus* and atypical molds) and CMV. EBB may be useful to establish airway infection caused by *Aspergillus.*

Reprinted from Harris B, Lowy FD, Stover DE, et al. Diagnostic bronchoscopy in solid-organ and hematopoietic stem cell transplantation. Ann Am Thorac Soc 2013;10(1):45; with permission.

Biomarkers

There is limited usefulness to nonspecific inflammatory biomarkers, such as C-reactive protein, in diagnosing PCs in HM and HCT patients. This lack is likely due to both test and patient characteristics, including highly varied and aberrant responses to inflammation. Serum procalcitonin may be useful in distinguishing bacterial from viral or fungal infection in the immunocompromised host, and may be considered for its negative predictive value in the neutropenic patient with persistent fever.[44] It generally has limited specificity in the critically ill HM patient,[45] or at the time of FN onset,[46] when it might be of greatest practical use. Furthermore, limited study in HCT recipients suggests that procalcitonin cannot distinguish between infectious and noninfectious pulmonary processes, but may indicate severity.[47] Few empiric treatment decisions are likely to be made or altered in the absence of more reliable, supportive data.

Other tests

Lung function testing is not indicated commonly in the evaluation of new pulmonary infiltrates. Pulmonary function tests may be valuable when there is suspicion of airways disease, such as bronchiolitis obliterans syndrome, which is a late complication, as well as monitoring response to therapy of the more common problems, such as chemotherapy toxicity. Last, echocardiography and measurement of serum B-natriuretic peptide may help to distinguish cardiogenic pulmonary edema from other causes of diffuse lung infiltrates.

Invasive Testing

Results of noninvasive testing may support a specific diagnosis, such as invasive aspergillosis in a patient with FN who presents with a halo sign on chest CT and elevated serum Aspergillus galactomannan antigen.[48] These results may be acceptable drivers of therapy in the high-risk or unstable patient who cannot safely undergo further diagnostic workup. However, for the clinically stable patient with a paucity of data supporting probable cause, diagnostic FOB is an important tool to consider early in PC management. The purpose of prompt lung sampling is as much to identify an infectious etiology on which to base or modify antimicrobial therapy, as it is to rule out an infectious process before empiric augmentation of immunosuppression for alternative causes.

Overview of fiberoptic bronchoscopy

Minimally invasive lung sampling via FOB is more likely to capture a snapshot of pulmonary process than expectorated sputum and tracheal aspirates, which are specimens highly contaminated by colonizing flora,[49] and may provide additional diagnostic information in more than one-half of patients.[50] Visual inspection of the airways may identify areas of focal hemorrhage, fungal plaques, purulence, and tumor. Specimens may be collected from the entire LRT via FOB, and most commonly include proximal and distal airway secretions collected via bronchial washing and bronchoalveolar lavage (BAL), and lung tissue via transbronchial lung biopsy (TBLB). Microbiologic, cytologic, and histopathologic studies of BAL and TBLB, when performed, are the primary sources of diagnostic information obtained via FOB.

Signs and symptoms warranting consideration of diagnostic FOB include fever, leukocytosis, hypoxemia, hemoptysis, and unexplained dyspnea, usually in association with new parenchymal opacities (see **Table 2**). The immediate period after recognition of symptoms may be a critical window for lung sampling in high-risk patients, including those with FN or early post-HCT, and for those who present acutely with multifocal or diffuse infiltrates. Once etiologies such as pulmonary embolism, cardiac abnormalities, and nonparenchymal infectious sources have been ruled out appropriately, FOB should be considered promptly. Empiric therapy may be warranted in the unstable patient (or in the stable but high-risk patient) in whom bronchoscopy cannot be performed urgently; however, the initiation of treatment should not preclude continued risk assessment to proceed with FOB in a timely manner (see **Fig. 3**).

Complications associated with FOB in HM and HCT patients are similar to those in the general population, and include hypoxemia, bleeding, bronchospasm, pneumothorax, and cardiac events.[51] Accordingly, contraindications to the procedure include severe hypoxemia, myocardial ischemia, hemodynamic instability, severe thrombocytopenia, or coagulopathy.[51] Bleeding is a common complication in HM and HCT subjects in the setting of prevalent cytopenias, and has been reported in up to 15% of HCT subjects who undergo diagnostic FOB.[52] A lower platelet threshold for BAL, for example, 20,000/μL, has been associated with only mild bleeding episodes,[53] and is a commonly used cutoff for performing BAL at our institution. Hypoxemia is another major concern in these patients, many of whom have diminished pulmonary reserve before FOB. In single-center retrospective studies of HCT recipients, the procedure has been associated with respiratory decline[54] and mortality.[55] Given that the likelihood of intubation after FOB in HCT recipients with acute respiratory failure may is greater, clinicians may favor a purely noninvasive diagnostic approach to PC diagnosis. However, data from a large cohort of HCT patients showed hypoxemia associated with FOB to occur in a small minority (1.8%), and led to mechanical ventilation in only 2% of that group.[52] The overall low rate of intubation in the HCT and neutropenic patients suggests that a low incidence of procedure-related hypoxemia may be an acceptable risk.[52,56–58]

In practice, myriad challenges face providers in determining the appropriate timing of FOB in HM and HCT patients, many of whom are too sick to undergo conscious sedation or general anesthesia for a diagnostic procedure. Provider preference has also been shown to be a barrier to FOB independent of clinical status,[59,60] and delay in diagnosis may have less to do with respiratory status than with physician choice.[61] Based on autopsy studies, PC diagnoses remain elusive before death in many HCT subjects,[12–14] suggesting that a 'wait and see' approach to empiric therapy is used commonly. As a result of these differences, rigorous study is difficult and there is limited prospective evidence on which to base decisions regarding optimal timing, modality, yield or impact of FOB on outcomes in these populations. The available literature regarding the role of diagnostic bronchoscopy in transplant recipients has been reviewed in detail previously[6] and is summarized briefly herein.

Yield and timing of fiberoptic bronchoscopy
Diagnostic yield commonly refers to the identification of a causative organism or other etiology in BAL, protected brush specimens (not routinely used in HM and HCT patients), and/or TBLB specimens. Using mostly retrospective data, the overall range for yield of FOB in HM and HCT is wide, from 30% to 67%.[15,56–58,62–65] Diagnostic yield may correlate with anatomic location and with radiographic patterns. For example, BAL return in the setting of reticular/nodular infiltrates is generally lower as compared with BAL performed in regions with hazy ground glass or consolidation.[42,66] FOB yield may be highest for multifocal infections, such as P jirovecii pneumonia, and lowest for mycobacterial or fungal etiologies.[67] Diagnostic yield may also be higher in febrile or symptomatic patients as compared with those who are asymptomatic.[57,66] In a retrospective review of 501 nonintubated allogeneic HCT recipients with new pulmonary infiltrates during the first 100 days after HCT, the diagnostic yield of FOB more than doubled during the first 4 days after symptom onset.[57] This same study showed a diagnostic yield of 75% if performed within 24 hours before the initiation of antimicrobials, and other studies suggest that optimal yield can still be achieved if FOB is performed within 1 to 3 days of the initiation of therapy.[58,68,69] Empirical antimicrobial therapy before lung sampling is an unavoidable reality in many high-risk patients and may reduce diagnostic yield for invasive fungal disease, in particular.[70] Accordingly, the yield of diagnostic FOB may be least in patients who would most greatly benefit from early treatment guidance, including critically ill HCT recipients[54] and those who have acute graft-versus-host disease.[71]

The importance of diagnostic yield lies in its direct impact on management, and on its indirect impact on PC-related outcomes, such as mortality. Although few studies have rigorously evaluated the impact of FOB on patient management or mortality using prospective methods, available data suggest that early FOB is more likely to provide a diagnosis (especially bacterial) upon which changes in management can be made.[72] FOB-guided changes in antimicrobial therapy have been reported in 20% to 70% of HM and HCT recipients,[52,54,57,58,62,65,73,74] including withdrawal of antimicrobial agents in nearly one-half of HCT subjects.[52,58] FOB results may also provide critical insight into the management of resistant pathogens. In 1 study, pathogens detected in BAL alone demonstrated antimicrobial resistance profiles integral to management, thus rendering inappropriate the choice of empiric therapy based on antimicrobial profiles identified in upper respiratory or peripheral specimens.[64] However, diagnostic yield may not always correlate with a change in management, as demonstrated in neutropenic intensive care unit patients, where a 50% diagnostic yield had little impact on treatment changes.[65]

The impact of diagnostic FOB on PC-related survival is also unclear. Several retrospective, single-center studies suggest that FOB has no discernible influence on mortality.[56,65,75] Although a prospective multicenter study of critically ill cancer patients, including a subset of HCT recipients, did not find FOB to influence mortality, FOB performed within 4 days of symptom onset was associated with a significant survival advantage at 30 days compared with subjects who underwent late FOB-associated antibiotic changes.[57] Another study showed FOB-driven changes in antimicrobial management within 7 days of presentation to be associated with lower mortality compared with patients in whom change was instituted beyond 1 week.[58] Thus, an inability to target treatment expediently may contribute to poor outcomes. Diagnostic delay or a lack of diagnosis has been shown to independently predict death in immunosuppressed hosts with pulmonary infiltrates, highest in critically ill HCT recipients and those with FN.[15,76] This finding highlights the importance of obtaining a correct microbiological diagnosis in the compromised patient, when possible.[77]

Recommended approach to diagnostic fiberoptic bronchoscopy

As a guiding principle, diagnostic FOB should be considered in the HM or HCT subject upon presentation with a new infiltrate on diagnostic chest imaging, and/or in the absence of clinical or radiographic response to at least 48 to 72 hours of empiric antimicrobial therapy (see **Fig. 3**). In the event that empiric therapy is instituted before sampling, whether based on the acuity of patient illness or high suspicion for opportunistic illness, timely investigation is critical to optimize yield and avoid masking a partially treated infection. If the clinical decision is to observe the effects of empiric therapy before lung sampling, this period should be limited to just a few days. The use of systematic institutional protocols for FOB in compromised hosts may be considered.[78]

Consideration of lung biopsy

There is controversy regarding the usefulness of lung biopsy in HM and HCT subjects. For some providers, BAL has historically been considered sufficient for diagnosis[65,79]; for others, the improved yield of combined BAL and TBLB as compared with BAL alone can also be justified by low reported complication rates.[80,81] In a more recent metaanalysis, similar rates of diagnosis were found in studies of BAL and lung biopsy from HCT recipients, although infection was identified more commonly from BAL and noninfectious etiologies were picked up on biopsy.[60] Upon suspicion of invasive fungal or viral infection, however, TBLB may improve diagnostic yield over BAL alone.[81] Overall, however, the impact of TBLB on management remains unclear.[82]

As an alternative to TBLB, CT-guided transthoracic lung biopsy may be preferred for sampling peripheral lung lesions (unless BAL would be contributory) and can be high yield in the HM or HCT patient.[42] A specificity of 100% for diagnosis of invasive fungal disease using CT-guided sampling has been reported.[83] There is an increased risk of pneumothorax using this approach as compared with TBLB; thus, it is important to choose a large enough nodule for improved sampling yield in the face of elevated procedural risk.[42]

Surgical lung biopsy (SLB), whether open or video assisted, is generally kept as a last resort owing to increased procedural risk. Although TBLB, transthoracic lung biopsy, and SLB have

not be compared head to head, the decision to proceed to SLB generally follows a nondiagnostic TBLB or an unrelenting course despite empiric therapy.[67] In a retrospective study from our institution, open lung biopsy in HM subjects demonstrated a specific diagnosis in 62%, led to a change in management in 69%, and correlated with an improved overall survival.[84] Although the diagnostic yield of SLB can be high,[85] its impact on management is difficult to ascertain, and associated mortality limits SLB as a first-line diagnostic modality in transplant recipients. Furthermore, SLB has been on the decrease in recent years as diagnostics for invasive fungal disease improve.[86]

Diagnostic testing of lung specimens

Table 3 summarizes the applications of assays to lung specimens for the diagnosis of infectious PCs. Culture-dependent and -independent methods for identifying common respiratory pathogens and opportunistic organisms in bronchoscopic specimens are similar to those applied to upper respiratory specimens; however, their interpretation requires caution. Contamination of LRT specimens by oral and upper airway flora or colonizers needs to be considered when interpreting the results of microbiological investigations in BAL. Furthermore, the identification of a potential pathogen, such as cytomegalovirus or methicillin-resistant *Staphylococcus aureus*, or fungal antigen, such as beta-D glucan, in BAL, does not always imply causation, emphasizing the importance of clinical context in the interpretation of results. BAL cytology continues to be useful to suggest processes involving tissue invasion (such as *P jirovecii* pneumonia and cytomegalovirus disease) in the absence of biopsy specimens, and may also identify malignant cells (eg, lymphoma), hemorrhage, and alveolar proteinosis. BAL cell count is generally nonspecific, although it may be useful in diffuse alveolar hemorrhage or organizing pneumonia. Lung tissue histopathology is important not only for definitive diagnosis of invasive fungal or viral infections, but also malignancy, organizing pneumonia, and interstitial diseases associated with drug toxicity.

SUMMARY

Early diagnosis of PCs is challenging owing to heterogeneous patient, clinical, and provider factors. A delay in PC diagnosis limits the opportunity for targeted treatment, which may contribute to poor outcomes. Thus, an integrated clinicoradiologic approach can provide crucial insight into the nature of PCs, and provide guidance for further diagnostic testing in HM and HCT patients. Although controversy persists, available data suggest an advantage to early FOB in terms of diagnostic yield, targeted management, and mortality for high-risk HM and HCT recipients, perhaps with exception in the critically ill population. A low threshold for minimally invasive lung sampling should therefore be a guiding principle in high-risk patients, including those with FN and recipients of HCT. This practice may become especially important as advances are made in the sensitivity and specificity of next-generation sequencing applications for infectious disease diagnosis. Empirical treatment is important for the neutropenic or febrile patient presenting with signs or symptoms of pneumonia, however FOB within 72 hours of intubation and empiric treatment is nonetheless encouraged. After careful assessment of risk, lung biopsy via TBLB or transthoracic lung biopsy should be considered when there is concern for invasive fungal or viral disease and in the absence of supportive data from noninvasive sources. SLB should be reserved for cases where diagnoses remain elusive despite investigations of BAL or lung tissue obtain via minimally invasive modalities, and where increased procedural risk is warranted in favor of diagnostic results that would impact key aspects of management. Although prospective study is needed to determine optimal the strategy for lung sampling, close attention to individual risk/benefit profiles will always remain integral to management.

REFERENCES

1. Harris B, Morjaria SM, Littmann ER, et al. Gut microbiota predict pulmonary infiltrates after allogeneic hematopoietic cell transplantation. Am J Respir Crit Care Med 2016;194(4):450–63.
2. Choi MH, Jung JI, Chung WD, et al. Acute pulmonary complications in patients with hematologic malignancies. Radiographics 2014;34(6):1755–68.
3. Gooley TA, Chien JW, Pergam SA, et al. Reduced mortality after allogeneic hematopoietic-cell transplantation. N Engl J Med 2010;363(22):2091–101.
4. Joos L, Tamm M. Breakdown of pulmonary host defense in the immunocompromised host: cancer chemotherapy. Proc Am Thorac Soc 2005;2(5):445–8.
5. Evans SE, Ost DE. Pneumonia in the neutropenic cancer patient. Curr Opin Pulm Med 2015;21(3):260–71.
6. Harris B, Lowy FD, Stover DE, et al. Diagnostic bronchoscopy in solid-organ and hematopoietic stem cell transplantation. Ann Am Thorac Soc 2013;10(1):39–49.
7. Afessa B, Abdulai RM, Kremers WK, et al. Risk factors and outcome of pulmonary complications after autologous hematopoietic stem cell transplant. Chest 2012;141(2):442–50.
8. Peters SG, Afessa B. Acute lung injury after hematopoietic stem cell transplantation. Clin Chest Med 2005;26:561–9.
9. Benz R, Schanz U, Maggiorini M, et al. Risk factors for ICU admission and ICU survival after allogeneic hematopoietic SCT. Bone Marrow Transplant 2014;49(1):62–5.
10. Garcia JB, Lei X, Wierda W, et al. Pneumonia during remission induction chemotherapy in patients with acute leukemia. Ann Am Thorac Soc 2013;10(5):432–40.
11. Mayer S, Pastores SM, Riedel E, et al. Short- and long-term outcomes of adult allogeneic hematopoietic stem cell transplant patients admitted to the intensive care unit in the peritransplant period. Leuk Lymphoma 2017;58(2):382–90.
12. Sharma S, Nadrous HF, Peters SG, et al. Pulmonary complications in adult blood and marrow transplant recipients: autopsy Findings. Chest 2005;128(3):1385–92.
13. Roychowdhury M, Pambuccian SE, Aslan DL, et al. Pulmonary complications after bone marrow transplantation: an autopsy study from a large transplantation center. Arch Pathol Lab Med 2005;129(3):366–71.
14. Pastores SM, Dulu A, Voigt L, et al. Premortem clinical diagnoses and postmortem autopsy findings: discrepancies in critically ill cancer patients. Crit Care 2007;11(2):R48.
15. Gruson D, Hilbert G, valentine R, et al. Utility of fiberoptic bronchoscopy in neutropenic patients admitted to the intensive care unit with pulmonary infiltrates. Crit Care Med 2000;28(7):2224–30.
16. Rano A, Agusti C, Natividada B, et al. Prognostic factors of non-HIV immunocompromised patients with pulmonary infiltrates. Chest 2002;122(1):253–61.
17. White DA. Drug-induced pulmonary infection. Clin Chest Med 2004;25(1):179–87.
18. Safdar A, Armstrong D. Infections in patients with hematologic neoplasms and hematopoietic stem cell transplantation: neutropenia, humoral, and splenic defects. Clin Infect Dis 2011;53(8):798–806.
19. Bennett CL, Djulbegovic B, Norris LB, et al. Colony-stimulating factors for febrile neutropenia during cancer therapy. N Engl J Med 2013;368(12):1131–9.
20. Neuberger S, Maschmeyer G. Update on management of infections in cancer and stem cell transplant patients. Ann Hematol 2006;85:346–56.
21. Marr KA. Delayed opportunistic infections in hematopoietic stem cell transplantation patients: a surmountable challenge. Hematology Am Soc Hematol Educ Program 2012;2012:265–70.

22. Carreras E, Diaz-Ricart M. The role of the endothelium in the short-term complications of hematopoietic SCT. Bone Marrow Transplant 2011;46(12): 1495–502.

23. Spira D, Wirths S, Skowronski F, et al. Diffuse alveolar hemorrhage in patients with hematological malignancies: HRCT patterns of pulmonary involvement and disease course. Clin Imaging 2013;37(4):680–6.

24. Panoskaltsis-Mortari A, Griese M, Madtes DK, et al, on behalf of the American Thoracic Society Committee on Idiopathic Pneumonia Syndrome. An official American Thoracic Society research statement: noninfectious lung injury after hematopoietic stem cell transplantation: idiopathic pneumonia syndrome. Am J Respir Crit Care Med 2011;183: 1262–79.

25. Pene F, Aubron C, Azoulay E, et al. Outcome of critically ill allogeneic hematopoietic stem cell transplantation recipients: a reappraisal of indications for organ failure supports. J Clin Oncol 2006;24(4): 643–9.

26. Azoulay E, Lemiale V, Mokart D, et al. Acute respiratory distress syndrome in patients with malignancies. Intensive Care Med 2014;40(8):1106–14.

27. Hanajiri R, Kakihana K, Kobayashi T, et al. Tobacco smoking is associated with infectious pulmonary complications after allogeneic hematopoietic stem cell transplantation. Bone Marrow Transplant 2015; 50(8):1141–3.

28. Sethi S, Maloney J, Grove L, et al. Airway inflammation and bronchial bacterial colonization in chronic obstructive pulmonary disease. Am J Respir Crit Care Med 2006;173:991–8.

29. Van Vliet MJ, Harmsen HJ, de Bont ES, et al. The role of intestinal microbiota in the development and severity of chemotherapy-induced mucositis. PLoS Pathog 2010;6(5):e1000879.

30. Ho VT, Weller E, Lee SJ, et al. Prognostic factors for early severe pulmonary complications after hematopoietic stem cell transplantation. Biol Blood Marrow Transplant 2001;7(4):223–9.

31. Sorror ML. Comorbidities and hematopoietic cell transplantation outcomes. Hematology Am Soc Hematol Educ Program 2010;2010:237–47.

32. Bayraktar UD, Shpall EJ, Liu P, et al. Hematopoietic cell transplantation-specific comorbidity index predicts inpatient mortality and survival in patients who received allogeneic transplantation admitted to the intensive care unit. J Clin Oncol 2013;31(33):4207–14.

33. Taur Y, Xavier JB, Lipuma L, et al. Intestinal domination and the risk of bacteremia in patients undergoing allogeneic hematopoietic stem cell transplantation. Clin Infect Dis 2012;55(7):905–14.

34. Taur Y, Jenq R, Perales M, et al. The effects of intestinal tract bacterial diversity on mortality following allogeneic hematopoietic stem cell transplantation. Blood 2014;124(7):1174–82.

35. Bergeron A. The pulmonologist's point of view on lung infiltrates in haematological malignancies. Diagn Interv Imaging 2013;94(2):216–20.

36. Maschmeyer G, Donnelly JP. How to manage lung infiltrates in adults suffering from haematological malignancies outside allogeneic haematopoietic stem cell transplantation. Br J Haematol 2016; 173(2):179–89.

37. Heussel CP, Kauczor HU, Heussel GE, et al. Pneumonia in febrile neutropenic patients and in bone marrow and blood stem-cell transplant recipients: use of high-resolution computed tomography. J Clin Oncol 1999;17(3):796–805.

38. Cereser L, Zuiani C, Graziani G, et al. Impact of clinical data on chest radiography sensitivity in detecting pulmonary abnormalities in immunocompromised patients with suspected pneumonia. Radiol Med 2010;115(2):205–14.

39. Wijers SC, Boelens JJ, Raphael MF, et al. Does high-resolution CT has diagnostic value in patients presenting with respiratory symptoms after hematopoietic stem cell transplantation? Eur J Radiol 2011; 80(3):e536–43.

40. Tanaka N, Kunihiro Y, Yujiri T, et al. High-resolution computed tomography of chest complications in patients treated with hematopoietic stem cell transplantation. Jpn J Radiol 2011;29(4):229–35.

41. Brodoefel H, Faul C, Salih H, et al. Therapy-related noninfectious complications in patients with hematologic malignancies: high-resolution computed tomography findings. J Thorac Imaging 2013;28(1): W5–11.

42. Wingard JR, Hiemenz JW, Jantz MA. How I manage pulmonary nodular lesions and nodular infiltrates in patients with hematologic malignancies or undergoing hematopoietic cell transplantation. Blood 2012; 120(9):1791–800.

43. Azoulay E, Guigue N, Darmon M, et al. (1, 3)-β-D-glucan assay for diagnosing invasive fungal infections in critically ill patients with hematological malignancies. Oncotarget 2016;7(16): 21484–95.

44. Koya J, Nannya Y, Ichikawa M, et al. The clinical role of procalcitonin in hematopoietic SCT. Bone Marrow Transplant 2012;47(10):1326–31.

45. Bele N, Darmon M, Coquet I, et al. Diagnostic accuracy of procalcitonin in critically ill immunocompromised patients. BMC Infect Dis 2011;11:224.

46. Robinson JO, Lamoth F, Bally F, et al. Monitoring procalcitonin in febrile neutropenia: what is its utility for initial diagnosis of infection and reassessment in persistent fever? PLoS One 2011; 6(4):e18886.

47. Lucena CM, Rovira M, Gabarrús A, et al. The clinical value of biomarkers in respiratory complications in hematopoietic SCT. Bone Marrow Transplant 2016. [Epub ahead of print].

48. Marom EM, Kontoyiannis DP. Imaging studies for diagnosing invasive fungal pneumonia in immuno-compromised patients. Curr Opin Infect Dis 2011; 24(4):309–14.

49. Lentino JR, Lucks DA. Nonvalue of sputum culture in the management of lower respiratory tract infections. J Clin Microbiol 1987;25(5):758–62.

50. Habtes I, Shah P, Harris B, et al. Bronchoalveolar lavage among hematopoietic stem cell transplant recipients: diagnostic yield and change in management. Poster presented at the ATS International Conference. San Francisco (CA), May 15, 2016.

51. British Thoracic Society Bronchoscopy Guidelines Committee, a Subcommittee of the Standards of Care Committee of the British Thoracic Society. British Thoracic Society guidelines on diagnostic flexible bronchoscopy. Thorax 2001;56(Suppl 1): i1–21.

52. Yanik GA, Ho VT, Levine JE, et al. The impact of soluble tumor necrosis factor receptor etanercept on the treatment of idiopathic pneumonia syndrome after allogenic hematopoietic stem cell transplantation. Blood 2008;112(8):3073–81.

53. Carr IM, Koefelenberg CF, von Groote-Bidlingmaier F, et al. Blood loss during flexible bronchoscopy: a prospective observational study. Respiration 2012; 84(4):312–8.

54. Azoulay E, Mokart D, Rabbat A, et al. Diagnostic bronchoscopy in hematology and oncology patients with acute respiratory failure: prospective multicenter data. Crit Care Med 2008;1(36):100–7.

55. Burger CD. Utility of positive bronchoalveolar lavage in predicting respiratory failure after hematopoietic stem cell transplantation: a retrospective analysis. Transplant Proc 2007;39:1623–5.

56. Kuehnhardt D, Hannemann M, Schmidt B, et al. Therapeutic implication of BAL in patients with neutropenia. Ann Hematol 2009;88:1249–56.

57. Shannon VR, Andersson BS, Lei X, et al. Utility of early versus late fiberoptic bronchoscopy in the evaluation of new pulmonary infiltrates following hematopoietic stem cell transplantation. Bone Marrow Transplant 2010;45:647–65.

58. Rano A, Agusti C, Jiminez P, et al. Pulmonary infiltrates in non-HIV immunocompromised patients: a diagnostic approach using non-invasive and bronchoscopic procedures. Thorax 2001;56: 379–87.

59. Wahidi MM, Rocha AT, Hollingsworth JW, et al. Contraindications and safety of transbronchial lung biopsy via flexible bronchoscopy. A survey of pulmonologists and review of the literature. Respiration 2005;72:285–95.

60. Chellapandian D, Lehrnbecher T, Phillips B, et al. Bronchoalveolar lavage and lung biopsy in patients with cancer and hematopoietic stem-cell transplantation recipients: a systematic review and meta-analysis. J Clin Oncol 2015;33(5): 501–9.

61. Wahla AS, Chatterjee A, Khan II, et al. Survey of academic pulmonologists, oncologists, and infectious disease physicians on the role of bronchoscopy in managing hematopoietic stem cell transplantation patients with pulmonary infiltrates. J Bronchology Interv Pulmonol 2014;21(1):32–9.

62. Kim SW, Rhee CK, Kang HS, et al. Diagnostic value of bronchoscopy in patients with hematologic malignancy and pulmonary infiltrates. Ann Hematol 2015; 94(1):153–9.

63. Hummel M, Rudert S, Hof H, et al. Diagnostic yield of bronchoscopy with bronchoalveolar lavage in febrile patients with hematologic malignancies and pulmonary infiltrates. Ann Hematol 2008;87(4):291–7.

64. Hohenadel IA, Kiworr M, Genitsariotis R, et al. Role of bronchoalveolar lavage in immunocompromised patients with pneumonia treated with a broad spectrum antibiotic and antifungal regimen. Thorax 2001; 56:115–20.

65. Hofmeister CC, Czerlanis C, Forsythe S, et al. Retrospective utility of bronchoscopy after hematopoietic stem cell transplant. Bone Marrow Transplant 2006; 38:693–8.

66. Brownback KR, Simpson SQ. Association of bronchoalveolar lavage yield with chest computed tomography findings and symptoms in immunocompromised patients. Ann Thorac Med 2013; 8(3):153–9.

67. Baughman RP, Lower EE. Diagnosis of pneumonia in immunocompromised patient. In: Agusti C, Torres A, editors. Pulmonary infection in the immunocompromised patient: strategies for management. West Sussex, United Kingdom: Wiley-Blackwell; 2009. p. 53–93.

68. Pereira Gomes JC, Pedreira JW Jr, Araujo EM, et al. Impact of BAL in the management of pneumonia with treatment failure: positivity of BAL culture under antibiotic therapy. Chest 2000;118(6):1739–46.

69. Yacoub AT, Thomas D, Yuan C, et al. Diagnostic value of bronchoalveolar lavage in leukemic and bone marrow transplant patients: the impact of antimicrobial therapy. Mediterr J Hematol Infect Dis 2015;7(1):e2015002.

70. Reinwald M, Hummel M, Kovalevskaya E, et al. Therapy with antifungals decreases the diagnostic performance of PCR for diagnosing invasive aspergillosis in bronchoalveolar lavage samples of patients with haematological malignancies. J Antimicrob Chemother 2012;67:2260–7.

71. Kasow KA, King E, Rochester R, et al. Diagnostic yield of bronchoalveolar lavage is low in allogeneic hematopoietic stem cell recipients receiving immunosuppressive therapy or with acute-graft-versus-host disease: the St. Jude experience. Biol Blood Marrow Transplant 2007;13:831–7.

72. Lucena CM, Torres A, Rovira M, et al. Pulmonary complications in hematopoietic SCT: a prospective study. Bone Marrow Transplant 2014;49(10):1293–9.

73. Gilbert CR, Lerner A, Baram M, et al. Utility of flexible bronchoscopy in the evaluation of pulmonary infiltrates in the hematopoietic stem cell transplant population – a single center fourteen year experience. Arch Bronconeumol 2013;49(5):189–95.

74. Gupta S, Sultenfuss M, Romaguera JE, et al. CT-guided percutaneous lung biopsies in patients with haematologic malignancies and undiagnosed pulmonary lesions. Hematol Oncol 2010;28(2):75–81.

75. Dunagan DP, Baker AM, Hurd DD, et al. Bronchoscopic evaluation of pulmonary infiltrates following bone marrow transplantation. Chest 1997;111(1):135–41.

76. Azoulay E, Mokart D, Lambert J, et al. Diagnostic strategy for hematology and oncology patients with acute respiratory failure: randomized controlled trial. Am J Respir Crit Care Med 2010;182(8):1038–46.

77. Kontoyiannis DP. Rational approach to pulmonary infiltrates in leukemia and transplantation. Best Pract Res Clin Haematol 2013;26(3):301–6.

78. Sampsonas F, Kontoyiannis DP, Dickey BF, et al. Performance of a standardized bronchoalveolar lavage protocol in a comprehensive cancer center: a prospective 2-year study. Cancer 2011;117(15):3424–33.

79. White P, Bonacum JT, Miller CB. Utility of fiberoptic bronchoscopy in bone marrow transplant patients. Bone Marrow Transplant 1997;20(8):681–7.

80. Jain P, Sandur S, Meli Y, et al. Role of flexible bronchoscopy in immunocompromised patients with lung infiltrates. Chest 2004;125(2):712–22.

81. Cazzadori A, DiPerri G, Todeschini G, et al. Transbronchial biopsy in the diagnosis of pulmonary infiltrates in immunosuppressed patients. Chest 1995;197:101–6.

82. Peikert T, Rana S, Edell ES. Safety, diagnostic yield, and therapeutic implications of flexible bronchoscopy in patients with febrile neutropenia and pulmonary infiltrates. Mayo Clin Proc 2005;80(11):1414–20.

83. Carrafiello G, Laganà D, Nosari AM, et al. Utility of computed tomography (CT) and of fine needle aspiration biopsy (FNAB) in early diagnosis of fungal pulmonary infections. Study of infections from filamentous fungi in haematologically immunodeficient patients. Radiol Med 2006;111(1):33–41.

84. White DA, Wong PW, Downey R. The utility of open lung biopsy in patients with hematologic malignancies. Am J Respir Crit Care Med 2000;161(3 Pt 1):723–9.

85. Zihlif M, Khanchandani G, Ahmed HP, et al. Surgical lung biopsy in patients with hematological malignancy or hematopoietic stem cell transplantation and unexplained pulmonary infiltrates: improved outcome with specific diagnosis. Am J Hematol 2005;78(2):94–9.

86. Cheng GS, Stednick ZJ, Madtes DK, et al. Decline in the use of surgical biopsy for diagnosis of pulmonary disease in hematopoietic cell transplantation recipients in an era of improved diagnostics and empirical therapy. Biol Blood Marrow Transplant 2016;22(12):2243–9.

Critical Care of the Patient with Malignancy

Critical Care Prognosis and Outcomes in Patients with Cancer

Ayman O. Soubani, MD

KEYWORDS

- Cancer • Intensive care unit • Outcomes • Patient admission/standards
- Multiple organ dysfunction

KEY POINTS

- There has been a steady increase in the use of intensive care services for critically ill patients with cancer associated with improvement in short- and long-term outcomes.
- Baseline cancer characteristics, neutropenia, and severity of illness scores have minimal effect on outcome and should not be used as reasons to deny admission to the intensive care unit.
- Poor performance status, progressive cancer despite treatment, allogeneic hematopoietic stem cell transplantation with refractory graft-versus-host disease, and persistent or worsening multiorgan failure are associated with poor outcome.
- There is a need for high-quality, multicenter studies that provide better outcome predictive models.

INTRODUCTION

Cancer survival has been steadily improving over the last few decades owing to earlier detection, advances in surgical and medical options for treatment, and better supportive care.[1,2] This in turn has led to more patients admitted to the intensive care unit (ICU) for the management of critical illnesses that are related either directly or indirectly to cancer. Historically, the prognosis of patients with cancer admitted to the ICU was extremely poor and patients were discouraged from using such services. However, in the last 2 decades, there has been a steady improvement in outcome of most critically ill patients with cancer. This report reviews the epidemiology related to the use of the ICU in this patient population, changes in outcome and factors—both system practices and patient clinical variables—that affect the outcome of these patients. It also provides an overview of the long-term outcome of patients with cancer who required intensive care.

CRITICAL CARE USE BY PATIENTS WITH CANCER

Several studies have shown increased the use of critical care services for patients with cancer. In a study of 36 ICUs in Denmark from 2004 to 2012, there was a steady annual increase in admission rates of 6% and 10% for patients with hematologic malignancies (HM) and solid tumors, respectively.[3] An analysis of 15-day surveillance study of septic patients admitted to 198 European ICUs, 15% of those patients had cancer.[4] Another study of 22 ICUs in Brazil showed that 20% of patients admitted to the ICU had cancer.[5] Also, in a retrospective analysis of the Surveillance, Epidemiology, and End Results database, the ICU admission for patients with lung cancer increased from around 135 per 1000 hospitalized patients in 1992 to around 200 per 1000 hospitalized patients in 2006, which was statistically significant.[6] In a retrospective analysis of a national cancer registry in England, 5.2% of patients with cancer developed a

Division of Pulmonary, Critical Care and Sleep Medicine, Wayne State University School of Medicine, 3990 John R- 3 Hudson, Detroit, MI 48201, USA
E-mail address: asoubani@med.wayne.edu

Clin Chest Med 38 (2017) 333–353
http://dx.doi.org/10.1016/j.ccm.2016.12.011
0272-5231/17/© 2016 Elsevier Inc. All rights reserved.

critical illness within 2 years of diagnosis requiring ICU admission.[7] The risk of ICU admission for patients with cancer increased significantly in the first 100 days after diagnosis and continued to increase thereafter, but at a slower rate.[7] In the case of allogeneic hematopoietic stem cell transplantation (HSCT), it is estimated that 20% of these patients may require ICU admission at 1 point after transplantation.[8] **Box 1** summarizes the main reasons for patients with cancer to require ICU admission.

OUTCOME OF PATIENTS WITH CANCER ADMITTED TO THE INTENSIVE CARE UNIT

Earlier reports have emphasized the poor outcome of patients with cancer admitted to the ICU

Box 1
Main causes of admission to the intensive care unit in patients with cancer

- Postoperative care—elective or emergency
- Acute respiratory failure
  - Infectious—bacteria, viral, fungal
  - Noninfectious
    - Diffuse alveolar hemorrhage
    - Idiopathic pneumonia syndrome
    - Pulmonary drug toxicity
    - Transfusion-related acute lung injury
- Severe sepsis and septic shock
- Bleeding—tumor erosion, coagulopathy, thrombocytopenia
- Alteration of mental status
  - Metabolic—sepsis, effect of medications, multiorgan system failure
  - Central nervous system bleeding
  - Tumor effect
  - Posterior reversible encephalopathy syndrome
- Oncologic emergencies
  - Tumor lysis syndrome
  - Leukostasis
  - Superior vena cava syndrome
  - Cardiac tamponade
  - Hypercalcemia
- Initiation of chemotherapy
- Comorbid illnesses—chronic obstructive pulmonary disease, pulmonary embolism, cardiac, renal, hepatic

---

(**Tables 1–3**). Reports from the 1980s and early 1990s have shown hospital mortality of patients with cancer admitted to the ICU to be as high as 80% and more than 90% in those who require mechanical ventilation.[9–12] The dismal outcome led many experts and clinicians to discourage ICU care for patients with cancer.[13,14] The presence of cancer was the second most common cause of denying ICU admission by intensivists.[15]

The experience with critically ill patients with cancer has shifted significantly in the last 2 decades, with multiple studies showing improved short-term outcomes as can be seen in **Tables 1–3**. Although the improved outcome is universal, there are variations in the degree of improvement between the different types of cancer. Generally, critically ill HM patients have higher mortality than those with solid cancers; however, the outcomes in HM patients have also been improving. A recent study of 1011 patients with HM showed an overall ICU mortality of 27.6% and hospital mortality of 39.3%.[16] In another study of patients admitted to Dutch ICUs, the risk-adjusted mortality rate for patients with HM was around 45%, which was similar to those with solid cancers (40%) and approaching others with severe comorbid illnesses.[3] More recent data show overall hospital mortality for HM patients to be 45.3% and in non-HSCT patients as low as 22.8%.[17]

In the case of solid cancers, many of these patients have similar outcomes to patients without cancer (see **Table 3**). In a well-designed systematic review of the literature of ICU patients with solid cancers, the overall average ICU mortality was 31.2% (95% confidence interval [CI], 24.0%–39.0%), whereas the average hospital mortality was 38.2% (95% CI, 33.8%–42.7%).[7] The mortality of critically ill patients with solid cancers also varies widely depending on the specific tumor site. Generally, patients with lung cancer have the highest mortality (average ICU mortality, 40.1%; 95% CI, 28.6%–52.2%), whereas patients with gynecologic malignancies have the lowest mortality (average ICU mortality, 12.0%; 95% CI, 7.4%–104%). Even in the case of lung cancer, recent reports continue to show improvement in short-term outcomes. In a study of 139 patients with lung cancer admitted to the ICU, 49% required mechanical ventilation. The ICU and hospital mortality were 22% and 40%, respectively.[18]

Traditionally, HSCT recipients admitted to the ICU had very poor outcome. However, there has also been modest improvement in outcome in this patient population (see **Table 2**). Autologous HSCT recipients have favorable ICU and hospital outcomes, and should not be denied ICU admission in case of critical illness.[19–22] Currently, the

Table 1
Major studies addressing short-term and long-term outcome of critically ill patients with hematologic malignancies

Author/Year	Study Type	Malignancy Type	Patient #	Mortality			MV Patient #	Mortality			Predictors of Mortality
				ICU	Hospital	≥6 mo		ICU	Hospital	≥6 mo	
Schuster & Marion,[9] 1983	R	HM	77	60%	80%	NR	52	NR	92%	NR	• Acute respiratory failure owing to infection • Prolonged MV
Lloyd-Thomas et al,[10] 1988	R	HM	60	63%	78%	NR	45	NR	87%	NA	• APACHE II >26 • Pneumonia with shock • Persistent neutropenia • Unresponsive malignancy • Multiorgan dysfunction
Peters et al,[11] 1988	R	HM on MV	116	NA	NA	NA	116	NR	82%	NR	• Non-Hodgkin lymphoma • Acute leukemia
Brunet et al,[104] 1990	R	HM	260	43%	57%	81%	111	85%	NR	NR	• High SAPS • Multiorgan failure • Intractable sepsis • Combination of mechanical ventilation and dialysis
Sculier & Markiewicz,[105] 1991	R	Predominant HM	1413	10%	22%	NR	64	72%	NR	NR	• MV
Epner et al,[62] 1996	R	HM on MV	157	NR	NR	NR	157	NR	83%	NR	• Stage beyond first complete remission • Duration of neutropenia >30 d • Treatment with HSCT

(continued on next page)

Table 1
(continued)

Author/Year	Study Type	Malignancy Type	Patient #	Mortality ICU	Mortality Hospital	Mortality ≥6 mo	MV Patient #	Mortality ICU	Mortality Hospital	Mortality ≥6 mo	Predictors of Mortality
Ewig et al,[106] 1998	R	HM	89	NR	70 (79%)	NR	76	NR	68 (90%)	NR	• Severe pulmonary complications • MV • HSCT • <90 d from HSCT to ICU admission
Kress et al,[44] 1999	R	Predominant HM	348	NR	41%	NR	153	NR	67%	NR	• MV • Hepatic failure • Cardiovascular failure
Groeger et al,[47] 1999	P	Predominant HM on MV	782	NR	NR	NR	782	NR	76%	NR	• Intubation after 24 h, leukemia • Progression or recurrence of cancer • Allogeneic HSCT • Cardiac arrhythmias • DIC • Vasopressor therapy
Staudinger et al,[42] 2000	R	Predominant HM	414	47%	77%	NR	NR	NR	NR	NR	• MV • Septic shock
Kroschinsky et al,[107] 2002	R	HM	104	44%	NR	67%	54	74%	NR	82%	• SAPS score >50 • MV
Larche et al,[25] 2003	R	Predominant HM	88	66%	NR	NR	68	71%	NR	NR	• Time to antibiotics • Need for MV
Benoit et al,[50] 2003	R	HM	124	42%	54%	66%	88	59%	69%	79%	• Leukopenia • Vasopressor use • Urea >0.75 g/L • MV

Study	Design	Population	N				N				Factors
Depuydt et al,[45] 2004	R	HM	166	62%	71%	NR	120	NR	70%	NR	• Female sex • MV <24 h • Bacteremia <48 h • AML • SAPS of >0.08
Soares et al,[43] 2005	P	Predominantly HM on MV	463	NR	NR	NR	463	50%	64%	NR	• Age >70 y • Poor Performance status • Pao_2/Fio_2 <150 • Cancer status • Severity of organ failure
Benoit et al,[71] 2006	R	HM	37	32%	43%	67%	23	54%	61%	74%	• MV
Lamia et al,[90] 2006	R	HM	92	NR	58%	NR	58	NR	79%	NR	• SAPS II, LODS and SOFA scores
Hampshire et al,[108] 2009	R	HM	7689	43%	59%	NR	NR	NR	NR	NR	• LOS in hospital before ICU • Severe sepsis • Low hematocrit
Taccone et al,[4] 2009	R	Predominant HM	473	23%	32%	NR	301	NR	NR	NR	• SAPS II, ALI/ARDS, sepsis, and MV for solid patients with cancer • SAPS II and ALI/ARDS for hematologic patients
Soares et al,[5] 2010	P	Predominant HM	717	21%	30%	NR	NR	NR	NR	NR	• Severity of organ failure • MV • Performance status
McGrath et al,[58] 2010	Both	Predominant HM	185	29%	NR	75%	NR	47.3%	NR	NR	• APACHE II and SOFA scores • Multiorgan failure
Hill et al,[99] 2012	R	HM	147	56%	73%	79%	88	NR	NR	NR	• HM • Greater age • MV • APACHE II

(continued on next page)

Table 1
(continued)

Author/Year	Study Type	Malignancy Type	Patient #	Mortality			MV Patient #	Mortality			Predictors of Mortality
				ICU	Hospital	≥6 mo		ICU	Hospital	≥6 mo	
Bird et al,[109] 2012	R	HM	199	33.7%	45.7%	59.3%	95	NR	64%	NR	• MV • Failure of >2 organ systems
Azoulay et al,[16] 2013	P	HM	1011	27.6%	39.3%	56.7%	484	NR	60.5%	NR	• Poor Performance status at admission • Charlson comorbidity index • Allogeneic HSCT • SOFA score • Admission for cardiac arrest or acute respiratory failure • Invasive pulmonary aspergillosis • Organ Infiltration by Malignancy
Azevedo et al,[81] 2014	P	Predominant HM on MV	263	54%	67%	NR	223	NR	72%	NR	• Newly diagnosed malignancy • Recurrent or progressive malignancy • Performance status • NIV followed by MV • MV • SOFA score

Abbreviations: ALI/ARDS, acute lung injury/acute respiratory distress syndrome; AML, acute myeloid leukemia; APACHE, Acute Physiology and Chronic Health Evaluation; DIC, disseminated intravascular coagulation; HM, hematologic malignancy; HSCT, hematopoietic stem cell transplantation; ICU, intensive care unit; LODS, logistic organ dysfunction system; LOS, length of stay; MV, mechanical ventilation; NA, not applicable; NIV, noninvasive ventilation; NR, not reported; R, retrospective; SAPS, Simplified Acute Physiology Score; SOFA, sequential organ failure assessment.

hospital mortality in autologous HSCT recipients admitted to the ICU is as low as 18.8% and in mechanically ventilated patients, it is around 40%.[17] In allogeneic HSCT recipients, in contrast, although improved, prognosis remains poor with a hospital mortality of greater than 60%, especially in mechanically ventilated patients and those with refractory acute graft-versus-host disease (GVHD), where mortality may be as high as 90%.[17]

SYSTEM PRACTICES IN THE INTENSIVE CARE UNIT INFLUENCING THE OUTCOME OF CRITICALLY ILL PATIENTS WITH CANCER

Several factors related to ICU care and system practices have contributed to the general improvement in outcome of patients with cancer admitted to the ICU. These are discussed below.

Improvement in Overall Care in the Intensive Care Unit

The recent advances in general ICU care have probably impacted the short-term outcome of critically ill patients with cancer as well. These include ventilator and supportive management of patients with acute respiratory distress syndrome, early use of noninvasive ventilation (NIV), and better management of sepsis and septic shock.[21,23–25] Also, a better understanding and management of multiorgan failure has contributed to improved outcomes in this patient population.[26] The availability of less invasive methods has led to improved diagnosis of opportunistic infections such as invasive pulmonary aspergillosis. Other measures including effective infection control procedures and the routine use of bedside ultrasonography have had a positive influence on outcome of critically ill patients in general, including patients with cancer.[27]

Multidisciplinary Care in the Intensive Care Unit

A high-quality multidisciplinary approach is an important factor in outcome of critically ill patients in general.[28] This concept is even more applicable to critically ill patients with cancer who have complex medical issues. The hematologist–oncologist provides expertise on the course and prognosis of the disease, the side effects of chemotherapeutic agents, and types of illnesses these patients are likely to face. The intensivists, in contrast, are more equipped to resuscitate these patients, support their organ functions, and monitor their progress during ICU care. Collaboration between these specialists is also paramount in discussing goals of care with patients and families and providing

professional advice from both their perspectives. Specialists in infectious diseases, nephrology, palliative care, and others may play a vital role depending on the specific situation of the patient. In a recent survey of 70 ICUs, the presence of clinical pharmacist, number of protocols implemented in the ICU, and daily meetings between oncologists and intensivists for care planning were associated with lower mortality in critically ill patients with cancer. Also these factors were associated independently with a more efficient use of resources.[29] However, it is also important to note that multispecialty involvement in the care of these patients may be a cause for conflict and contradictions, so it is essential that there is high degree of coordination between these specialists.

Timing of Admission to the Intensive Care Unit

The early identification of organ dysfunction and initiation of therapy have been shown to improve the outcome of critically ill patients in general.[30] Several studies have shown that a delay in ICU admission, especially in patients with multiple organ failure, is associated with an high risk of death.[30] Also it has been reported that the management of severely ill patients before transfer to the ICU tends to be suboptimal with an increased risk of multiorgan dysfunction and death.[31] Similar findings have been reported in patients with cancer.[32–34] In 1 study of 219 patients with cancer with acute respiratory failure, time between respiratory symptoms onset and ICU admission of greater than 2 days was associated with worse outcome (odds ratio, 2.50; 95% CI, 1.25–5.02; $P = .01$).[35] Increased awareness about the importance of timing in the care of critically ill patients with cancer is likely to influence the outcome for these patients.

Admission Policies in the Intensive Care Unit

There are wide variations between hospitals around the world regarding ICU admission policies for patients with cancer. The changes in ICU policies to increased accommodation of patients with cancer have shown positive impact on survival. In a study of 103 critically ill lung patients with cancer, only one-third of patients were referred for ICU admission.[36] The hospital mortality for those who were admitted to the ICU was 63% as compared with 94% in those who were not admitted to the ICU. In this regard, the clinical evaluation alone as a tool to determine whether an acutely ill patient with cancer needs ICU admission has not been shown to be specific or sensitive. In a prospective study to evaluate the outcome of

Table 2
Major studies addressing short-term and long-term outcome of critically ill HSCT recipients

Author/Year	Study Type	Patients Type	Patient #	Mortality			MV Patient#	Mortality			Predictors of Mortality
				ICU	Hospital	≥6 mo		ICU	Hospital	≥6 mo	
Torrecilla et al,[63] 1988	R	HSCT	25	83%	NR	NR	NR	NR	NR	NR	• MV >7 d • ICU LOS >10 d • Failure of >3 organ systems • Septic shock • Severe neutropenia on admission
Crawford et al,[12] 1988	R	HSCT	1089	NR	NR	40%	232	NR	NR	84%	• NR
Denardo et al,[110] 1989	R	HSCT	50	NR	82%	NR	NR	NR	NR	NR	• MV >4 d • ICU LOS
Afessa et al,[111] 1992	R	HSCT	35	NR	77%	NR	27	NR	93%	NR	• MV • Multiple organ failure
Crawford & Petersen,[112] 1992	R	HSCT on MV	348	NR	NR	NR	348	NR	96%	97%	• NR
Paz et al,[113] 1993	R	HSCT	36	66%	NR	NR	28	96%	NR	NR	• MV • APACHE II score
Faber-Langendoen et al,[114] 1993	R	HSCT on MV	191	NR	NR	NR	191	91%	NR	97%	• MV and reason for MV • Age >40 y • BMT to ICU <90 d
Price et al,[20] 1998	P	HSCT	115	NR	54%	NR	48	NR	81%	NR	• MV • Allogeneic HSCT • Infection, respiratory rate, days since transplant, heart rate and, bilirubin level
Jackson et al,[100] 1998	R	HSCT	116	77%	83%	86%	92	62%	83%	NR	• Year of HSCT • Hemodynamic support • Bilirubin level
Huaringa et al,[19] 2000	R	HSCT on MV	60	NR	NR	NR	60	82%	NR	95%	• Prolonged MV >15 d • Respiratory failure >30 d after HSCT

Study		Population									
Khassawneh et al,[85] 2002	R	Autologous HSCT on MV	78	NR	NR	NR	78	NR	74%	83%	• Lung injury with vasopressor use • Hepatic and renal failure
Soubani et al,[115] 2004	R	HSCT	85	39%	59%	72%	51	63%	NR	NR	• Elevated Lactate level • MV • Failure of >1 organ system
Pene et al,[21] 2006	R	Allogeneic HSCT	209	51.7%	67.5%	72.8%	122	82%	83.4%	86%	• MV • Steroids for the treatment of GVHD • Elevated bilirubin • Multiple organ failure if mechanically ventilated
Scales et al,[22] 2008	R	HSCT	504	NR	NR	67%	258	NR	NR	87%	• MV • Hemodialysis
Trinkaus et al,[67] 2009	R	Autologous HSCT	34	38%	NR	NR	11	55%	NR	NR	• Multiorgan failure • MV • Inotropic support >4 h • Gram-negative sepsis
Depuydt et al,[116] 2011	P	Allogeneic HSCT	44	61%	75%	80%	32	NR	NR	NR	• Bacterial infection was associated with lower mortality
Townsend et al,[117] 2013	R	Allogeneic HSCT	164	68%	NR	NR	NR	NR	NR	NR	• MV • Elevated urea • Intensity of chemotherapy before HSCT
Benz et al,[118] 2014	R	Allogeneic HSCT	33	64%	NR	85%	21	NR	NR	NR	• Failure of >1 organ system
Allareddy et al,[119] 2014	R	HSCT on MV	6074	NR	NR	NR	6074	NR	50.6%	NR	• MV for >96 h
Platon et al,[120] 2016	R	Allogeneic HSCT	73	40%	63%	NR	29	62%	NR	NR	• Worsening SOFA from day 1 to day 3 • MV • Active GVHD

Abbreviations: APACHE, Acute Physiology and Chronic Health Evaluation; BMT, bone marrow transplantation; GVHD, graft-versus-host disease; HSCT, hematopoietic stem cell transplantation; ICU, intensive care unit; LOS, length of stay; MV, mechanical ventilation; NR, not reported; R, retrospective; SOFA, sequential organ failure assessment.

Table 3
Major studies addressing short-term and long-term outcome of critically ill patients with solid cancers

Author/Year	Study Type	Patients Type	Patient #	Mortality			MV Patient #	Mortality			Predictors of Mortality
				ICU	Hospital	≥6 mo		ICU	Hospital	≥6 mo	
Jennens et al,[121] 2002	R	Lung cancer	20	85%	NR	NR	9	NR	NR	NR	NR
Reichner et al,[122] 2006	R	Lung cancer	47	43%	60%	NR	NR	74%	NR	NR	MV SOFA Stage IV lung cancer
Christodoulou et al,[86] 2007	R	Solid cancers	69	46.3%	66.6%	NR	44	NR	81.8%	NR	Performance status
Soares et al,[87] 2007	P	Head and neck cancer	121	39%	56%	72%	100	NR	64%	NR	Performance status Advanced cancer Number of organ failure
Soares et al,[56] 2007	R	Lung cancer	143	42%	59%	NR	100	56%	69%	NR	Airway infiltration by tumor Number of organ failure Cancer progression or recurrence Severity of comorbidities
Mendoza et al,[80] 2008	R	Solid cancers	147	28.5%	39.4%	NR	93	NR	51%	NR	Vasopressors Metastatic disease
Adam & Soubani,[18] 2008	R	Lung cancer	139	22%	40%	NR	68	38%	53%	NR	Vasopressor >2 organ failure
Roques et al,[88] 2009	P	Lung cancer	105	43%	54%	73%	43	NR	70%	NR	Performance status MV Cancer progression

Study		Cancer type	N									
Aldawood,[123] 2010	P	Lung cancer	51	49%	60%	NR	NR	NR	NR	NR	NR	Thrombocytopenia SAPS II
Caruso et al,[124] 2010	R	Solid cancers	83	55.4%	28.9%	12%	NR	NR	NR	NR	NR	Vasopressors APACHE II
Namendys-Silva et al,[125] 2010	P	Solid cancers	177	21.4%	NR	NR	141	NR	NR	NR	NR	Vasopressors MV Thrombocytopenia
Andrejak et al,[126] 2011	R	Lung cancer	76	47%	64.5%	NR	57	59%	NR	59%	NR	SOFA score Performance status
Namendys-Silva et al,[89] 2013	P	Gynecologic cancers	92	41.2%	NA	NR	NR	NR	NR	NR	NR	Performance status Metastasis on admission Worsening LODS
Toffart et al,[127] 2011	R	Lung cancer	103	31%	48%	NR	41	NR	NR	NR	NR	Sepsis MV
Bonomi et al,[101] 2012	R	Lung cancer	1134	NR	33%	90%	NR	NR	NR	NR	NR	Medical indication
Bos et al,[128] 2012	R	Solid cancers	15,211	30.4%	40.6%	NR	NR	NR	NR	NR	NR	SOFA score
Chou et al,[129] 2012	R	Lung cancer	70	NR	58.6%	NR	70	58.6%	NR	58.6%	NR	MV
Slatore et al,[130] 2012	R	Lung cancer	49,373	NR	34%	65%	10,463	59%	85%	59%	85%	Vasopressors MV >2 organ failure Septic conditions
Anisoglou et al,[82] 2013	R	Lung cancer	105	44.7%	56.1%	77.1%	NR	NR	NR	NR	NR	Age Male Organ support Socioeconomic deprivation
Puxty et al,[131] 2015	R	Solid cancers	118541	14.1%	24.6%	NR	NR	NR	NR	NR	NR	

Abbreviations: APACHE, Acute Physiology and Chronic Health Evaluation; ICU, intensive care unit; LODS, logistic organ dysfunction system; MV, mechanical ventilation; NR, not reported; R, retrospective; SAPS, Simplified Acute Physiology Score; SOFA, sequential organ failure assessment.

patients evaluated for admission to the ICU, 20% of those considered to be too well died during their hospitalization, whereas 25% of patients not admitted to the ICU because there were too sick survived.[37] These observations suggest that updating admission policies to allow for ICU admission (unlimited or ICU trial, discussed below) for most patients with cancer is warranted and should result in better outcomes for many of these patients.

Case Volume of Patients with Cancer

There is a correlation between outcome of critically ill patients with cancer and the volume of such patients cared for in these units. Most of the studies have shown that patients with cancer treated in ICUs with a high cancer case volume had better outcomes,[38,39] although this has not been shown consistently.[3] Patients with cancer with acute respiratory failure or septic shock have a mortality between 34% and 50% in specialized ICU with an high volume of patients with cancer , as compared with 66% to 68% in general ICUs.[40] There are number of factors that explain why case volume may play a role in outcome of critically ill patients with cancer, including greater experience, knowledge, and comfort in dealing with this patient population. Also, there is a tendency for these ICUs to be in academic or tertiary centers with access to specialized services that can assist in the management of complex situations in patients with cancer. Dissemination of knowledge about the management of critically ill patient with cancer and following standardized protocols are important steps that may bridge the gap between high- and low-volume ICUs.[41]

CLINICAL VARIABLES AND THE ASSOCIATION WITH SHORT-TERM OUTCOMES IN THE INTENSIVE CARE UNIT

Although the outcome of patients with cancer admitted to the ICU has been improving, not all patients benefit from such care and, for some, ICU admission is associated with an high physical and emotional toll on patients and their families, and results in an inappropriate use of critical resources. The main clinical variables that have been reported in the literature to influence the outcome of critically ill patients with cancer are discussed.

Clinical Variables with Minimal Effect on Outcome

Age
Aging is associated with a reduction in physiologic capacity and a greater prevalence of chronic illnesses. Although some studies have suggested that age is associated with relatively worse outcome,[42,43] most have not shown age to be an independent predictor of death in critically ill patients with cancer.[44–48] Elderly patients with multiple comorbidities should have the goals of care addressed if they develop critical illness and an assessment should be made on whether ICU admission is likely to prolong their life. This process should start ideally with patients and their families early, before a critical illness develops.

Cancer characteristics (type, stage, status, therapy)
Most studies show that patients with HM have worse outcome than those with solid malignancies. However, recent studies on mechanically ventilated patients show no difference between the 2 groups.[43,45,49–52] Also, the type of malignancy does not seem to have impact on short-term outcome of critical illness.[43,48] Cancer types that are generally considered to be high risk such as lung cancer or acute leukemia have shown significant improvements in survival.[18,53] The short-term outcome is also generally not affected by tumor stage at diagnosis nor by the disease status (relapse vs remission).[54] Also failure of first-line chemotherapy with the availability of other options for treatment should not be a reason against ICU admission.[55] However, progressive disease with no further treatment options is associated with poor outcomes.[43,47]

There are few exceptions where certain tumor characteristics remain to be associated with poor outcomes. Most of these factors are related to solid tumors with acute respiratory failure caused by direct invasion of the airways or lymphangitic spread by tumor.[43,56,57] Also, although tumor characteristics do not seem to affect the short-term outcome of critically ill patients with cancer, they do impact the long-term prognosis of these patients.[58]

Initial physiologic severity scores
General severity of illness scores such as Acute Physiology and Chronic Health Evaluation (APACHE), Simplified Acute Physiology Score (SAPS), and Mortality Prediction Model (MPM) have not been shown to predict outcome of critically ill patients with cancer owing to inadequate calibration and underestimation of mortality.[47,59,60] Although these scores are useful in clinical studies, evaluation of ICU performance, quality improvement projects, and for benchmarking purposes, they should not be used to assess the prognosis of individual patients with cancer or in the decision making for admission to the ICU. There are models

that are specific to patients with cancer that have been tested and suggested to be useful in predicting outcome of patients upon admission to the ICU, such as the Hematopoietic Cell Transplantation–Specific Comorbidity Index (HCT-CI) and the ICU Cancer Mortality Model (CMM).[60,61] However prospective, multicenter trials to validate these tools are lacking.

Neutropenia

Initial studies have suggested that the presence of neutropenia in critically ill patients with cancer was associated with worse outcomes.[10,50,62,63] However, more recent studies have shown that this was no longer valid.[35,64,65] A recent metaanalysis of 38 studies addressing the outcome of critically ill neutropenic patients showed that those patients had 11% higher mortality; however, when adjusted to severity of illness, the effect of neutropenia disappeared.[66]

Autologous hematopoietic stem cell transplantation

Autologous HSCT may be associated with a brief critical illness related to high-dose chemotherapy, neutropenia, and organ failure. Previous studies have shown high mortality in these patients.[63] However, with advances in ICU and supportive care, the prognosis of these patients has improved significantly, and several studies have shown that autologous HSCT recipients admitted to the ICU had the same prognosis as the general ICU population.[17,19,22,67]

Tumor lysis syndrome

Tumor lysis syndrome is a major complication of a variety of HM and occasionally in patients with solid cancers. It could happen spontaneously or with the onset of chemotherapy. Tumor lysis syndrome is associated with significant electrolyte abnormalities and organ failure, especially acute renal failure, which may lead to admission to the ICU. With the appropriate supportive care in the ICU, the prognosis of these patients is generally good, with survival exceeding 70%.[68,69] There is even evidence that patients at high risk for tumor lysis syndrome have better outcomes if they are admitted to the ICU prophylactically.[69]

Chemotherapy in the intensive care unit

Studies have shown the feasibility of giving chemotherapy in the ICU to critically ill patients and that this was associated with a reasonable outcome. Chemotherapy actually may improve the outcome of critically ill patients in situations where the underlying malignancy is the main reason for the critical illness, such as tumor infiltration of the lung by cancer.[68,70,71] Some studies have even suggested that sepsis associated with recent chemotherapy has a better prognosis than in those who have not received recent chemotherapy.[72] Furthermore, there is evidence that admitting high-risk patients to receive chemotherapy in the ICU may result in better outcomes and fewer complications, given the high-quality care and close monitoring in this environment.[70]

Clinical Variables with Significant Impact on Outcome

Acute respiratory failure requiring mechanical ventilation

Acute respiratory failure (ARF) develops in 10% to 50% of patients with cancer and is an important cause of admission to the ICU in this patient population.[73] Invasive mechanical ventilation for ARF has been associated traditionally with a high mortality, exceeding 90%.[10,11,62] Although more recent studies have documented a significant improvement in survival, mortality remains between 55% and 83%, with an average of 66%.[74] In acute respiratory distress syndrome, mortality in patients with cancer decreased from 89% to around 55% with and odds ratio of 2.54 (95% CI, 1.570–4.120) when compared with patients without cancer.[23,24]

NIV is reported to be associated commonly with a better outcome in patients with cancer with ARF.[75,76] However, recent large well-designed multicenter trials suggest that early NIV was not superior to other forms of oxygen supplementation.[77] Failure of NIV in patients with ARF is associated with an even higher mortality when compared with primary mechanical ventilation.[75,78] Thus, it is imperative that patients be selected carefully for NIV and that invasive mechanical ventilation is not delayed.

Type and number of organ failure

The higher the number of organ failure upon admission to the ICU, the worse the outcome of critically ill patients. In a study of patients newly diagnosed with cancer and admitted to the ICU, there was good correlation between the number of organ failures and short-term mortality (<20% with 1 organ failure and >80% for 6 organ failures).[70]

Also, the type of organ failure is an important factor influencing the outcome of critically ill patients with cancer, as mentioned in the case of ARF. Similarly, the development of acute renal failure in these patients is associated with high mortality. In a study of 1009 patients with cancer admitted to an ICU in Europe, 671 patients (66.5%) developed acute renal failure during their ICU stay. Their hospital mortality was 44.3% compared with 25.4% for patients without acute renal failure (P<.0001). Those who required renal replacement therapy had even higher mortality compared with those who did not (57.2% vs 31.2%, respectively; P<.0001).[79] Hemodynamic instability requiring vasopressor therapy has also been reported in some studies to be associated with poor outcome. However, other studies have not confirmed this association.[18,50,80–82]

Although the number and type of organ failure on admission to the ICU are important considerations in predicting the outcome of these patients, the reports in the literature show inconsistent results and overall there seems to be improvement in outcome over the years. The number and type of organ failure should not be the determining factor in admitting patients to the ICU; rather, these patients should be given appropriate ICU care to monitor their response. Persistence and/or worsening of organ failure during the ICU stay seems to be a much more significant predictor of a poor outcome.

Allogeneic hematopoietic stem cell transplantation

Allogeneic HSCT is associated with a variety of infectious and noninfectious complications that may lead to critical illness.[83] The improvements in supportive care, prophylactic measures, and treatment of GVHD have decreased the need for ICU care. Before 1995, around 20% of patients with allogeneic HSCT required ICU admission, and this has decreased to less than 12% of patients.[84] Earlier reports have indicated mortality rates exceeding 80%, especially in mechanically ventilated patients.[19,21,85] Although more recent studies show better outcomes, hospital mortality remains in the range of 60% to 70% and the 6-month mortality is around 70% (see **Table 2**). The primary reasons for the high mortality in this patient population are related to ARF requiring mechanical ventilation, especially for noninfectious etiologies that generally do not have effective therapies. Another important factor is ongoing GVHD with the need for immunosuppressive therapy. Despite the high mortality in allogeneic HSCT recipients, it is recommended that these patients be admitted to the ICU for the management of critical illness and consider full care, especially if the admission is in the first 30 days after transplantation.[21] The goals of care should be readdressed if the patient develops progressive or persistent multiorgan failure, especially in the setting of refractory GVHD.

Clinical Variables Associated with Poor Outcome

Poor performance status

Several studies have shown that baseline performance status is an independent factor predicting outcome in critically ill patients with cancer.[5,16,43,81,86–89] In a prospective, multicenter study of 717 patients with cancer admitted to the ICU, performance status was the most important predictor of hospital outcome (odds ratio, 3.40; 95% CI, 2.19–5.26).[5] In a systematic review of critically ill solid patients with cancer, poor performance status (Eastern Cooperative Oncology Group 3 or 4) was associated with a 4- to 7-fold increase in ICU mortality and 2- to 3-fold increase in 90-day mortality.[7]

Performance status may be a composite reflection of advanced age, severe comorbid illnesses, or refractory malignancy, all of which are factors that lead to poor outcome in critically ill patients. Highly dependent or bedridden patients with cancer (Eastern Cooperative Oncology Group performance status of 3–4) should have the goals of care addressed early before critical illness and are generally discouraged from referral for admission to the ICU. Having said that, there are unique situations where the patient may have poor performance owing to a specific type of malignancy that is newly diagnosed or may be associated with severe organ dysfunction but has the potential of reversibility with appropriate treatment. Examples include limited activity associated with bone pain or neurologic deficits related to multiple myeloma, respiratory compromise related to large malignant pleural effusion, and acute renal failure associated with tumor lysis syndrome or urinary obstruction. These patients may present with poor performance status that could potentially improve with aggressive therapy of the underlying malignancy. Such situations should be individualized and some of these patients may still benefit from ICU admission during critical illness.

No cancer treatment options

One of the important goals of admission to the ICU in critically ill patients with cancer is stabilization of patients' conditions and improving their short-term prognosis so they can undergo further treatment of the underlying malignancy. If the cancer is progressive or refractory to chemotherapy with limited treatment options, then it is unlikely that ICU care is going to change the overall outcome. For such patients, there should be an early discussion to avoid a prolonged and potentially painful dying process.

Persistent or progressive multiorgan failure

As mentioned, although the presence of multiorgan failure on admission to the ICU is associated with a worse outcome, the prognosis of these patients has been improving. A better indicator of outcome is the response of organ failure to adequate and appropriate ICU care. Patients with cancer who have persistent or progressive multi-organ failure have a particularity poor prognosis.[25,90–92] In a study of 188 patients with cancer admitted to the ICU, there was no difference between survivors and nonsurvivors in relation to the number of organ failure on admission to the ICU; however, there was strong correlation between survival and number of organ failures on day 6. Mortality was 26% in patients with 1 organ failure on day 6, 55% in patients with 2 organ failures, and 95% in patients with 6 organ failures.[91]

The duration of the aggressive therapy before determining futility of care is not clear. Some studies have suggested that persistent multiorgan failure after 3 to 5 days is associated with a poor outcome.[91] This is the basis of "ICU trial" that has been proposed as a strategy of managing critically ill patients with cancer. This approach suggests that aggressive and appropriate ICU care should be offered to the majority of critically ill patients with cancer for 3 to 5 days, followed by reevaluation of the futility of such care. If the number and/or severity of organ failure persists or worsens, then it is unlikely the patient will benefit from continuing aggressive care and serious consideration should be given to comfort measures. This concept may be discussed and agreed on by the patient, family, and treating physicians upon admission to the ICU. It is likely that the duration of ICU trial needs to be individualized and may be different from 1 patient to another.

Allogeneic hematopoietic stem cell transplantation with severe acute graft-versus-host disease resistant to immunosuppressive therapy

GVHD is a primary cause of morbidity and mortality in allogeneic HSCT recipients. Many of those with controlled or stable GVHD who develop critical illness benefit from ICU care and should be considered for admission to the ICU.[84] However, progressive acute GVHD that is refractory to immunosuppressive therapy is associated particularly with a poor prognosis and it is less likely that such patients will benefit from ICU care.[8,21,40]

Multiple readmissions to the intensive care unit

Patients who require multiple readmissions for decompensated organ dysfunction after an initial ICU care tend to have a poor prognosis and decreased quality of life. Studies have indicated that patients readmitted to the ICU have mortality rates up to 6 times higher than those not readmitted and are 11 times more likely to die in hospital.[93,94] These patients may also not be candidates for further therapy for the underlying

malignancy. A multidisciplinary discussion that includes the patient, family, and the different specialties involved in the care are warranted in these situations to address the potential benefits and harms of further ICU admissions and consider changing the goals of care.

After cardiopulmonary resuscitation

Patients with cancer who achieve return of circulation after cardiac arrest and cardiopulmonary resuscitation (CPR) have a poor prognosis and further ICU care is likely to be futile. In a review of 5196 admissions to an ICU of a large tertiary care cancer center over an 8-year period, 406 patients (8%) underwent CPR, with return of spontaneous circulation in 37%. Only 7 patients (2%) survived to hospital discharge.[95] In a metaanalysis investigating the survival to hospital discharge of adult patients with cancer undergoing in-hospital CPR, the overall survival to discharge was 6.2%. In those patients who were in the ICU when they had the cardiac arrest, the hospital survival was 2.2%.[96]

Although the overall prognosis of patients with cancer who suffer cardiac arrest and undergo CPR is clearly poor, there is at least 1 study that showed a reasonably positive outcome,[97] so further management of these patients should be assessed on a case-by-case basis.

LONG-TERM SURVIVAL

Although the improvement in the short-term outcomes of critically ill patients with cancer is well-established, the long-term survival (>6 months) is less well-studied and there are many more variations than with short-term survival. **Tables 1–3** show that the long-term mortality in ranges between 59% to 81% critically ill patients with HM, 40% to 86% in HSCT recipients, and 12% to 90% in patients with a solid cancer.

The long-term outcome of critically ill patients is more complex than short-term survival. It is influenced by the prognosis of underlying malignancy, comorbid illnesses, long-term effects of critical illness, and ability to undergo further cancer treatment. In a prospective, multicenter study of 1011 critically ill patients with HM, the hospital survival was 60.7% and the 1-year survival rate was 43.3%. At 6 months, 80% of survivors had no change in treatment intensity compared with similar patients not admitted to the ICU, and 80% were in remission.[16] However, such findings were not confirmed by other studies.[98–101]

Another important aspect of long-term survival of critically ill patients with cancer is quality of life. There are few studies that address this vital issue and most of these suggested poor quality of life in this patient population.[16,102] In a well-designed study from Brazil, 792 patients were followed prospectively for 24 months. The 12- and 18-month survivals were 42.4% and 38.1%, respectively. There were significant differences in survival time and quality-adjusted life-years according to all assessed baseline characteristics (ICU admission after elective surgery, emergency surgery, or medical admission; Simplified Acute Physiology Score III; cancer extension; cancer status; previous surgery; previous chemotherapy; previous radiotherapy; performance status; and previous health-related quality of life). Only the previous health-related quality of life and performance status were associated with the health-related quality of life during the 18-month follow-up. In summary, the long-term survival, health-related quality of life, and quality-adjusted life-year expectancy of patients with cancer admitted to the ICU were limited. Nevertheless, these clinical outcomes exhibit wide variability among patients and are associated with simple characteristics present at the time of ICU admission, which may help health care professionals to estimate patients' prognosis early in the course of their illness.[103]

More studies are needed to address the long-term prognosis of critically ill patients with cancer, including the variables that affect outcome differentiating the role of cancer versus critical illness on the outcome. Also, more insight is needed onto the physical and emotional burden of critical illness on the patients and their families.

FUTURE DIRECTIONS

The improvement in the outcome of critically ill patients with cancer is real and promising. However, this progress has opened the door for further questions and challenges. These challenges revolve around the fact that not all patients with cancer will benefit from intensive care and that we need better predictive modeling to help clinicians and patients when determining goals of care. It is also clear that there is variability in outcome between different types of cancer, so it would be useful to provide specific data on more homogenous groups of patients. Although the short-term outcome studies seem to be robust, the data on long-term outcomes are scarce and sometimes conflicting. Longitudinal studies that address the long-term outcome of critically ill patients with cancer including quality of life; cognitive, emotional, and physical impact on the patient; and the ability to treat the underlying malignancy are essential.

REFERENCES

1. Henley SJ, Singh SD, King J, et al. Invasive cancer incidence and Survival–United States, 2012. MMWR Morb Mortal Wkly Rep 2015;64(49):1353–8.
2. Aberle DR, Adams AM, Berg CD, et al. Reduced lung-cancer mortality with low-dose computed tomographic screening. N Engl J Med 2011; 365(5):395–409.
3. van Vliet M, Verburg IW, van den Boogaard M, et al. Trends in admission prevalence, illness severity and survival of haematological patients treated in Dutch intensive care units. Intensive Care Med 2014;40(9):1275–84.
4. Taccone FS, Artigas AA, Sprung CL, et al. Characteristics and outcomes of cancer patients in European ICUs. Crit Care 2009;13(1):R15.
5. Soares M, Caruso P, Silva E, et al. Characteristics and outcomes of patients with cancer requiring admission to intensive care units: a prospective multicenter study. Crit Care Med 2010;38(1):9–15.
6. Cooke CR, Feemster LC, Wiener RS, et al. Aggressiveness of intensive care use among patients with lung cancer in the Surveillance, Epidemiology, and End Results-Medicare Registry. Chest 2014; 146(4):916–23.
7. Puxty K, McLoone P, Quasim T, et al. Survival in solid cancer patients following intensive care unit admission. Intensive Care Med 2014;40(10): 1409–28.
8. Pene F, Salluh JI, Staudinger T. Has survival increased in cancer patients admitted to the ICU? No. Intensive Care Med 2014;40(10):1573–5.
9. Schuster DP, Marion JM. Precedents for meaningful recovery during treatment in a medical intensive care unit. Outcome in patients with hematologic malignancy. Am J Med 1983;75(3):402–8.
10. Lloyd-Thomas AR, Wright I, Lister TA, et al. Prognosis of patients receiving intensive care for lifethreatening medical complications of haematological malignancy. Br Med J 1988;296(6628):1025–9.
11. Peters SG, Meadows JA 3rd, Gracey DR. Outcome of respiratory failure in hematologic malignancy. Chest 1988;94(1):99–102.
12. Crawford SW, Schwartz DA, Petersen FB, et al. Mechanical ventilation after marrow transplantation. Risk factors and clinical outcome. Am Rev Respir Dis 1988;137(3):682–7.
13. Schapira DV, Studnicki J, Bradham DD, et al. Intensive care, survival, and expense of treating critically ill cancer patients. JAMA 1993;269(6):783–6.
14. Guidelines for intensive care unit admission, discharge, and triage. Task force of the American College of Critical Care Medicine, Society of Critical Care Medicine. Crit Care Med 1999;27(3):633–8.
15. Garrouste-Orgeas M, Montuclard L, Timsit JF, et al. Predictors of intensive care unit refusal in French

intensive care units: a multiple-center study. Crit Care Med 2005;33(4):750–5.

16. Azoulay E, Mokart D, Pene F, et al. Outcomes of critically ill patients with hematologic malignancies: prospective multicenter data from France and Belgium–a Groupe de Recherche Respiratoire en Reanimation Onco-Hematologique study. J Clin Oncol 2013;31(22):2810–8.

17. Al-Zubaidi N, Soubani AO. Predictors of mortality in patients with hematologic malignances admitted to the ICU - a prospective observational study. Am J Respir Crit Care Med 2016;193:A3657.

18. Adam AK, Soubani AO. Outcome and prognostic factors of lung cancer patients admitted to the medical intensive care unit. Eur Respir J 2008; 31(1):47–53.

19. Huaringa AJ, Leyva FJ, Giralt SA, et al. Outcome of bone marrow transplantation patients requiring mechanical ventilation. Crit Care Med 2000;28(4): 1014–7.

20. Price KJ, Thall PF, Kish SK, et al. Prognostic indicators for blood and marrow transplant patients admitted to an intensive care unit. Am J Respir Crit Care Med 1998;158(3):876–84.

21. Pene F, Aubron C, Azoulay E, et al. Outcome of critically ill allogeneic hematopoietic stem-cell transplantation recipients: a reappraisal of indications for organ failure supports. J Clin Oncol 2006; 24(4):643–9.

22. Scales DC, Thiruchelvam D, Kiss A, et al. Intensive care outcomes in bone marrow transplant recipients: a population-based cohort analysis. Crit Care 2008;12(3):R77.

23. Azoulay E, Lemiale V, Mokart D, et al. Acute respiratory distress syndrome in patients with malignancies. Intensive Care Med 2014;40(8):1106–14.

24. Soubani AO, Shehada E, Chen W, et al. The outcome of cancer patients with acute respiratory distress syndrome. J Crit Care 2014;29(1):183. e7-12.

25. Larche J, Azoulay E, Fieux F, et al. Improved survival of critically ill cancer patients with septic shock. Intensive Care Med 2003;29(10):1688–95.

26. Maccariello E, Valente C, Nogueira L, et al. Outcomes of cancer and non-cancer patients with acute kidney injury and need of renal replacement therapy admitted to general intensive care units. Nephrol Dial Transplant 2011;26(2):537–43.

27. Frankel HL, Kirkpatrick AW, Elbarbary M, et al. Guidelines for the appropriate use of bedside general and cardiac ultrasonography in the evaluation of critically III patients-part I: general ultrasonography. Crit Care Med 2015;43(11):2479–502.

28. Weled BJ, Adzhigirey LA, Hodgman TM, et al. Critical care delivery: the importance of process of care and ICU structure to improved outcomes: an update from the American College of Critical Care medicine task force on models of critical care. Crit Care Med 2015;43(7):1520–5.

29. Soares M, Bozza FA, Azevedo LC, et al. Effects of organizational characteristics on outcomes and resource use in patients with cancer admitted to intensive care units. J Clin Oncol 2016;34(27): 3315–24.

30. Sprung CL, Geber D, Eidelman LA, et al. Evaluation of triage decisions for intensive care admission. Crit Care Med 1999;27(6):1073–9.

31. McQuillan P, Pilkington S, Allan A, et al. Confidential inquiry into quality of care before admission to intensive care. BMJ 1998;316(7148):1853–8.

32. Lengline E, Raffoux E, Lemiale V, et al. Intensive care unit management of patients with newly diagnosed acute myeloid leukemia with no organ failure. Leuk Lymphoma 2012;53(7):1352–9.

33. Song JU, Suh GY, Park HY, et al. Early intervention on the outcomes in critically ill cancer patients admitted to intensive care units. Intensive Care Med 2012;38(9):1505–13.

34. de Montmollin E, Tandjaoui-Lambiotte Y, Legrand M, et al. Outcomes in critically ill cancer patients with septic shock of pulmonary origin. Shock 2013;39(3):250–4.

35. Mokart D, Lambert J, Schnell D, et al. Delayed intensive care unit admission is associated with increased mortality in patients with cancer with acute respiratory failure. Leuk Lymphoma 2013; 54(8):1724–9.

36. Toffart AC, Pizarro CA, Schwebel C, et al. Selection criteria for intensive care unit referral of lung cancer patients: a pilot study. Eur Respir J 2015;45(2): 491–500.

37. Thiery G, Azoulay E, Darmon M, et al. Outcome of cancer patients considered for intensive care unit admission: a hospital-wide prospective study. J Clin Oncol 2005;23(19):4406–13.

38. Zuber B, Tran TC, Aegerter P, et al. Impact of case volume on survival of septic shock in patients with malignancies. Crit Care Med 2012;40(1):55–62.

39. Lecuyer L, Chevret S, Guidet B, et al. Case volume and mortality in haematological patients with acute respiratory failure. Eur Respir J 2008;32(3): 748–54.

40. Benoit DD, Soares M, Azoulay E. Has survival increased in cancer patients admitted to the ICU? We are not sure. Intensive Care Med 2014;40(10): 1576–9.

41. Soubani AO, Decruyenaere J. Improved outcome of critically ill patients with hematological malignancies: what's next? Intensive Care Med 2014; 40(9):1377–80.

42. Staudinger T, Stoiser B, Mullner M, et al. Outcome and prognostic factors in critically ill cancer patients admitted to the intensive care unit. Crit Care Med 2000;28(5):1322–8.

43. Soares M, Salluh JI, Spector N, et al. Characteristics and outcomes of cancer patients requiring mechanical ventilatory support for >24 hrs. Crit Care Med 2005;33(3):520–6.

44. Kress JP, Christenson J, Pohlman AS, et al. Outcomes of critically ill cancer patients in a university hospital setting. Am J Respir Crit Care Med 1999; 160(6):1957–61.

45. Depuydt PO, Benoit DD, Vandewoude KH, et al. Outcome in noninvasively and invasively ventilated hematologic patients with acute respiratory failure. Chest 2004;126(4):1299–306.

46. Depuydt PO, Benoit DD, Roosens CD, et al. The impact of the initial ventilatory strategy on survival in hematological patients with acute hypoxemic respiratory failure. J Crit Care 2010;25(1):30–6.

47. Groeger JS, White P Jr, Nierman DM, et al. Outcome for cancer patients requiring mechanical ventilation. J Clin Oncol 1999;17(3):991–7.

48. Azoulay E, Alberti C, Bornstain C, et al. Improved survival in cancer patients requiring mechanical ventilatory support: impact of noninvasive mechanical ventilatory support. Crit Care Med 2001;29(3): 519–25.

49. Azoulay E, Moreau D, Alberti C, et al. Predictors of short-term mortality in critically ill patients with solid malignancies. Intensive Care Med 2000;26(12): 1817–23.

50. Benoit DD, Vandewoude KH, Decruyenaere JM, et al. Outcome and early prognostic indicators in patients with a hematologic malignancy admitted to the intensive care unit for a life-threatening complication. Crit Care Med 2003;31(1):104–12.

51. Massion PB, Dive AM, Doyen C, et al. Prognosis of hematologic malignancies does not predict intensive care unit mortality. Crit Care Med 2002; 30(10):2260–70.

52. Shimabukuro-Vornhagen A, Boll B, Kochanek M, et al. Critical care of patients with cancer. CA Cancer J Clin 2016;66:496–517.

53. Park HY, Suh GY, Jeon K, et al. Outcome and prognostic factors of patients with acute leukemia admitted to the intensive care unit for septic shock. Leuk Lymphoma 2008;49(10):1929–34.

54. Peigne V, Rusinova K, Karlin L, et al. Continued survival gains in recent years among critically ill myeloma patients. Intensive Care Med 2009; 35(3):512–8.

55. Azoulay E, Pene F, Darmon M, et al. Managing critically Ill hematology patients: time to think differently. Blood Rev 2015;29(6):359–67.

56. Soares M, Darmon M, Salluh JI, et al. Prognosis of lung cancer patients with life-threatening complications. Chest 2007;131(3):840–6.

57. Azoulay E, Thiery G, Chevret S, et al. The prognosis of acute respiratory failure in critically ill cancer patients. Medicine 2004;83(6):360–70.

58. McGrath S, Chatterjee F, Whiteley C, et al. ICU and 6-month outcome of oncology patients in the intensive care unit. QJM 2010;103(6):397–403.

59. Soares M, Salluh JI. Validation of the SAPS 3 admission prognostic model in patients with cancer in need of intensive care. Intensive Care Med 2006;32(11):1839–44.

60. Soares M, Fontes F, Dantas J, et al. Performance of six severity-of-illness scores in cancer patients requiring admission to the intensive care unit: a prospective observational study. Crit Care 2004; 8(4):R194–203.

61. Bayraktar UD, Shpall EJ, Liu P, et al. Hematopoietic cell transplantation-specific comorbidity index predicts inpatient mortality and survival in patients who received allogeneic transplantation admitted to the intensive care unit. J Clin Oncol 2013; 31(33):4207–14.

62. Epner DE, White P, Krasnoff M, et al. Outcome of mechanical ventilation for adults with hematologic malignancy. J Investig Med 1996;44(5):254–60.

63. Torrecilla C, Cortes JL, Chamorro C, et al. Prognostic assessment of the acute complications of bone marrow transplantation requiring intensive therapy. Intensive Care Med 1988;14(4):393–8.

64. Legrand M, Max A, Peigne V, et al. Survival in neutropenic patients with severe sepsis or septic shock. Crit Care Med 2012;40(1):43–9.

65. Mokart D, Darmon M, Resche-Rigon M, et al. Prognosis of neutropenic patients admitted to the intensive care unit. Intensive Care Med 2015;41(2):296–303.

66. Bouteloup M, Perinel S, Bourmaud A, et al. Outcomes in adult critically Ill cancer patients with and without neutropenia: a systematic review and meta-analysis of the Groupe de Recherche en Reanimation Respiratoire du patient d'Onco-Hematologie (GRRR-OH). Oncotarget 2017;8(1): 1860–70.

67. Trinkaus MA, Lapinsky SE, Crump M, et al. Predictors of mortality in patients undergoing autologous hematopoietic cell transplantation admitted to the intensive care unit. Bone Marrow Transplant 2009; 43(5):411–5.

68. Wohlfarth P, Staudinger T, Sperr WR, et al. Prognostic factors, long-term survival, and outcome of cancer patients receiving chemotherapy in the intensive care unit. Ann Hematol 2014;93(10): 1629–36.

69. Lameire N, Vanholder R, Van Biesen W, et al. Acute kidney injury in critically ill cancer patients: an update. Crit Care 2016;20(1):209.

70. Darmon M, Thiery G, Ciroldi M, et al. Intensive care in patients with newly diagnosed malignancies and a need for cancer chemotherapy. Crit Care Med 2005;33(11):2488–93.

71. Benoit DD, Depuydt PO, Vandewoude KH, et al. Outcome in severely ill patients with hematological

malignancies who received intravenous chemo-therapy in the intensive care unit. Intensive Care Med 2006;32(1):93–9.

72. Vandijck DM, Benoit DD, Depuydt PO, et al. Impact of recent intravenous chemotherapy on outcome in severe sepsis and septic shock patients with he-matological malignancies. Intensive Care Med 2008;34(5):847–55.

73. Pastores SM, Voigt LP. Acute respiratory failure in the patient with cancer: diagnostic and manage-ment strategies. Crit Care Clin 2010;26(1):21–40.

74. Soares M, Depuydt PO, Salluh JI. Mechanical ventilation in cancer patients: clinical character-istics and outcomes. Crit Care Clin 2010;26(1): 41–58.

75. Hilbert G, Gruson D, Vargas F, et al. Noninvasive ventilation in immunosuppressed patients with pul-monary infiltrates, fever, and acute respiratory fail-ure. N Engl J Med 2001;344(7):481–7.

76. Antonelli M, Conti G, Bufi M, et al. Noninvasive ventilation for treatment of acute respiratory failure in patients undergoing solid organ transplantation: a randomized trial. JAMA 2000;283(2):235–41.

77. Lemiale V, Mokart D, Resche-Rigon M, et al. Effect of noninvasive ventilation vs oxygen therapy on mortality among immunocompromised patients with acute respiratory failure: a randomized clinical trial. JAMA 2015;314(16):1711–9.

78. Adda M, Coquet I, Darmon M, et al. Predictors of noninvasive ventilation failure in patients with he-matologic malignancy and acute respiratory fail-ure. Crit Care Med 2008;36(10):2766–72.

79. Darmon M, Vincent F, Canet E, et al. Acute kidney injury in critically ill patients with haematological malignancies: results of a multicentre cohort study from the Groupe de Recherche en Reanimation Respiratoire en Onco-Hematologie. Nephrol Dial Transplant 2015;30(12):2006–13.

80. Mendoza V, Lee A, Marik PE. The hospital-survival and prognostic factors of patients with solid tumors admitted to an ICU. Am J Hosp Palliat Care 2008; 25(3):240–3.

81. Azevedo LC, Caruso P, Silva UV, et al. Outcomes for patients with cancer admitted to the ICU requiring ventilatory support: results from a pro-spective multicenter study. Chest 2014;146(2): 257–66.

82. Anisoglou S, Asteriou C, Barbetakis N, et al. Outcome of lung cancer patients admitted to the intensive care unit with acute respiratory failure. Hippokratia 2013;17(1):60–3.

83. Chi AK, Soubani AO, White AC, et al. An update on pulmonary complications of hematopoietic stem cell transplantation. Chest 2013;144(6):1913–22.

84. Afessa B, Azoulay E. Critical care of the hemato-poietic stem cell transplant recipient. Crit Care Clin 2010;26(1):133–50.

85. Khassawneh BY, White P Jr, Anaissie EJ, et al. Outcome from mechanical ventilation after autolo-gous peripheral blood stem cell transplantation. Chest 2002;121(1):185–8.

86. Christodoulou C, Rizos M, Galani E, et al. Perfor-mance status (PS): a simple predictor of short-term outcome of cancer patients with solid tumors admitted to the intensive care unit (ICU). Anti-cancer Res 2007;27(4c):2945–8.

87. Soares M, Salluh JI, Toscano L, et al. Outcomes and prognostic factors in patients with head and neck cancer and severe acute illnesses. Intensive Care Med 2007;33(11):2009–13.

88. Roques S, Parrot A, Lavole A, et al. Six-month prognosis of patients with lung cancer admitted to the intensive care unit. Intensive Care Med 2009;35(12):2044–50.

89. Namendys-Silva SA, Gonzalez-Herrera MO, Texco-cano-Becerra J, et al. Outcomes of critically ill gy-necological cancer patients admitted to intensive care unit. Am J Hosp Palliat Care 2013;30(1):7–11.

90. Lamia B, Hellot MF, Girault C, et al. Changes in severity and organ failure scores as prognostic fac-tors in onco-hematological malignancy patients admitted to the ICU. Intensive Care Med 2006; 32(10):1560–8.

91. Lecuyer L, Chevret S, Thiery G, et al. The ICU trial: a new admission policy for cancer patients requiring mechanical ventilation. Crit Care Med 2007;35(3):808–14.

92. Guiguet M, Blot F, Escudier B, et al. Severity-of-illness scores for neutropenic cancer patients in an intensive care unit: which is the best predictor? Do multiple assessment times improve the predic-tive value? Crit Care Med 1998;26(3):488–93.

93. Elliott M. Readmission to intensive care: a review of the literature. Aust Crit Care 2006;19(3):96–8, 100–4.

94. Kaben A, Correa F, Reinhart K, et al. Readmission to a surgical intensive care unit: incidence, outcome and risk factors. Crit Care 2008;12(5): R123.

95. Wallace S, Ewer MS, Price KJ, et al. Outcome and cost implications of cardiopulmonary resuscitation in the medical intensive care unit of a comprehen-sive cancer center. Support Care Cancer 2002; 10(5):425–9.

96. Reisfield GM, Wallace SK, Munsell MF, et al. Sur-vival in cancer patients undergoing in-hospital car-diopulmonary resuscitation: a meta-analysis. Resuscitation 2006;71(2):152–60.

97. Champigneulle B, Merceron S, Lemiale V, et al. What is the outcome of cancer patients admitted to the ICU after cardiac arrest? Results from a multicenter study. Resuscitation 2015;92:38–44.

98. Oeyen SG, Benoit DD, Annemans L, et al. Long-term outcomes and quality of life in critically ill

patients with hematological or solid malignancies: a single center study. Intensive Care Med 2013; 39(5):889–98.

99. Hill QA, Kelly RJ, Patalappa C, et al. Survival of patients with hematological malignancy admitted to the intensive care unit: prognostic factors and outcome compared to unselected medical intensive care unit admissions, a parallel group study. Leuk Lymphoma 2012;53(2):282–8.

100. Jackson SR, Tweeddale MG, Barnett MJ, et al. Admission of bone marrow transplant recipients to the intensive care unit: outcome, survival and prognostic factors. Bone Marrow Transplant 1998; 21(7):697–704.

101. Bonomi MR, Smith CB, Mhango G, et al. Outcomes of elderly patients with stage IIIB-IV non-small cell lung cancer admitted to the intensive care unit. Lung Cancer 2012;77(3):600–4.

102. Shih CY, Hung MC, Lu HM, et al. Incidence, life expectancy and prognostic factors in cancer patients under prolonged mechanical ventilation: a nationwide analysis of 5,138 cases during 1998-2007. Crit Care 2013;17(4):R144.

103. Normilio-Silva K, de Figueiredo AC, Pedroso-de-Lima AC, et al. Long-term survival, quality of life, and quality-adjusted survival in critically ill patients with cancer. Crit Care Med 2016;44(7):1327–37.

104. Brunet F, Lanore JJ, Dhainaut JF, et al. Is intensive care justified for patients with haematological malignancies? Intensive Care Med 1990;16(5):291–7.

105. Sculier JP, Markiewicz E. Medical cancer patients and intensive care. Anticancer Res 1991;11(6): 2171–4.

106. Ewig S, Torres A, Riquelme R, et al. Pulmonary complications in patients with haematological malignancies treated at a respiratory ICU. Eur Respir J 1998;12(1):116–22.

107. Kroschinsky F, Weise M, Illmer T, et al. Outcome and prognostic features of intensive care unit treatment in patients with hematological malignancies. Intensive Care Med 2002;28(9):1294–300.

108. Hampshire PA, Welch CA, McCrossan LA, et al. Admission factors associated with hospital mortality in patients with haematological malignancy admitted to UK adult, general critical care units: a secondary analysis of the ICNARC Case Mix Programme Database. Crit Care 2009;13(4):R137.

109. Bird GT, Farquhar-Smith P, Wigmore T, et al. Outcomes and prognostic factors in patients with haematological malignancy admitted to a specialist cancer intensive care unit: a 5 yr study. Br J Anaesth 2012;108(3):452–9.

110. Denardo SJ, Oye RK, Bellamy PE. Efficacy of intensive care for bone marrow transplant patients with respiratory failure. Crit Care Med 1989;17(1):4–6.

111. Afessa B, Tefferi A, Hoagland HC, et al. Outcome of recipients of bone marrow transplants who require intensive-care unit support. Mayo Clin Proc 1992; 67(2):117–22.

112. Crawford SW, Petersen FB. Long-term survival from respiratory failure after marrow transplantation for malignancy. Am Rev Respir Dis 1992;145(3): 510–4.

113. Paz HL, Crilley P, Weinar M, et al. Outcome of patients requiring medical ICU admission following bone marrow transplantation. Chest 1993;104(2): 527–31.

114. Faber-Langendoen K, Caplan AL, McGlave PB. Survival of adult bone marrow transplant patients receiving mechanical ventilation: a case for restricted use. Bone Marrow Transplant 1993;12(5): 501–7.

115. Soubani AO, Kseibi E, Bander JJ, et al. Outcome and prognostic factors of hematopoietic stem cell transplantation recipients admitted to a medical ICU. Chest 2004;126(5):1604–11.

116. Depuydt P, Kerre T, Noens L, et al. Outcome in critically ill patients with allogeneic BM or peripheral haematopoietic SCT: a single-centre experience. Bone Marrow Transplant 2011;46(9):1186–91.

117. Townsend WM, Holroyd A, Pearce R, et al. Improved intensive care unit survival for critically ill allogeneic haematopoietic stem cell transplant recipients following reduced intensity conditioning. Br J Haematol 2013;161(4):578–86.

118. Benz R, Schanz U, Maggiorini M, et al. Risk factors for ICU admission and ICU survival after allogeneic hematopoietic SCT. Bone Marrow Transplant 2014; 49(1):62–5.

119. Allareddy V, Roy A, Rampa S, et al. Outcomes of stem cell transplant patients with acute respiratory failure requiring mechanical ventilation in the United States. Bone Marrow Transplant 2014; 49(10):1278–86.

120. Platon L, Amigues L, Ceballos P, et al. A reappraisal of ICU and long-term outcome of allogeneic hematopoietic stem cell transplantation patients and reassessment of prognosis factors: results of a 5-year cohort study (2009-2013). Bone Marrow Transplant 2016;51(2):256–61.

121. Jennens RR, Rosenthal MA, Mitchell P, et al. Outcome of patients admitted to the intensive care unit with newly diagnosed small cell lung cancer. Lung Cancer 2002;38(3):291–6.

122. Reichner CA, Thompson JA, O'Brien S, et al. Outcome and code status of lung cancer patients admitted to the medical ICU. Chest 2006;130(3): 719–23.

123. Aldawood AS. Prognosis and resuscitation status of critically ill patients with lung cancer admitted to the intensive care unit. Anaesth Intensive Care 2010;38(5):920–3.

124. Caruso P, Ferreira AC, Laurienzo CE, et al. Short- and long-term survival of patients with metastatic solid

cancer admitted to the intensive care unit: prognostic factors. Eur J Cancer Care 2010;19(2):260–6.

125. Namendys-Silva SA, Texcocano-Becerra J, Herrera-Gomez A. Prognostic factors in critically ill patients with solid tumours admitted to an oncological intensive care unit. Anaesth Intensive Care 2010; 38(2):317–24.

126. Andrejak C, Terzi N, Thielen S, et al. Admission of advanced lung cancer patients to intensive care unit: a retrospective study of 76 patients. BMC Cancer 2011;11:159.

127. Toffart AC, Minet C, Raynard B, et al. Use of intensive care in patients with nonresectable lung cancer. Chest 2011;139(1):101–8.

128. Bos MM, de Keizer NF, Meynaar IA, et al. Outcomes of cancer patients after unplanned admission to general intensive care units. Acta Oncol 2012;51(7):897–905.

129. Chou KT, Chen CS, Su KC, et al. Hospital outcomes for patients with stage III and IV lung cancer admitted to the intensive care unit for sepsis-related acute respiratory failure. J Palliat Med 2012;15(11):1234–9.

130. Slatore CG, Cecere LM, Letourneau JL, et al. Intensive care unit outcomes among patients with lung cancer in the Surveillance, Epidemiology, and End Results-Medicare registry. J Clin Oncol 2012; 30(14):1686–91.

131. Puxty K, McLoone P, Quasim T, et al. Risk of Critical illness among patients with solid cancers: a population-based observational study. JAMA Oncol 2015;1(8):1078–85.

Acute Respiratory Failure in Patients with Hematologic Malignancies

Anne-Sophie Moreau, MD[a], Olivier Peyrony, MD[b],
Virginie Lemiale, MD[b], Lara Zafrani, MD, PhD[b],
Elie Azoulay, MD, PhD[b],*

KEYWORDS

- High-resolution computed tomography • Immunocompromised • Noninvasive tests
- Bronchoalveolar lavage

KEY POINTS

- Acute respiratory failure in patients with hematologic malignancies is frequent and associated with high mortality.
- Early recognition of acute respiratory failure in this population is necessary for improving outcomes.
- The diagnostic strategy for critically ill patients with hematologic malignancies differs from that in patients not admitted to the intensive care unit because of a different risk/benefit ratio of bronchoscopy and bronchoalveolar lavage (BAL) in deeply hypoxemic patients.
- Noninvasive diagnostic tests have a high diagnostic yield, whereas fiberoptic bronchoscopy with BAL adds limited diagnostic information.

INTRODUCTION

In immunosuppressed patients with cancer, the development of acute respiratory failure (ARF) is a common event. Overall, 15% of patients with hematologic malignancies present with a pulmonary event during the course of the disease and up to half the patients with prolonged neutropenia (ie, induction of acute leukemia or recipients of allogeneic hematopoietic stem cell transplants) have a pulmonary complication.[1] ARF is the leading cause of admission to the intensive care unit (ICU) for patients treated for hematologic malignancies, followed by shock and neurologic failure.[2–4] Etiologies of ARF are numerous and include pulmonary infections, complications of chemotherapy or of new anticancer drugs, or specific pulmonary involvement by the malignancy. In 20% of the cases, more than 1 cause is identified.

In critically ill hematology patients, survival after ICU management has greatly improved over the last 2 decades, thanks to a better selection of the patients eligible for intensive care and improvements in cancer treatments and in ICU management.[5–9] However, the need for intubation and invasive mechanical ventilation remains, and is associated with a 60% in-hospital mortality because it may reflect the subset of the sickest patients who also have several associated organ dysfunctions, including shock or renal, brain, or liver dysfunction.[2] Great hopes were prompted by the use of noninvasive mechanical ventilation (NIV) in this population,[5,10] but subsequent studies

Disclosure: The authors have no conflicts of interest to declare.
[a] Centre de réanimation, Hôpital Salengro, CHU-Lille, Lille F-59000, France; [b] Medical Intensive Care Unit, Hôpital Saint-Louis, Paris, France
* Corresponding author. ECSTRA Team, Biostatistics and Clinical Epidemiology, UMR 1153 (Center of Epidemiology and Biostatistics Sorbonne Paris Cité, CRESS), INSERM, Paris Diderot Sorbonne University.
E-mail address: elie.azoulay@sls.aphp.fr

Clin Chest Med 38 (2017) 355–362
http://dx.doi.org/10.1016/j.ccm.2017.02.001
0272-5231/17/© 2017 Elsevier Inc. All rights reserved.

showed controversial results.[11-13] Recently, NIV was shown not to be superior to standard oxygen therapy in a multicenter prospective randomized study,[14] and NIV may be associated with an increased risk of intubation and death.[15]

Survival after ICU management is also linked to the early recognition of ARF and early transfer to the ICU.[3,16,17] Studies have shown that ARF from an undetermined cause was associated with higher mortality.[18,19] However, in this population, causes of ARF can be multifactorial and making an appropriate diagnosis may be very difficult. In an autopsy series of hematopoietic stem cell transplant recipients, only 28% of diagnoses were made before death.[20] Rapid and appropriate treatment of all possible causes of ARF is the key to improved outcome.

This article focuses on the clinical approach and diagnostic strategies for ARF in patients with non-pulmonary malignancy, specifically those with hematologic malignancies.

CLINICAL APPROACH

The first step is to recognize early signs of ARF in the hematology ward so early transfer to the ICU may be considered. Early recognition of ARF in this population is the key for improving outcomes.[16,17].

Some investigators described early criteria to diagnose early acute lung injury (EALI) before the onset of ARF and acute lung injury and in order to start a specific treatment as early as possible.[21] The EALI score is based on oxygen requirement (1 point for an oxygen requirement >2–6 L/min or 2 points for >6 L/min), respiratory rate (1 point for a respiratory rate ≥30 breaths/min), and immune suppression (1 point for baseline immune suppression). A score greater than or equal to 2 identified patients who progressed to acute lung injury requiring positive pressure noninvasive ventilation with 89% sensitivity and 75% specificity. This score could be easily used by clinicians for patients in hematology wards. More complex scores have been described but are difficult to use in practice.[22]

The second step is to make a rapid and accurate diagnosis of the underlying cause. However, the clinical lung examination is not specific and additional pulmonary signs should be carefully screened. Therefore, a systematic and rationalized approach is necessary to narrow the differential diagnosis.

The authors previously described a clinical approach described by the mnemonic, DIRECT[1] (**Box 1**), to assist clinicians in determining ARF cause and guide initial treatment and complementary investigations.[23] It is based on the analysis of the delay since the onset of malignancy or

---

Box 1
DIRECT criteria for identifying the most likely causes of acute respiratory failure in patients with cancer

Delay since malignancy onset or HSCT

Immune deficiency pattern

Radiographic appearance

Experience and knowledge of the literature

Clinical picture

HRCT findings

Abbreviations: HRCT, high-resolution computed tomography; HSCT, hematopoietic stem cell transplantation.

---

hematopoietic stem cell transplant, or the delay since initial effective antibiotic therapy or chemoprophylaxis; the pattern of immune deficiency; the radiographic appearance; the experience and knowledge of the literature; the clinical picture (ie, septic shock, skin rash, or associated extrapulmonary symptoms); and patterns observed on the computed tomography (CT) scan.

Also, given advances in patient management and the many new anticancer and antiinflammatory drugs, managing patients in perfect synchrony with hematologists is an obvious requirement. Some of the adverse events of these recently developed agents are still to be described. For example, idelalisib is now described to be responsible for acute pneumonitis[24] and anti–tumor necrosis factor drugs have been associated with an increased risk of nocardiosis.[25]

DIAGNOSTIC STRATEGIES

After a careful clinical examination, patients can be classified based on the clinical pulmonary pattern (focal consolidation vs diffuse crackles, cardiac insufficiency vs noncardiac pulmonary involvement, pleural effusions, extrathoracic findings). A careful approach to additional diagnostic studies must be guided by the clinical findings and the DIRECT screening.

Transthoracic Echocardiography

This test should be obtained in order to rule out cardiogenic pulmonary edema.[26] Performing echocardiography also allows examination of the lungs and pleura, which is helpful when it is not feasible for the patient to undergo lung high-resolution computed tomography (HRCT).[26,27] Note that, because of vascular toxicity from chemotherapy and diastolic cardiac insufficiency, only a complete assessment by a cardiologist or a trained intensivist can rule out cardiac pulmonary edema. Moreover, biomarkers well validated in the emergency department to distinguish between cardiac and noncardiac ARF have a high negative predictive value (NPV) but a low diagnostic yield. The authors discourage their use in this setting.

High-resolution Computed Tomography

In febrile neutropenic patients, the diagnostic value of conventional chest radiographs is very low. In contrast, in neutropenic patients with fever and a normal chest radiograph, lung HRCT identifies 60% to 100% of abnormalities.[28,29] In patients with allogeneic stem cell transplant, lung HRCT had a significantly higher sensitivity (89%) and NPV (80%) than chest radiograph (68% and 47%, respectively).[29,30] However, given a NPV of 80%, a lung HRCT considered as normal is not sufficient to rule out an infection in this population of patients.

Lung HRCT can also differentiate fungal from nonfungal lung infiltrates.[31,32] Specific radiographic patterns have been part of the European Organization for Research and Treatment of Cancer (EORTC) definitions of pulmonary aspergillosis since 2002.[33] Nodular or cavitary lesions are suggestive of invasive fungal infection (IFI), whereas consolidations are suggestive of bacterial infections and ground-glass opacities of viral

pneumonia or *Pneumocystis jiroveci* pneumonia. However, CT patterns are not pathognomonic of any given cause and should be interpreted according to the clinical context and in comparison with previous HRCTs when available.

Microbiological Analysis

Noninvasive tests, which include culture-based and non–culture-based tests (**Table 1**), should be performed routinely. In a previous study, the authors showed that noninvasive tests could yield a diagnosis in 55% of cases.[34]

Culture-based tests

These tests include blood cultures, assisted or induced sputum analysis, and nasopharyngeal aspirates or swabs. These tests require 48 to 72 hours of culture, but have a low diagnostic yield because the patients often are heavily pretreated by antiinfective agents.

Direct sputum examination may allow detection of fungus in patients with airway invasive infections in nonneutropenic patients. Blood cultures remain the best investigation for the diagnosis of candidemia, but may take 48 to 96 hours to grow, which can lead a delayed start of an appropriate treatment and increased mortality.[35] Analysis of high-quality induced sputa by routine staining is able to identify *Pneumocystis* in most patients.

Table 1 Noninvasive diagnostic tests used in evaluating acute respiratory failure		
Radiography		
Chest radiography		
Thin-section HRCT		
Echocardiography or pleural ultrasonography		
Microbiology		
Bacteria	Blood culture Sputum analysis culture Serology: *Chlamydia, Mycoplasma, Legionella* Urine tests: *Pneumococcus* and *Legionella* antigens	
Virus	Serum: herpes consensus PCR test Cytomegalovirus PCR Nasopharyngeal aspiration with multiplex PCR test	
Fungi	Sputum analysis (*Aspergillus*) Circulating *Aspergillus* antigen galactomannan Serum beta1,3-D-glucan Sputum (induced): tests for *P jiroveci* (Grocott-Gomori silver staining and immunofluorescence), PCR for *P jiroveci*	
Biological markers		
BNP or proBNP C-reactive protein Procalcitonin		

Abbreviations: BNP, brain natriuretic peptide; PCR, polymerase chain reaction.

Virus detection

Viruses are easily detected with polymerase chain reaction (PCR) analysis of various noninvasive (nasopharyngeal aspirates or swabs) or invasive (bronchoalveolar lavage [BAL]) samples. Multiplex molecular assays can be performed on respiratory samples and are more sensitive in detecting viruses than immunofluorescence in immunocompromised patients.[36] They provide a specific diagnosis in half the patients in whom other investigations yielded no diagnoses. Specific serum PCR should systematically include cytomegalovirus PCR.

Fungal markers

Galactomannan Galactomannan (GM) is a component of the *Aspergillus* cell membrane. GM level is a robust marker and is part of the revised EORTC/MSG (European Organization for Research and Treatment of Cancer/Mycoses Study Group) criteria for aspergillosis.[34] It can be sampled in serum and pulmonary fluids.

BAL fluid analysis is more sensitive when guided by HRCT, particularly regarding GM detection, which is more sensitive and specific than GM detection in serum to diagnose invasive pulmonary aspergillosis.[37–39] GM level was also correlated to the outcome.[40] The authors consider BAL galactomannan not properly assessed in our ICU hematologic populations, and therefore we are reluctant to recommend its usage.

β-(1,3)-D-Glucan Serum β-(1,3)-D-glucan is an early marker for IFI, with a sensitivity of 78% depending on the clinical context and the type of fungal infection (68% aspergillosis, 85% candidemia, and 100% *Pneumocystis*) and a specificity of 70%. It has a very good NPV (80%–100%) and a good positive predictive value (PPV) for pneumocystis pneumonia when levels are higher than 500 pg/mL.[41] It was included in EORTC/MSG criteria for aspergillosis in 2008.[42] However, the benefit of this test is controversial because of low specificity and high cost.[43] Furthermore, it was recently tested in unselected immunocompromised hematology patients admitted to the ICU, but showed only moderate diagnostic performance, with a low specificity and sensitivity.[44] The NPV was high (94%), making it potentially useful in ruling out IFI and possibly in antifungal deescalation.

Fungal polymerase chain reaction

Aspergillus polymerase chain reaction Aspergillus PCR is a recent method used to diagnose invasive pulmonary aspergillosis. It is not yet included in EORTC/MSG criteria but may be a useful marker with an NPV ranging from 92% to 99% and a 98% specificity.[45,46] PPV is only 75%, and

sensitivity 66%, making it impossible to be used alone. When combined with GM, sensitivity increases to 88%.

Pneumocystis polymerase chain reaction *P jiroveci* pneumonia is based on the identification on a respiratory sample of cysts using various stains (toluidine blue O, Grocott-Gomori silver stain, or Giemsa stains) or indirect immunofluorescence.[35] However, because of the specific pathophysiology of *P jiroveci* pneumonia in hematology patients, the sensitivity of classic staining and immunofluorescence in patients without human immunodeficiency virus (HIV) is lower than in HIV-related *P jiroveci* pneumonia. *Pneumocystis* PCR in respiratory samples is a very sensitive method, but issues are raised about the threshold between colonization and infection.[35,47] However, a negative PCR rules out a pneumocystis pneumonia.

Procalcitonin

Procalcitonin (PCT) level may be useful to exclude bacterial sepsis when less than usual thresholds. However, in immunocompromised patients, association of PCT with mortality is controversial.[48] Moreover, interventional studies are necessary to confirm its utility in reducing antibiotic consumption and multidrug-resistant bacteria in patients with cancer.[49] However, based on current evidence, the value of PCT is mostly based on its high NPV. Otherwise, high PCT concentrations have been observed in nonbacterial and even noninfectious diseases.

Does Bronchoalveolar Lavage Need to be Performed?

Fiberoptic bronchoscopy with BAL (FO-BAL) is a cornerstone for investigating lung infiltrates in immunosuppressed patients, allowing direct visualization of the bronchial tree and sampling of pulmonary secretions and distal alveoli via lavage. However, its diagnostic yield varies across published studies.[10,34,50–52] Moreover, FO-BAL has been described as responsible for respiratory deterioration in immunosuppressed patients with ARF.[19,34,51] More recently, FO-BAL was proved to be safe when performed early after admission to the ICU in patients with spontaneous breathing and receiving NIV.[53] High-flow oxygen can also be applied in this setting. However, many studies show a low diagnostic yield of this procedure[34,50,51] and, in a randomized study, BAL added diagnostic information to noninvasive tests in only 18% of patients and was less helpful when performed later in the course of respiratory failure.[53] Given this evidence, the authors recommend avoiding

FO-BAL in specific settings, such as pulmonary infiltration from malignancies, P jiroveci pneumonia, and drug-related pulmonary toxicity, as well as for the diagnosis of new clinical scenarios or new pulmonary toxicities.[53]

Lung Biopsy

Lung biopsy can be considered when no diagnosis is obtained after all the previous explorations, or when a minimally invasive CT-guided biopsy can easily be performed by a trained radiologist in the setting of ensured hemostasis on stable patients. Only few data are available, because the procedure is not commonly performed in this population of immunosuppressed patients in poor condition. Three modalities exist: transbronchial, CT scan–guided, and surgical biopsies.

Transbronchial lung biopsies

Transbronchial lung biopsy (TBLB) along with BAL obtain a higher diagnostic yield than BAL alone in immunocompromised patients, and seems to be a safe procedure.[54,55] A recent study tested cryo-transbronchial biopsies in very selected patients with good results, few complications, and a change in therapy in 80% of the cases.[56] However, studies to assess the risk/benefit ratio in these patients, who are frequently thrombocytopenic or with hemostasis disorders, are warranted.

Computed tomography scan–guided lung biopsies[57,58]

This technique has a high diagnostic yield, with a sensitivity of 94%, specificity of 100%, and NPV of 73%. It is less sensitive for infectious or inflammatory process than malignancy, with 60% specific diagnoses and 20% to 30% of infectious diagnoses,[58,59] and induced a change of therapy in 80% of the cases when a specific diagnosis was made. Major complications include pneumothorax (21%), requiring drainage in 2.0% of cases.[60]

Surgical biopsies[61]

Video-assisted thoracoscopic biopsies in trained hands and safe conditions have a high diagnostic yield, but have not yet been properly evaluated in hematology patients with ARF of undetermined cause. Open lung biopsy can lead to a diagnosis in 60% of cases.[61] In a series of hematopoietic stem cell transplant recipients, an infectious cause was found in one-third of the cases (mainly cytomegalovirus) and a specific cause in two-thirds of the cases.[62] It induced change of therapy in two-thirds of the cases.

In patients with acute respiratory distress syndrome receiving mechanical ventilation, open lung biopsies at bedside were reported to be safe (26% of immediate complications: pneumothorax, minimal bleeding) and resulted in major changes in management in 89% of the patients, with a decision to limit care in 12 of 17 patients who died.[63]

SUMMARY

Significant advances have been made in the management and diagnosis of ARF in immunocompromised patients. However, the cause of ARF remains undiagnosed in many individuals, leading to increased mortality. Improvements are still needed to better characterize the role of fungal PCR, new biomarkers, and the appropriate timing and circumstance for pulmonary biopsies. Particular attention should be given to new anticancer drugs and their potential pulmonary toxicities that are yet to be described and documented.

REFERENCES

1. Azoulay É, Schlemmer B. Diagnostic strategy in cancer patients with acute respiratory failure. Intensive Care Med 2006;32(6):808–22.
2. Azoulay E, Mokart D, Pene F, et al. Outcomes of critically ill patients with hematologic malignancies: prospective multicenter data from France and Belgium–A Groupe de Recherche Respiratoire en Reanimation Onco-Hematologique study. J Clin Oncol 2013;31(22):2810–8.
3. Thiery G. Outcome of cancer patients considered for intensive care unit admission: a hospital-wide prospective study. J Clin Oncol 2005;23(19):4406–13.
4. Benoit DD, Vandewoude KH, Decruyenaere JM, et al. Outcome and early prognostic indicators in patients with a hematologic malignancy admitted to the intensive care unit for a life-threatening complication. Crit Care Med 2003;31(1):104–12.
5. Azoulay E, Alberti C, Bornstain C, et al. Improved survival in cancer patients requiring mechanical ventilatory support: impact of noninvasive mechanical ventilatory support. Crit Care Med 2001;29(3):519–25.
6. Peigne V, Rusinová K, Karlin L, et al. Continued survival gains in recent years among critically ill myeloma patients. Intensive Care Med 2009;35(3):512–8.
7. Khassawneh BY, White P, Anaissie EJ, et al. Outcome from mechanical ventilation after autologous peripheral blood stem cell transplantation. Chest 2002;121(1):185–8.
8. Legrand M, Max A, Peigne V, et al. Survival in neutropenic patients with severe sepsis or septic shock. Crit Care Med 2012;40(1):43–9.

9. Zuber B, Tran T-C, Aegerter P, et al. Impact of case volume on survival of septic shock in patients with malignancies. Crit Care Med 2012;40(1):55–62.

10. Hilbert G, Gruson D, Vargas F, et al. Noninvasive ventilation in immunosuppressed patients with pulmonary infiltrates, fever, and acute respiratory failure. N Engl J Med 2001;344(7):481–7.

11. Schnell D, Timsit J-F, Darmon M, et al. Noninvasive mechanical ventilation in acute respiratory failure: trends in use and outcomes. Intensive Care Med 2014;40(4):582–91.

12. Gristina GR, Antonelli M, Conti G, et al. Noninvasive versus invasive ventilation for acute respiratory failure in patients with hematologic malignancies: a 5-year multicenter observational survey. Crit Care Med 2011;39(10):2232–9.

13. Azoulay E, Lemiale V. Non-invasive mechanical ventilation in hematology patients with hypoxemic acute respiratory failure: a false belief? Bone Marrow Transplant 2012;47(4):469–72.

14. Lemiale V, Mokart D, Resche-Rigon M, et al. Effect of noninvasive ventilation vs oxygen therapy on mortality among immunocompromised patients with acute respiratory failure: a randomized clinical trial. JAMA 2015;314(16):1711.

15. Frat J-P, Ragot S, Girault C, et al. Effect of non-invasive oxygenation strategies in immunocompromised patients with severe acute respiratory failure: a post-hoc analysis of a randomised trial. Lancet Respir Med 2016;4(8):646–52.

16. Mokart D, Lambert J, Schnell D, et al. Delayed intensive care unit admission is associated with increased mortality in patients with cancer with acute respiratory failure. Leuk Lymphoma 2013;54(8):1724–9.

17. Song J-U, Suh GY, Park HY, et al. Early intervention on the outcomes in critically ill cancer patients admitted to intensive care units. Intensive Care Med 2012;38(9):1505–13.

18. Chaoui D, Legrand O, Roche N, et al. Incidence and prognostic value of respiratory events in acute leukemia. Leukemia 2004;18(4):670–5.

19. Azoulay É, Thiéry G, Chevret S, et al. The prognosis of acute respiratory failure in critically ill cancer patients. Medicine (Baltimore) 2004;83(6):360–70.

20. Sharma S, Nadrous HF, Peters SG, et al. Pulmonary complications in adult blood and marrow transplant recipients: autopsy findings. Chest 2005;128(3):1385–92.

21. Levitt JE, Calfee CS, Goldstein BA, et al. Early acute lung injury: criteria for identifying lung injury prior to the need for positive pressure ventilation. Crit Care Med 2013;41(8):1929–37.

22. Gajic O, Dabbagh O, Park PK, et al. Early identification of patients at risk of acute lung injury: evaluation of lung injury prediction score in a multicenter cohort study. Am J Respir Crit Care Med 2011;183(4):462–70.

23. Schnell D, Mayaux J, Lambert J, et al. Clinical assessment for identifying causes of acute respiratory failure in cancer patients. Eur Respir J 2013;42(2):435–43.

24. Haustraete E, Obert J, Diab S, et al. Idelalisib-related pneumonitis. Eur Respir J 2016;47(4):1280–3.

25. Abreu C. Nocardia infections among immunomodulated inflammatory bowel disease patients: a review. World J Gastroenterol 2015;21(21):6491.

26. Blanco PA, Cianciulli TF. Pulmonary edema assessed by ultrasound: impact in cardiology and intensive care practice. Echocardiography 2016;33(5):778–87.

27. Frankel HL, Kirkpatrick AW, Elbarbary M, et al. Guidelines for the appropriate use of bedside general and cardiac ultrasonography in the evaluation of critically ill patients—Part I: general ultrasonography. Crit Care Med 2015;43(11):2479–502.

28. Rámila E, Sureda A, Martino R, et al. Bronchoscopy guided by high-resolution computed tomography for the diagnosis of pulmonary infections in patients with hematologic malignancies and normal plain chest X-ray. Haematologica 2000;85(9):961–6.

29. Heussel CP, Kauczor HU, Heussel GE, et al. Pneumonia in febrile neutropenic patients and in bone marrow and blood stem-cell transplant recipients: use of high-resolution computed tomography. J Clin Oncol 1999;17(3):796–805.

30. Schueller G, Matzek W, Kalhs P, et al. Pulmonary infections in the late period after allogeneic bone marrow transplantation: chest radiography versus computed tomography. Eur J Radiol 2005;53(3):489–94.

31. Caillot D, Latrabe V, Thiébaut A, et al. Computer tomography in pulmonary invasive aspergillosis in hematological patients with neutropenia: an useful tool for diagnosis and assessment of outcome in clinical trials. Eur J Radiol 2010;74(3):e172–175.

32. Beigelman-Aubry C, Godet C, Caumes E. Lung infections: the radiologist's perspective. Diagn Interv Imaging 2012;93(6):431–40.

33. Ascioglu S, Rex JH, de Pauw B, et al. Defining opportunistic invasive fungal infections in immunocompromised patients with cancer and hematopoietic stem cell transplants: an international consensus. Clin Infect Dis 2002;34(1):7–14.

34. Azoulay E, Mokart D, Rabbat A, et al. Diagnostic bronchoscopy in hematology and oncology patients with acute respiratory failure: prospective multicenter data. Crit Care Med 2008;36(1):100–7.

35. Arvanitis M, Anagnostou T, Fuchs BB, et al. Molecular and nonmolecular diagnostic methods for invasive fungal infections. Clin Microbiol Rev 2014;27(3):490–526.

36. Schnell D, Legoff J, Mariotte E, et al. Molecular detection of respiratory viruses in immunocompromised ICU patients: incidence and meaning. Respir Med 2012;106(8):1184–91.

37. Becker MJ, Lugtenburg EJ, Cornelissen JJ, et al. Galactomannan detection in computerized tomography-based broncho-alveolar lavage fluid and serum in haematological patients at risk for invasive pulmonary aspergillosis. Br J Haematol 2003;121(3): 448–57.

38. Meersseman W, Lagrou K, Maertens J, et al. Galactomannan in bronchoalveolar lavage fluid: a tool for diagnosing aspergillosis in intensive care unit patients. Am J Respir Crit Care Med 2008;177(1): 27–34.

39. Schroeder M, Simon M, Katchanov J, et al. Does galactomannan testing increase diagnostic accuracy for IPA in the ICU? A prospective observational study. Crit Care 2016;20(1):139.

40. Bergeron A, Porcher R, Menotti J, et al. Prospective evaluation of clinical and biological markers to predict the outcome of invasive pulmonary aspergillosis in hematological patients. J Clin Microbiol 2012; 50(3):823–30.

41. Ostrosky-Zeichner L, Alexander BD, Kett DH, et al. Multicenter clinical evaluation of the (1−>3) beta-D-glucan assay as an aid to diagnosis of fungal infections in humans. Clin Infect Dis 2005;41(5):654–9.

42. De Pauw B, Walsh TJ, Donnelly JP, et al. Revised definitions of invasive fungal disease from the European Organization for Research and Treatment of Cancer/Invasive Fungal Infections Cooperative Group and the National Institute of Allergy and Infectious Diseases Mycoses Study Group (EORTC/MSG) Consensus Group. Clin Infect Dis 2008; 46(12):1813–21.

43. Sulahian A, Porcher R, Bergeron A, et al. Use and limits of (1-3)-β-d-glucan assay (Fungitell), compared to galactomannan determination (Platelia Aspergillus), for diagnosis of invasive aspergillosis. J Clin Microbiol 2014;52(7):2328–33.

44. Azoulay E, Guigue N, Darmon M, et al. (1, 3)-β-D-glucan assay for diagnosing invasive fungal infections in critically ill patients with hematological malignancies. Oncotarget 2016;7(16):21484–95.

45. Imbert S, Gauthier L, Joly I, et al. Aspergillus PCR in serum for the diagnosis, follow-up and prognosis of invasive aspergillosis in neutropenic and nonneutropenic patients. Clin Microbiol Infect 2016;22(6):562. e1-8.

46. White PL, Wingard JR, Bretagne S, et al. Aspergillus polymerase chain reaction: systematic review of evidence for clinical use in comparison with antigen testing. Clin Infect Dis 2015;61(8):1293–303.

47. Fauchier T, Hasseine L, Gari-Toussaint M, et al. Detection of Pneumocystis jirovecii by quantitative PCR to differentiate colonization and pneumonia in immunocompromised HIV-positive and HIV-negative patients. J Clin Microbiol 2016;54(6): 1487–95.

48. Bele N, Darmon M, Coquet I, et al. Diagnostic accuracy of procalcitonin in critically ill immunocompromised patients. BMC Infect Dis 2011;11:224.

49. Sedef AM, Kose F, Mertsoylu H, et al. Procalcitonin as a biomarker for infection-related mortality in cancer patients. Curr Opin Support Palliat Care 2015; 9(2):168–73.

50. Rabbat A, Chaoui D, Lefebvre A, et al. Is BAL useful in patients with acute myeloid leukemia admitted in ICU for severe respiratory complications? Leukemia 2008;22(7):1361–7.

51. White P, Bonacum JT, Miller CB. Utility of fiberoptic bronchoscopy in bone marrow transplant patients. Bone Marrow Transplant 1997;20(8):681–7.

52. Gruson D, Hilbert G, Valentino R, et al. Utility of fiberoptic bronchoscopy in neutropenic patients admitted to the intensive care unit with pulmonary infiltrates. Crit Care Med 2000;28(7): 2224–30.

53. Azoulay É, Mokart D, Lambert J, et al. Diagnostic strategy for hematology and oncology patients with acute respiratory failure: randomized controlled trial. Am J Respir Crit Care Med 2010;182(8):1038–46.

54. Cazzadori A, Di Perri G, Todeschini G, et al. Transbronchial biopsy in the diagnosis of pulmonary infiltrates in immunocompromised patients. Chest 1995;107(1):101–6.

55. Mulabecirovic A, Gaulhofer P, Auner HW, et al. Pulmonary infiltrates in patients with haematologic malignancies: transbronchial lung biopsy increases the diagnostic yield with respect to neoplastic infiltrates and toxic pneumonitis. Ann Hematol 2004; 83(7):420–2.

56. Fruchter O, Fridel L, Rosengarten D, et al. Transbronchial cryobiopsy in immunocompromised patients with pulmonary infiltrates: a pilot study. Lung 2013; 191(6):619–24.

57. Lass-Flörl C, Resch G, Nachbaur D, et al. The value of computed tomography-guided percutaneous lung biopsy for diagnosis of invasive fungal infection in immunocompromised patients. Clin Infect Dis 2007;45(7):e101–104.

58. Kothary N, Bartos JA, Hwang GL, et al. Computed tomography-guided percutaneous needle biopsy of indeterminate pulmonary pathology: efficacy of obtaining a diagnostic sample in immunocompetent and immunocompromised patients. Clin Lung Cancer 2010;11(4):251–6.

59. Gupta S, Sultenfuss M, Romaguera JE, et al. CT-guided percutaneous lung biopsies in patients with haematologic malignancies and undiagnosed pulmonary lesions. Hematol Oncol 2010;28(2): 75–81.

60. Muehlstaedt M, Bruening R, Diebold J, et al. CT/fluoroscopy-guided transthoracic needle biopsy: sensitivity and complication rate in 98 procedures. J Comput Assist Tomogr 2002;26(2):191–6.

61. White DA, Wong PW, Downey R. The utility of open lung biopsy in patients with hematologic malignancies. Am J Respir Crit Care Med 2000;161(3):723–9.

62. Wang J-Y, Chang Y-L, Lee L-N, et al. Diffuse pulmonary infiltrates after bone marrow transplantation: the role of open lung biopsy. Ann Thorac Surg 2004;78(1):267–72.

63. Charbonney E, Robert J, Pache J-C, et al. Impact of bedside open lung biopsies on the management of mechanically ventilated immunocompromised patients with acute respiratory distress syndrome of unknown etiology. J Crit Care 2009; 24(1):122–8.

Palliative and End-of-Life Care for Patients with Malignancy

Kathleen M. Akgün, MD, MS

KEYWORDS

- Palliative care • End-of-life (EOL) • Hospice • Cancer • Life-sustaining treatments (LST)
- Symptoms • Patient-centered and family-centered outcomes

KEY POINTS

- Palliative and end-of-life (EOL) care needs for patients living with cancer and their families are substantial and include distressing symptoms, psychosocial suffering, and existential and/or spiritual suffering.
- Palliative care referral is associated with improved symptoms, decreased intensity of non-palliative EOL care, and higher family-rated satisfaction with EOL care.
- Provider attitudes and perceptions continue to be important barriers to referral to specialty palliative care.
- Disparities in referral to palliative care persist for nonwhite populations of patients with malignancy.
- Palliative care delivery may be improved by addressing attitudes and knowledge about palliative care among health care providers and patients.

INTRODUCTION

Many patients with cancer are living longer. Development of targeted, disease-specific cancer treatments has reshaped the way clinicians think about cancer.[1–7] When patients with cancer develop life-threatening complications from their disease or its treatments, improvements in the delivery of life-sustaining treatments (LSTs), usually delivered in an intensive care unit (ICU), have been instrumental in supporting patients through decompensations and complications. LSTs have improved survival for general ICU populations.[8–14] Although the efficacy of some LSTs has been mixed in patients with cancer, time-limited trials for many of these therapies are reasonable to consider for appropriate patients.[9,15–17]

Cancer remains a common and important life-limiting condition. Worldwide, cancer was responsible for 8.2 million deaths, or 13% of all deaths, in 2012. In the United States, cancer is the second most common cause of death following heart disease.[18] Given the prevalence of cancer, its associated symptoms, and its impact on quality of life and life expectancy, patients and their families are at risk for unmet palliative care (PC) needs from the time of diagnosis, during active cancer treatment, and up to the time of the patient's death. This article defines palliative and

Disclosure: There is no relevant commercial or financial conflict of interest to declare. No funding support was part of this article preparation.
Disclaimer: The views expressed in this article of those of the author and do not necessarily represent the views of the US government, the US Department of Veterans Affairs, or any of the author's affiliated hospitals and academic institutions.

Section of Pulmonary, Critical Care and Sleep Medicine, Department of Internal Medicine, VA Connecticut Healthcare System, Yale University School of Medicine, 950 Campbell Avenue, MS11 ACSLG, West Haven, CT 06516, USA
E-mail addresses: kathleen.akgun@yale.edu; kathleen.akgun@va.gov

Clin Chest Med 38 (2017) 363–376
http://dx.doi.org/10.1016/j.ccm.2016.12.010
0272-5231/17/Published by Elsevier Inc.

end-of-life (EOL) care. It then reviews causes and treatments of dyspnea for patients with cancer. Models and timing for palliative and EOL care delivery are discussed, including the promising role for technology in addressing unmet PC needs. In addition, common barriers to delivery of palliative and EOL care for patients living with cancer are identified.

DEFINING PALLIATIVE AND END-OF-LIFE CARE

The World Health Organization (WHO) defines PC as:

> A [team] approach that improves the quality of life of patients and their families facing the problem associated with life-threatening illness, through the prevention and relief of suffering by means of early identification and impeccable assessment and treatment of pain and other problems, physical, psychosocial and spiritual.[19]

PC teams address domains of physical, existential, spiritual, and social suffering and facilitate complex decision making at any stage of a disease (**Box 1**).[20–23] PC is an important aspect to delivering high-quality EOL care, defined as the last 6 months of life for hospice evaluation, but is not restricted to EOL care and decision making.

Clinical practice guidelines and expert opinion recommend incorporating PC into oncology practices or teams.[24] Patients with cancer frequently live with a high burden of physical symptoms. Existential, psychosocial, and spiritual suffering are also common and can be more difficult to identify and quantify. Weighing acceptable tradeoffs between quality of life and potential treatment options to achieve control or even cure contribute to

patients' uncertainty over their lives, their roles in their families, and their roles in society. High-quality PC can uncover priorities, preferences, and goals for patients as they consider these choices. Thus, PC plays a critical role in delivering patient-centered and family-centered care for patients living with cancer.

Inconsistent terminology is challenge in defining PC and understanding its impact on clinical and patient-centered and family-centered outcomes. In a systematic review, terms including "palliative care," "[best] supportive care," "terminal care," "end of life," "goals of care," and "transition of care" were used to discuss PC and associated interventions.[25] Furthermore, the type of journal also affects which terms are used, with "supportive care" more frequently used in oncology journals, whereas "palliative care" and "end of life" were more frequent in palliative medicine journals. Establishing a common language with consistent definitions for PC is necessary to better understand the impact of PC on the quality of care for patients with life-limiting conditions such as cancer.

PALLIATION OF DYSPNEA IN CANCER
Dyspnea Prevalence, Causes, and Significance

Symptom burden is substantial for patients with cancer. Fatigue, decreased appetite, pain, and dyspnea are frequently reported and are among the most bothersome symptoms to patients. Many of these symptoms worsen as patients approach the end of their lives (**Fig. 1**).[26] Although a review of all of the symptoms experienced by patients living with cancer is beyond the scope of this article, a brief review of dyspnea prevalence, its causes, and its association with outcomes is presented.

Respiratory symptoms are among the most common physical symptoms for patients living with cancer.[26] Moderate to severe dyspnea affects approximately 25% of patients with advanced cancer, with prevalence increasing during the last 6 months of life.[26–29] Seventy percent of patients with cancer report intense, episodic exacerbations of dyspnea with activity during the last 6 months of life.[26,27] Moreover, dyspnea can exacerbate other distressing symptoms such as pain and fatigue.[26]

Like pain assessment, there is no objective measurement tool for dyspnea. Vital signs, laboratory tests, or radiographic imaging should not be used to confirm the presence of dyspnea or gauge its severity. Patients with cancer frequently report significant, distressing dyspnea without typical signs of respiratory distress such as tachypnea

---

Box 1
Evidence-based domains of high-quality palliative care

Symptom relief

Emotional support to patient and families

Promote shared decision making and advanced care planning

Meeting the needs of patients and their families/caregivers

Addressing grief and spirituality

Preparation for the dying process

Coordination of care

Data from Refs.[20–23]

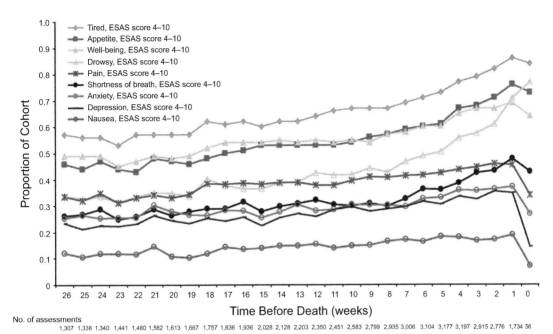

No. of assessments

1,307 1,338 1,340 1,441 1,480 1,582 1,613 1,667 1,757 1,836 1,936 2,028 2,128 2,203 2,350 2,451 2,583 2,799 2,935 3,006 3,104 3,177 3,197 2,915 2,776 1,734 56

Fig. 1. Prevalence of moderate-to-severe symptoms reported by patients with cancer using Edmonton Symptom Assessment System (ESAS) scores (ie, 4–10) during the last 6 months of life (from a cohort of 10,752 patients in a longitudinal cohort from Ontario, CA, between January 1, 2007, and March 31, 2009). (*Data from* Seow H, Barbera L, Sutradhar R, et al. Trajectory of performance status and symptom scores for patients with cancer during the last six months of life. J Clin Oncol 2011;29:1154; with permission from American Society of Clinical Oncology.)

or oxygen desaturation. Thus, dyspnea must be assessed directly by patient self-report. Dyspnea should be assessed for its quality (eg, increased effort to breathe, air hunger, chest tightness), its intensity, and its impact on overall activities.[30–32] Several disease-specific and symptom-specific tools have been developed and validated to assess dyspnea for patients with cancer, such as the numeric rating or visual analog scales.[33]

Multiple pulmonary and extrapulmonary causes of dyspnea should be considered for patients with cancer (**Table 1**). Comorbidities such as chronic obstructive pulmonary disease and pulmonary fibrosis are common causes for dyspnea and increase with age in patients living with cancer.[29,34] Dyspnea can also be caused by direct pulmonary involvement of tumor in the central airways, alveoli, interstitium, pleural spaces, or chest wall and ribs. In addition, pulmonary toxicity associated with treatment regimens can contribute to dyspnea. Frequently dyspnea has multiple pulmonary and extrapulmonary causes simultaneously, including paraneoplastic conditions, anemia, cardiac disease, neuromuscular disease, and psychiatric conditions.[32,35] Evaluation of dyspnea should be based on a detailed history, physical examination, and appropriately targeted laboratory and radiographic testing.

Dyspnea is associated with poor health outcomes. Dyspnea is closely related to other uncomfortable physical and psychological symptoms, including pain and anxiety.[29] Worsening dyspnea is associated with increased symptom burden over time and has a significant detrimental effect on performance status for patients living with malignancy.[29] Dyspnea also affects outcomes for patients who may be candidates for curative cancer surgery. Patients who reported dyspnea at rest or on exertion before lung cancer resection surgery had 4.2 and 2.0 increased odds for mortality respectively, after adjusting for other important demographic, clinical, and surgical risk factors.[36] In another single-center series of patients with cancer who presented to an emergency department, dyspnea was associated with 3-fold increased mortality at 90 and 180 days.[37] Dyspnea continues to be a common and uncomfortable symptom for patients living with malignancy that is also an important predictor for mortality.

Dyspnea Treatment and Management for Patients with Malignancy

While addressing underlying causes, dyspnea should be treated with best supportive care to

Table 1
Pulmonary causes of dyspnea and management for patients with cancer

Causes	Treatments, Management
Pneumonia (bacterial, viral, fungal)	Antibiotics, antivirals, antifungals as indicated, bronchodilators
Underlying pulmonary disease (COPD, asthma)	Bronchodilators, corticosteroids
Airway obstruction	Airway stents, surgical or minimally invasive laser surgery resection
Lymphangitic spread	Chemotherapy, corticosteroids, oxygen if hypoxemic
Pneumonitis (radiation, drug related, idiopathic)	Corticosteroids, discontinuing offending agent
Pleural effusion	Thoracentesis, chest tube/pleural catheter if recurrent and aligns with goals of care
Bronchorrhea[35]	Anticholinergic medications, octreotide (case reports)
Pulmonary embolism	Anticoagulation, inferior vena cava filter if indicated
Respiratory muscle weakness (paraneoplastic syndrome)	Noninvasive ventilation

Abbreviation: COPD, chronic obstructive pulmonary disease.

relieve symptoms. Cool air blown by a fan can relieve some degree of dyspnea. Although a therapeutic trial of oxygen is reasonable for patients with dyspnea who are approaching the end of their lives, oxygen prescription should be primarily reserved for patients with cancer who are hypoxemic.[38–41] In a randomized trial including 239 patients from Australia, the United States, and the United Kingdom, supplement oxygen was no more effective than room air in relieving refractory dyspnea in patients with life-limiting diseases who did not have hypoxemia.[40] High-flow oxygen and noninvasive ventilation can also be used to treat dyspnea and could be opioid sparing for dyspnea management in patients with malignancy.[42,43] However, both supplemental oxygen and noninvasive ventilation should be identified as LSTs.[44,45] Patients and their family members should engage in shared decision making about the role of these LSTs toward the EOL, including time-limited trials and the threshold for cessation.[44,45]

Opioids are the mainstay pharmacologic treatment of refractory dyspnea, and can be used to safely treat dyspnea for patients with cancer, often at doses lower than are typically used to treat cancer pain.[46–48] Benzodiazepines can be helpful for patients who also have anxiety.[49] Corticosteroids have also been used to treat dyspnea for patients with cancer, especially for patients with lymphangitic tumor spread or airway obstruction. Although the exact mechanisms are unclear, it is speculated that corticosteroids relieve dyspnea by reducing edema around the tumor. A recent randomized controlled pilot study suggested that 7 days of dexamethasone was associated with significantly improved dyspnea and was well tolerated by patients.[50] However, despite its frequent use for palliative purposes in cancer care, evidence supporting its broad use in managing dyspnea in malignancy is limited.[51–54]

Nasal and nebulized medications have been evaluated for management of dyspnea for patients with cancer. Nasal fentanyl decreased subjective dyspnea and increased walk distance compared with placebo in a pilot study of 24 patients with malignancy who reported exercise-induced dyspnea.[55] Nebulized opioids have been an attractive method for treating dyspnea, theoretically affecting mu-receptors in the airways while avoiding excessive sedation from systemic absorption. However, randomized studies failed to show the efficacy of nebulized morphine in controlling dyspnea in patients with malignancy.[53] Similarly, despite case reports that suggested nebulized furosemide could be used to treat cancer-related dyspnea, results could not be replicated in randomized trials.[33,56] Based on current data, there is no role for nebulized opioids or furosemide in the treatment of dyspnea.

Nonpharmacologic treatments are effective in relieving dyspnea for patients with cancer. Pulmonary rehabilitation and strength training are feasible and can improve dyspnea for patients with advanced lung cancer.[57–60] Cognitive behavior therapy may also improve dyspnea.[59,60] Participation in breathlessness support groups has been associated with improved symptoms management in a London-based randomized trial of patients with breathlessness caused by a variety of advanced diseases.[61] Complementary and alternative medicine may play a role in treating cancer-related dyspnea.[62] In patients with non–small cell lung cancer or mesothelioma, acupuncture improved patient-reported dyspnea scores compared with morphine alone.[63,64] Guided imagery and relaxing music have also shown promise at reducing dyspnea for patients with cancer toward the EOL.[65] However, larger-scale randomized controlled trials are necessary to determine the efficacy of complementary and alternative medicine to treat dyspnea for patients with malignancy.

WHAT OUTCOMES ARE AFFECTED BY PALLIATIVE AND END-OF-LIFE CARE?

PC interventions have been evaluated for efficacy across multiple clinical and patient-centered outcomes (**Box 2**).[66]

Palliative, EOL, and hospice care are associated with improvements in symptom management, quality of life, patient-reported and family-reported satisfaction, and survival outcomes for patients living with cancer.[67–69] PC may also help patients avoid nonbeneficial care as they approach

the end of their lives.[70,71] Medicare patients with poor-prognosis cancer who were referred to hospice were 33% less likely to be hospitalized, 47% less likely to receive invasive procedures, and 58% less likely to have an ICU admission compared with matched patients who were not enrolled in hospice.[71] Similarly, in a retrospective study of hospitalized patients in 2 Veterans' Affairs (VA) medical centers, PC referral during a terminal hospitalization was associated with 42% decreased likelihood for ICU admission compared with usual care.[72] However, PC is not necessarily associated with reduced intensity of care at the EOL. In a study by Bakitas and colleagues,[68] including 322 patients with solid organ tumors from rural New England in the United States, number of emergency department visits, hospital days, and ICU days were similar between patients randomized to a nurse-led PC intervention compared with usual care.

PC may be associated with improved survival for patients with cancer.[73,74] In the landmark study by Temel and colleagues,[74] 151 patients with metastatic non–small cell lung cancer were randomized to receive early PC in addition to usual cancer care or usual cancer care alone. Patients in the early PC group lived more than 2 months longer compared with patients who received usual cancer care alone ($P = .02$). This survival benefit was observed despite the patients in the early PC group receiving less aggressive EOL care. In another study, patients randomized to early PC, defined as PC at the time of study enrollment, had 1-year survival of 63% compared with 48% in the delayed group who received PC 3 months later.[73]

The associations between PC and patient-centered outcomes such as quality of life, mood, and depression are also inconsistent.[68,74,75] In the study by Bakitas and colleagues,[68] the nurse-led PC intervention was associated with improvements in quality of life and mood. Temel and colleagues[74] also showed that early referral to PC was associated with significantly improved quality of life and less depressive symptoms compared with usual care. However, in a systematic review of the effectiveness of specialty PC on mood and depression, few studies reported improvements in these domains.[75] Outcome heterogeneity and methodological limitations of these studies may partially explain the inconsistent association on patient-centered outcomes.

PC involvement is associated with improved family-reported satisfaction with the quality of cancer and EOL care.[67] Referral to hospice, avoiding ICU admissions, and death of a loved one outside of the hospital may be associated with improved family-rated quality of EOL care and satisfaction.[76]

Box 2
Outcomes used for measuring efficacy of palliative care interventions

Clinical

　Survival

　Emergency department visits

　Inpatient admissions

　Length of inpatient stay

　Intensity of EOL care

　ICU admissions

　Receiving chemotherapy at time of death

　Location of death

Patient centered

　Symptom severity scores

　Quality of life

　Code status changes

　Patient-reported satisfaction

Family centered

　Caregiver burden scales

　Complicated grief scales

　Quality of dying and death

　Psychological symptoms (anxiety, depression)

Among bereaved family members of patients with cancer, family-rated satisfaction was significantly higher 1 month after the death of their loved one for those randomized to PC compared with patients who received conventional care.[77] This effect was significant even after adjusting for the nature of the relationship between the patient and family member (eg, spouse, child, sibling) and demographics and clinical characteristics of the patient.[77] In surveys of bereaved family members of patients enrolled in hospice, family satisfaction is associated with perceived adequate symptom control and high-quality communication between the hospice team and family members.[78,79] Together, these data suggest that PC within the final months of life is associated with improved EOL care, including improved symptom control, avoiding nonbeneficial care, and comforting grieving families.

HOW CAN PALLIATIVE AND END-OF-LIFE CARE BE DELIVERED?

PC can be delivered in dichotomous, overlapping, and concurrent models (**Fig. 2**). In the dichotomous model, PC becomes the focus for the patient only after cancer treatment options are exhausted (see **Fig. 2**A). This approach is typically an all-or-nothing, only-cure or only-comfort approach. For the overlapping model, PC is increasingly focused on as the curative treatment options become more limited (see **Fig. 2**B). Concurrent PC includes PC from the moment of cancer diagnosis and symptoms, is maintained during active treatment, and continues to support the family during the bereavement period following the patient's death (see **Fig. 2**C).[80,81] Concurrent models of care have increasingly been embraced by oncology providers.[24,80] In building relationships with patients over time, concurrent PC models may play a role in helping patients keep their decision making in the context of what matters most to them, including identification of appropriate timing to transition to EOL care.

Primary Palliative Care Delivered by Oncology Clinicians and Specialty Palliative Care

Primary PC can be delivered by oncology providers for all patients with cancer throughout their disease trajectories.[82] Oncology providers should have at least a minimum competency and comfort level to address symptoms, use patient-centered communication and shared decision making, introduce advanced care planning, and anticipate and identify EOL needs for all patients with cancer.[82] Primary PC is especially important in settings with limited access to specialty PC.[83]

Sometimes patients with cancer have more complicated symptoms or struggle with uncertainty or feelings of ambivalence toward EOL decision making. Referral to specialty PC may be appropriate for patients with complex symptoms and other psychosocial and existential sources of suffering.[24,84] Symptoms, disease trajectory, prognosis, performance status, psychosocial distress, and EOL planning are common reasons for referral to specialty PC.[85] Although trigger tools for referral to PC have been developed, there is a lack of consensus for which criteria should be used to automatically refer patients to specialty PC.[85]

Specialty PC can be provided through integrative or consultative models. Integrated PC consists of PC teams embedded into outpatient cancer teams. Integrated PC may be less burdensome for patients because there is no need for separate appointments or travel to different offices to have comprehensive palliative cancer care. In a trial of 50 patients with advanced cardiopulmonary conditions or cancer in a general medicine clinic who were expected to live less than 5 years, integrated PC was associated with significant improvements in dyspnea, anxiety, sleep, quality of life, and spiritual well-being compared with usual care.[86]

In health systems unable to implement integrated palliative cancer care, consultative PC may be available to support patients with cancer and their families. However, demand for specialty PC exceeds supply, and access remains an issue for many patients and family members, particularly as patients approach the end of their lives.[84] Telemedicine may be an emerging alternative model for delivering palliative cancer care, especially to patients in rural areas with limited access to the nearest specialty PC services.[87,88] Telemedicine has been used to manage common distressing symptoms for patients with cancer. In a randomized trial of patients with cancer in rural and urban oncology practices in Indiana (United States), a semiautomated telecare assessment and management of pain and depression by a collaborative cancer care team was associated with improved symptom control 3 and 12 months after study enrollment.[87] Other studies have shown the feasibility and preliminary efficacy of using Web-based tools to transmit patient-reported symptoms to clinicians via email alerts to improve communication between patients and clinicians.[89,90] Qualitative studies suggest that telemedicine can successfully deliver empathic, patient-centered care for patients with cancer receiving home-based PC.[91] Personal computing devices and smartphones have become ubiquitous, so their role in facilitating delivery of PC for patients who might otherwise

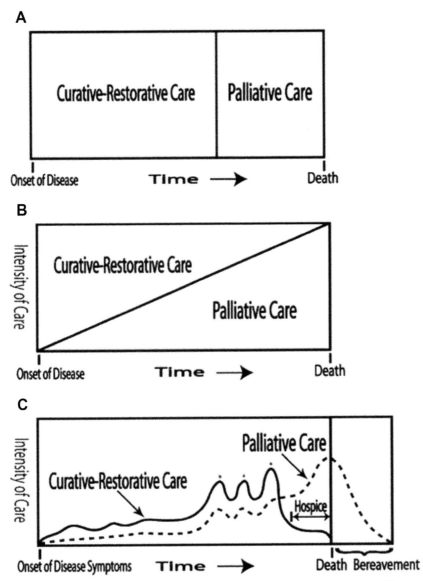

Fig. 2. Models for delivery of palliative care in the setting of serious, life-limiting disease like cancer. (*A*) Traditional dichotomous model of palliative care, in which patients first receive curative-restorative care and continue receiving it until it fails and then they receive palliative care. (*B*) Overlapping model of palliative care, in which patients receive a gradually increasing degree of palliative care while they receive a gradually decreasing degree of curative/restorative care. In both models (*A, B*), palliative care ends at the time of death. (*C*) Individualized integrated model of palliative care (which the original statement/reference and this article recommend as the preferred approach), in which the patient receives palliative care (*dashed line*) at the onset of symptoms from a progressive disease and then concurrently with curative/restorative care (*solid line*) in an individualized manner. Like curative/restorative care, the intensity of palliative care increases and decreases to reflect the needs and preferences of the patient and the patient's family. The asterisks indicate periods of high intensity of curative/restorative care (eg, hospitalizations for lower respiratory tract infections). Note that palliative care encompasses both hospice care and care during the period of bereavement for the family (which may begin before the death of the patient). (*From* Lanken PN, Terry PB, DeLisser HM, et al. An official American Thoracic Society clinical policy statement: palliative care for patients with respiratory diseases and critical illnesses. Am J Respir Crit Care Med 2008;177:914; with permission from the American Thoracic Society.)

have limited access to these services may make them effective tools for enhancing the quality of palliative cancer care.

What Is the Optimal Timing for Palliative Care Referral?

Many questions remain on the appropriate timing for PC referral.[73,74] Among patients who die with cancer, outpatient referral to PC more than 3 months before death was associated with approximately 50% fewer emergency department visits and hospital and ICU admissions and 18% fewer in-hospital deaths.[92] In another multicenter randomized trial of 207 patients with advanced cancer in New England (United States), early PC referral, defined as around the time of cancer diagnosis, was not associated with decreased chemotherapy or health care use during the last weeks of life compared with referral to PC 3 months later.[73] There were also no significant improvements in symptom burden, quality of life, or mood between the two groups.

Although ICU admission cannot always be anticipated, it provides an opportunity to address suffering and EOL care planning if PC has not previously been addressed with the patient and, more frequently, the family. However, patients with cancer admitted to the ICU may be less likely to receive PC. Among patients with cancer from MD Anderson Cancer Center in Texas (United States), 15% of patients admitted to the ICU had a PC referral compared with 52% of patients who were not admitted to the ICU ($P < .0001$).[93] These differences may be explained by improvements in ICU outcomes for patients with cancer and improvements in treatments and management of cancer complications, especially hematologic malignancies. When patients with cancer in the ICU are referred to PC, more than half already have multiple complex symptoms, including delirium, dyspnea, pain, fatigue, and anxiety.[94] Once referred to PC, most of these patients experience substantial improvement in their symptom distress through pharmacologic management and spiritual or emotional counseling.[94] Together, these studies show important challenges to optimal timing for referral to PC for patients living with malignancy. Given the ongoing PC needs for these patients and persistent shortages of the PC provider workforce, determining optimal timing for PC referral is a priority. PC domains can begin to be addressed by primary oncology clinicians at the time of diagnosis. In centers with access to specialty PC, referral within the first 3 months of diagnosis may help build rapport and establish PC as part of the team approach to cancer care.

BARRIERS TO PALLIATIVE AND END-OF-LIFE CARE FOR PATIENTS WITH MALIGNANCY
General Attitudes of Oncology Providers Toward Palliative and End-of-life Care

Gaps remain between guidelines recommendations for engagement with palliative and hospice care for patients approaching the end of their lives.[95] In addition to workforce limitations, clinician attitudes continue to be important barriers to palliative and hospice care services for patients living with cancer. Only 52% of patients receiving cancer care in centers participating in the National Comprehensive Cancer Network report were told about PC services and fewer than half of the patients who screen positive for requiring specialty PC were referred.[96]

Oncology providers may perceive referral to specialty PC as a sign of giving up hope.[97,98] Even patients with metastatic disease receiving palliative interventions are subject to poor quality of care at the end of their lives. Patients with cancer receiving palliative chemotherapy or radiation therapy are more likely to receive cardiopulmonary resuscitation and intubation/mechanical ventilation at the end of their lives and less frequent referral to hospice compared with patients who do not receive these palliative treatments.[99–101] These findings may reflect the tension and perceived opposing goals of active cancer treatment and PC. These data suggest that in-depth negotiations between the clinical team and patients and their families are required to determine PC needs and expectations for patients who agree to palliative interventions at the EOL.

Hematologic Malignancies and Hematopoietic Cell Transplant

Multiple observational studies have found that patients with hematologic tumors were less likely to be referred to palliative and hospice care.[97,102–105] A meta-analysis of 9 studies showed that patients with hematologic malignancies were approximately half as likely to receive PC or hospice referral during their treatment compared with other cancer populations.[102,105] Another study from a large US cancer institute reported that inpatient decedents with hematologic malignancy were much less likely to have access to PC services during inpatient admission compared with solid tumors (20% compared with 44%, respectively; $P < .0001$).[93] Among hematologic oncology patients admitted to the ICU, only 10% were referred to specialty PC.

Hematologists care for their patients for months, years, and even decades. They offer aggressive therapies, including hematopoietic cell transplant (HCT), that can be lifesaving for their patients, which may contribute to hematologists' perceptions that PC is not necessary and/or that it would interfere with ongoing aggressive care of the underlying hematologic disease.[97] In a random survey of 240 oncology clinicians at a single institution, patients under the care of hematologic specialists were 2.7 times more likely to receive cancer treatment during their last month of life compared with solid organ cancer specialists.[106] In addition, 46% of hematologic oncologists reported a sense of failure when the cancer progressed compared with 31% of solid organ oncologists ($P = .04$). In a multicenter mixed-methods study exploring attitudes to and perceptions of PC among cancer providers, 30% of hematologists reported never referring their patients to PC.[98] Hematology providers preferred to maintain control over their patients' PC needs and perceived referral to PC as EOL care. Improved education and communication are required to address ongoing perceptions of hematologists about PC and to determine how best to facilitate referral of hematologic patients to PC specialists.[107]

There are limited data about referral patterns to PC for patients who received HCT. In one series of 30 patients from New Zealand and Australia who relapsed following HCT, 14 were referred to PC.[108] HCT patients experienced several symptoms at the EOL and, when they were referred to PC, it usually occurred very late in their course. Similarly, in the pediatric population, HCT recipients who died were infrequently referred to PC and were referred a median of 0.7 months before death.[109] When pediatric HCT patients were referred to PC, they were more likely to die outside of the ICU and more likely to receive hospice care.

There are limited data on HCT patients' attitudes, knowledge, or receptivity toward PC. A quality improvement project from a single center that referred patients to PC early in the transplant process suggested that patients increased their knowledge of PC and reported feeling that they knew how to access PC in the future.[110] However, the PC team reported that patients were often overwhelmed by these meetings and did not remember the content of the initial referrals. These data suggest that HCT patients may benefit from PC referral but that a better understanding of the role and timing of PC in this population with unique PC needs is necessary. Integration of PC into routine care for hematologic oncology and HCT patients will require ongoing partnerships and communication between hematologists and PC providers.

Potential Health Care Disparities in Access to Palliative and End-of-Life Care

Poorer quality of EOL care has been reported for ethnic and racial minorities with advanced cancer. In-hospital deaths and intensity of care at the EOL are higher, whereas use of palliative and hospice care services is less, in nonwhite cancer populations.[111,112] In a study of more than 40,000 patients with cancer using the Surveillance Epidemiology and End-Results Medicare data, 37% of black patients, 32% of Asian patients, and 38% of Hispanic patients enrolled in hospice compared with 42% of white patients.[113] Nonwhite patients are more likely to be hospitalized and spend more days in the hospital, and are more likely to be admitted to the ICU during their last month of life compared with white patients.

Some of these differences may be influenced by differences in patients' preferences for EOL care. In a survey of Medicare beneficiaries asked about treatment preferences if they had a serious condition with less than 1 year to live, 18% of black patients and 15% of Hispanic patients wanted to die in a hospital, compared with 8% of white patients.[114] Similar differences in responses were reported for attitudes toward LSTs such as mechanical ventilation or life-prolonging drugs that may negatively affect quality of life. However, it is important to highlight that most older Medicare beneficiaries still prefer to avoid dying in the hospital, receiving medications with unpleasant side effects, and mechanical ventilation.

Undocumented immigrants face additional barriers to high-quality palliative and EOL care, including cultural and religious beliefs, language difficulties, social isolation, limited finances, and fear of deportation.[115] PC providers, with the assistance of professional interpreters when indicated, can explore cultural preferences and beliefs of patients, as well as perceived barriers to PC.[116]

In general populations, women with advanced cancer receive less aggressive EOL care as measured using hospital and ICU admissions compared with men.[117] However, women with gynecologic cancers are frequently referred to PC only after disease recurrence or hospital admissions for distressing symptoms or other complications of their disease.[118,119] Like most patients living with cancer, patients with gynecologic malignancies live with several symptoms. Approximately one-third experience moderate to severe pain and 47% report moderate to severe fatigue.[119] PC referral is associated with rapid relief of distressing symptoms for patients with gynecologic malignancies.[120] Additional studies are necessary to enhance primary PC from gynecologic oncologists as well as education and implementation of PC referral when necessary.

SUMMARY

Palliative and EOL care needs for patients living with malignancy are substantial. PC specialists can improve symptom management. PC interventions have also been associated with improvements in survival for patients living with cancer while avoiding nonbeneficial care that is misaligned with patients' EOL priorities. Optimal outcomes for determining efficacy of PC interventions have not been determined but likely require engagement with key stakeholders, including patients, their families, and oncology providers. As part of the comprehensive care for patients with cancer, clinicians should incorporate routine assessment of PC domains from the time of diagnosis. Comprehensive PC assessment should focus on patient-centered experiences to identify sources of physical, psychosocial, and spiritual suffering. Cancer clinicians should be prepared to consult with PC specialists as PC needs becomes more complex. Education and routine exposure to PC domains may help improve attitudes, knowledge, and comfort with PC among patients as well as clinicians. Future work is needed to determine how to improve delivery of PC to patients with limited access to this kind of care because of scarce resources.

REFERENCES

1. Bryan LJ, Gordon LI. Releasing the brake on the immune system: the PD-1 strategy for hematologic malignancies. Oncology 2015;29:431–9.

2. Burotto M, Manasanch EE, Wilkerson J, et al. Gefitinib and erlotinib in metastatic non-small cell lung cancer: a meta-analysis of toxicity and efficacy of randomized clinical trials. Oncologist 2015;20:400–10.

3. Dijkstra KK, Voabil P, Schumacher TN, et al. Genomics- and transcriptomics-based patient selection for cancer treatment with immune checkpoint inhibitors: a review. JAMA Oncol 2016;2(11):1490–5.

4. Matsuki E, Younes A. Checkpoint inhibitors and other immune therapies for Hodgkin and non-Hodgkin lymphoma. Curr Treat Options Oncol 2016;17:31.

5. McDermott DF, Drake CG, Sznol M, et al. Survival, durable response, and long-term safety in patients with previously treated advanced renal cell carcinoma receiving nivolumab. J Clin Oncol 2015;33: 2013–20.

6. Motzer RJ, Escudier B, McDermott DF, et al. Nivolumab versus everolimus in advanced renal-cell carcinoma. N Engl J Med 2015;373:1803–13.

7. Petrelli F, Borgonovo K, Cabiddu M, et al. Relationship between skin rash and outcome in non-small-cell lung cancer patients treated with anti-EGFR tyrosine kinase inhibitors: a literature-based meta-analysis of 24 trials. Lung Cancer 2012;78:8–15.

8. Levy MM, Rhodes A, Phillips GS, et al. Surviving Sepsis Campaign: association between performance metrics and outcomes in a 7.5-year study. Crit Care Med 2015;43:3–12.

9. Lee HY, Rhee CK, Lee JW. Feasibility of high-flow nasal cannula oxygen therapy for acute respiratory failure in patients with hematologic malignancies: a retrospective single-center study. J Crit Care 2015;30:773–7.

10. Frat JP, Thille AW, Mercat A, et al. High-flow oxygen through nasal cannula in acute hypoxemic respiratory failure. N Engl J Med 2015;372:2185–96.

11. Frat JP, Ragot S, Girault C, et al. Effect of non-invasive oxygenation strategies in immunocompromised patients with severe acute respiratory failure: a post-hoc analysis of a randomised trial. Lancet Respir Med 2016;4:646–52.

12. Coudroy R, Jamet A, Petua P, et al. High-flow nasal cannula oxygen therapy versus noninvasive ventilation in immunocompromised patients with acute respiratory failure: an observational cohort study. Ann Intensive Care 2016;6:45.

13. Frat JP, Coudroy R, Thille AW. Noninvasive ventilation and outcomes among immunocompromised patients. JAMA 2016;315:1901–2.

14. Lemiale V, Mokart D, Resche-Rigon M, et al. Effect of noninvasive ventilation vs oxygen therapy on mortality among immunocompromised patients with acute respiratory failure: a randomized clinical trial. JAMA 2015;314:1711–9.

15. Harada K, Kurosawa S, Hino Y, et al. Clinical utility of high-flow nasal cannula oxygen therapy for acute respiratory failure in patients with hematological disease. Springerplus 2016;5:512.

16. Azevedo LC, Caruso P, Silva UV, et al. Outcomes for patients with cancer admitted to the ICU requiring ventilatory support: results from a prospective multicenter study. Chest 2014;146:257–66.

17. Toffart AC, Minet C, Raynard B, et al. Use of intensive care in patients with nonresectable lung cancer. Chest 2011;139:101–8.

18. Five-year relative cancer survival rates for selected cancer sites, by race and sex: United States, selected geographic areas, selected years 1975-1977 through 2005-2011. Available at: http://www.cdc.gov/nchs/hus/contents2015.htm#019; http://globocan.iarc.fr/Pages/fact_sheets_cancer.aspx. Accessed August 18, 2016.

19. WHO Definition of Palliative Care. Available at: http://www.who.int/cancer/palliative/definition/en/. Accessed August 18, 2016.

20. American Academy of Hospice and Palliative Medicine, Center to Advance Palliative Care, Hospice

and Palliative Nurses Association, et al. National consensus project for quality palliative care: clinical practice guidelines for quality palliative care, executive summary. J Palliat Med 2004;7:611–27.

21. Teno JM, Connor SR. Referring a patient and family to high-quality palliative care at the close of life: "We met a new personality... with this level of compassion and empathy". JAMA 2009;301: 651–9.

22. Teno JM, Casey VA, Welch LC, et al. Patient-focused, family-centered end-of-life medical care: views of the guidelines and bereaved family members. J Pain Symptom Manage 2001;22:738–51.

23. Singer PA, Martin DK, Kelner M. Quality end-of-life care: patients' perspectives. JAMA 1999;281: 163–8.

24. Smith TJ, Temin S, Alesi ER, et al. American Society of Clinical Oncology provisional clinical opinion: the integration of palliative care into standard oncology care. J Clin Oncol 2012;30:880–7.

25. Hui D, Mori M, Parsons HA, et al. The lack of standard definitions in the supportive and palliative oncology literature. J Pain Symptom Manage 2012;43:582–92.

26. Seow H, Barbera L, Sutradhar R, et al. Trajectory of performance status and symptom scores for patients with cancer during the last six months of life. J Clin Oncol 2011;29:1151–8.

27. Mercadante S, Aielli F, Adile C, et al. Epidemiology and characteristics of episodic breathlessness in advanced cancer patients: an observational study. J Pain Symptom Manage 2016;51:17–24.

28. Currow DC, Smith J, Davidson PM, et al. Do the trajectories of dyspnea differ in prevalence and intensity by diagnosis at the end of life? A consecutive cohort study. J Pain Symptom Manage 2010;39: 680–90.

29. Ekstrom M, Johnson MJ, Schioler L, et al. Who experiences higher and increasing breathlessness in advanced cancer? The longitudinal EPCCS Study. Support Care Cancer 2016;24:3803–11.

30. Bausewein C, Farquhar M, Booth S, et al. Measurement of breathlessness in advanced disease: a systematic review. Respir Med 2007;101:399–410.

31. Mularski RA, Campbell ML, Asch SM, et al. A review of quality of care evaluation for the palliation of dyspnea. Am J Respir Crit Care Med 2010; 181:534–8.

32. Parshall MB, Schwartzstein RM, Adams L, et al. An official American Thoracic Society statement: update on the mechanisms, assessment, and management of dyspnea. Am J Respir Crit Care Med 2012;185:435–52.

33. Dorman S, Byrne A, Edwards A. Which measurement scales should we use to measure breathlessness in palliative care? A systematic review. Palliat Med 2007;21:177–91.

34. Akgun KM, Crothers K, Pisani M. Epidemiology and management of common pulmonary diseases in older persons. J Gerontol A Biol Sci Med Sci 2012;67:276–91.

35. Remi C, Remi J, Bausewein C. Pharmacological management of bronchorrhea in malignant disease: a systematic literature review. J Pain Symptom Manage 2016;51:916–25.

36. Jean RA, DeLuzio MR, Kraev AI, et al. Analyzing risk factors for morbidity and mortality after lung resection for lung cancer using the NSQIP database. J Am Coll Surg 2016;222:992–1000.e1.

37. Geraci JM, Tsang W, Valdres RV, et al. Progressive disease in patients with cancer presenting to an emergency room with acute symptoms predicts short-term mortality. Support Care Cancer 2006; 14:1038–45.

38. Bruera E, de Stoutz N, Velasco-Leiva A, et al. Effects of oxygen on dyspnoea in hypoxaemic terminal-cancer patients. Lancet 1993;342:13–4.

39. Booth S, Kelly MJ, Cox NP, et al. Does oxygen help dyspnea in patients with cancer? Am J Respir Crit Care Med 1996;153:1515–8.

40. Abernethy AP, McDonald CF, Frith PA, et al. Effect of palliative oxygen versus room air in relief of breathlessness in patients with refractory dyspnoea: a double-blind, randomised controlled trial. Lancet 2010;376:784–93.

41. Campbell ML, Yarandi H, Dove-Medows E. Oxygen is nonbeneficial for most patients who are near death. J Pain Symptom Manage 2013;45: 517–23.

42. Hui D, Morgado M, Chisholm G, et al. High-flow oxygen and bilevel positive airway pressure for persistent dyspnea in patients with advanced cancer: a phase II randomized trial. J Pain Symptom Manage 2013;46:463–73.

43. Nava S, Ferrer M, Esquinas A, et al. Palliative use of non-invasive ventilation in end-of-life patients with solid tumours: a randomised feasibility trial. Lancet Oncol 2013;14:219–27.

44. Quill CM, Quill TE. Palliative use of noninvasive ventilation: navigating murky waters. J Palliat Med 2014;17:657–61.

45. Halpern SD, Hansen-Flaschen J. Terminal withdrawal of life-sustaining supplemental oxygen. JAMA 2006;296:1397–400.

46. Ben-Aharon I, Gafter-Gvili A, Paul M, et al. Interventions for alleviating cancer-related dyspnea: a systematic review. J Clin Oncol 2008;26:2396–404.

47. Hallenbeck J. Pathophysiologies of dyspnea explained: why might opioids relieve dyspnea and not hasten death? J Palliat Med 2012;15:848–53.

48. Ben-Aharon I, Gafter-Gvili A, Leibovici L, et al. Interventions for alleviating cancer-related dyspnea: a systematic review and meta-analysis. Acta Oncol 2012;51:996–1008.

49. Clemens KE, Klaschik E. Dyspnoea associated with anxiety–symptomatic therapy with opioids in combination with lorazepam and its effect on ventilation in palliative care patients. Support Care Cancer 2011;19:2027–33.

50. Hui D, Kilgore K, Frisbee-Hume S, et al. Dexamethasone for dyspnea in cancer patients: a pilot double-blind, randomized, controlled trial. J Pain Symptom Manage 2016;52:8–16.e1.

51. Lin RJ, Adelman RD, Mehta SS. Dyspnea in palliative care: expanding the role of corticosteroids. J Palliat Med 2012;15:834–7.

52. Matsuo N, Morita T, Iwase S. Efficacy and undesirable effects of corticosteroid therapy experienced by palliative care specialists in Japan: a nationwide survey. J Palliat Med 2011;14:840–5.

53. Viola R, Kiteley C, Lloyd NS, et al. The management of dyspnea in cancer patients: a systematic review. Support Care Cancer 2008;16:329–37.

54. Elsayem A, Bruera E. High-dose corticosteroids for the management of dyspnea in patients with tumor obstruction of the upper airway. Support Care Cancer 2007;15:1437–9.

55. Hui D, Kilgore K, Park M, et al. Impact of prophylactic fentanyl pectin nasal spray on exercise-induced episodic dyspnea in cancer patients: a double-blind, randomized controlled trial. J Pain Symptom Manage 2016;52(4):459–68.e1.

56. Wilcock A, Walton A, Manderson C, et al. Randomised, placebo controlled trial of nebulised furosemide for breathlessness in patients with cancer. Thorax 2008;63:872–5.

57. Molassiotis A, Charalambous A, Taylor P, et al. The effect of resistance inspiratory muscle training in the management of breathlessness in patients with thoracic malignancies: a feasibility randomised trial. Support Care Cancer 2015;23: 1637–45.

58. Henke CC, Cabri J, Fricke L, et al. Strength and endurance training in the treatment of lung cancer patients in stages IIIA/IIIB/IV. Support Care Cancer 2014;22:95–101.

59. Donesky D, Nguyen HQ, Paul SM, et al. The affective dimension of dyspnea improves in a dyspnea self-management program with exercise training. J Pain Symptom Manage 2014;47:757–71.

60. Riesenberg H, Lubbe AS. In-patient rehabilitation of lung cancer patients–a prospective study. Support Care Cancer 2010;18:877–82.

61. Higginson IJ, Bausewein C, Reilly CC, et al. An integrated palliative and respiratory care service for patients with advanced disease and refractory breathlessness: a randomised controlled trial. Lancet Respir Med 2014;2:979–87.

62. Pan CX, Morrison RS, Ness J, et al. Complementary and alternative medicine in the management of pain, dyspnea, and nausea and vomiting near the end of life. A systematic review. J Pain Symptom Manage 2000;20:374–87.

63. Minchom A, Punwani R, Filshie J, et al. A randomised study comparing the effectiveness of acupuncture or morphine versus the combination for the relief of dyspnoea in patients with advanced non-small cell lung cancer and mesothelioma. Eur J Cancer 2016;61:102–10.

64. Filshie J, Penn K, Ashley S, et al. Acupuncture for the relief of cancer-related breathlessness. Palliat Med 1996;10:145–50.

65. Lai WS, Chao CS, Yang WP, et al. Efficacy of guided imagery with theta music for advanced cancer patients with dyspnea: a pilot study. Biol Res Nurs 2010;12:188–97.

66. Singer AE, Goebel JR, Kim YS, et al. Populations and interventions for palliative and end-of-life care: a systematic review. J Palliat Med 2016;19: 995–1008.

67. Wachterman MW, Pilver C, Smith D, et al. Quality of end-of-life care provided to patients with different serious illnesses. JAMA Intern Med 2016;176: 1095–102.

68. Bakitas M, Lyons KD, Hegel MT, et al. Effects of a palliative care intervention on clinical outcomes in patients with advanced cancer: the Project ENABLE II randomized controlled trial. JAMA 2009;302:741–9.

69. Teno JM, Clarridge BR, Casey V, et al. Family perspectives on end-of-life care at the last place of care. JAMA 2004;291:88–93.

70. Khandelwal N, Kross EK, Engelberg RA, et al. Estimating the effect of palliative care interventions and advance care planning on ICU utilization: a systematic review. Crit Care Med 2015;43:1102–11.

71. Obermeyer Z, Makar M, Abujaber S, et al. Association between the Medicare hospice benefit and health care utilization and costs for patients with poor-prognosis cancer. JAMA 2014;312:1888–96.

72. Penrod JD, Deb P, Luhrs C, et al. Cost and utilization outcomes of patients receiving hospital-based palliative care consultation. J Palliat Med 2006;9: 855–60.

73. Bakitas MA, Tosteson TD, Li Z, et al. Early versus delayed initiation of concurrent palliative oncology care: patient outcomes in the ENABLE III randomized controlled trial. J Clin Oncol 2015;33:1438–45.

74. Temel JS, Greer JA, Muzikansky A, et al. Early palliative care for patients with metastatic non-small-cell lung cancer. N Engl J Med 2010;363:733–42.

75. Zimmermann C, Riechelmann R, Krzyzanowska M, et al. Effectiveness of specialized palliative care: a systematic review. JAMA 2008;299:1698–709.

76. Wright AA, Keating NL, Ayanian JZ, et al. Family perspectives on aggressive cancer care near the end of life. JAMA 2016;315:284–92.

77. Ringdal GI, Jordhoy MS, Kaasa S. Family satisfaction with end-of-life care for cancer patients in a cluster randomized trial. J Pain Symptom Manage 2002;24:53–63.

78. Ong J, Brennsteiner A, Chow E, et al. Correlates of family satisfaction with hospice care: general inpatient hospice care versus routine home hospice care. J Palliat Med 2016;19:97–100.

79. Rhodes RL, Mitchell SL, Miller SC, et al. Bereaved family members' evaluation of hospice care: what factors influence overall satisfaction with services? J Pain Symptom Manage 2008; 35:365–71.

80. Mor V, Joyce NR, Cote DL, et al. The rise of concurrent care for veterans with advanced cancer at the end of life. Cancer 2016;122:782–90.

81. LeBlanc TW. Addressing end-of-life quality gaps in hematologic cancers: the importance of early concurrent palliative care. JAMA Intern Med 2016;176: 265–6.

82. Bickel KE, McNiff K, Buss MK, et al. Defining high-quality palliative care in oncology practice: an American Society of Clinical Oncology/American Academy of Hospice and Palliative Medicine guidance statement. J Oncol Pract 2016;12:e828–38.

83. Van Vorst RF, Crane LA, Barton PL, et al. Barriers to quality care for dying patients in rural communities. J Rural Health 2006;22:248–53.

84. Quill TE, Abernethy AP. Generalist plus specialist palliative care–creating a more sustainable model. N Engl J Med 2013;368:1173–5.

85. Hui D, Meng YC, Bruera S, et al. Referral criteria for outpatient palliative cancer care: a systematic review. Oncologist 2016;21:895–901.

86. Rabow MW, Dibble SL, Pantilat SZ, et al. The comprehensive care team: a controlled trial of outpatient palliative medicine consultation. Arch Intern Med 2004;164:83–91.

87. Kroenke K, Theobald D, Wu J, et al. Effect of telecare management on pain and depression in patients with cancer: a randomized trial. JAMA 2010;304:163–71.

88. Whitten P, Doolittle G, Mackert M. Telehospice in Michigan: use and patient acceptance. Am J Hosp Palliat Care 2004;21:191–5.

89. Abernethy AP, Ahmad A, Zafar SY, et al. Electronic patient-reported data capture as a foundation of rapid learning cancer care. Med Care 2010;48: S32–8.

90. Dy SM, Roy J, Ott GE, et al. Tell Us: a Web-based tool for improving communication among patients, families, and providers in hospice and palliative care through systematic data specification, collection, and use. J Pain Symptom Manage 2011;42: 526–34.

91. van Gurp J, van Selm M, Vissers K, et al. How outpatient palliative care teleconsultation facilitates empathic patient-professional relationships: a qualitative study. PLoS One 2015;10:e0124387.

92. Hui D, Kim SH, Roquemore J, et al. Impact of timing and setting of palliative care referral on quality of end-of-life care in cancer patients. Cancer 2014;120:1743–9.

93. Fadul N, Elsayem A, Palmer JL, et al. Predictors of access to palliative care services among patients who died at a comprehensive cancer center. J Palliat Med 2007;10:1146–52.

94. Delgado-Guay MO, Parsons HA, Li Z, et al. Symptom distress, interventions, and outcomes of intensive care unit cancer patients referred to a palliative care consult team. Cancer 2009;115: 437–45.

95. Gidwani R, Joyce N, Kinosian B, et al. Gap between recommendations and practice of palliative care and hospice in cancer patients. J Palliat Med 2016;19:957–63.

96. Simoff MJ, Lally B, Slade MG, et al. Symptom management in patients with lung cancer: diagnosis and management of lung cancer, 3rd ed: American College of Chest Physicians evidence-based clinical practice guidelines. Chest 2013; 143:e455S–497.

97. Morikawa M, Shirai Y, Ochiai R, et al. Barriers to the collaboration between hematologists and palliative care teams on relapse or refractory leukemia and malignant lymphoma patients' care: a qualitative study. Am J Hosp Palliat Care 2015; 33(10):977–84.

98. LeBlanc TW, O'Donnell JD, Crowley-Matoka M, et al. Perceptions of palliative care among hematologic malignancy specialists: a mixed-methods study. J Oncol Pract 2015;11:e230–8.

99. Zhang Z, Gu XL, Chen ML, et al. Use of palliative chemo- and radiotherapy at the end of life in patients with cancer: a retrospective cohort study. Am J Hosp Palliat Care 2016. [Epub ahead of print].

100. Wu CC, Hsu TW, Chang CM, et al. Palliative chemotherapy affects aggressiveness of end-of-life care. Oncologist 2016;21:771–7.

101. Wright AA, Zhang B, Keating NL, et al. Associations between palliative chemotherapy and adult cancer patients' end of life care and place of death: prospective cohort study. BMJ 2014;348: g1219.

102. Calton BA, Alvarez-Perez A, Portman DG, et al. The current state of palliative care for patients cared for at leading US cancer centers: the 2015 NCCN Palliative Care Survey. J Natl Compr Cancer Netw 2016;14:859–66.

103. Cheng HW, Li CW, Chan KY, et al. End-of-life characteristics and palliative care provision for elderly patients suffering from acute myeloid leukemia. Support Care Cancer 2015;23:111–6.

104. Sexauer A, Cheng MJ, Knight L, et al. Patterns of hospice use in patients dying from hematologic malignancies. J Palliat Med 2014;17:195–9.

105. Howell DA, Shellens R, Roman E, et al. Haematological malignancy: are patients appropriately referred for specialist palliative and hospice care? A systematic review and meta-analysis of published data. Palliat Med 2011;25:630–41.

106. Hui D, Bansal S, Park M, et al. Differences in attitudes and beliefs toward end-of-life care between hematologic and solid tumor oncology specialists. Ann Oncol 2015;26:1440–6.

107. Manitta VJ, Philip JA, Cole-Sinclair MF. Palliative care and the hemato-oncological patient: can we live together? A review of the literature. J Palliat Med 2010;13:1021–5.

108. Button EB, Gavin NC, Keogh SJ. Exploring palliative care provision for recipients of allogeneic hematopoietic stem cell transplantation who relapsed. Oncol Nurs Forum 2014;41:370–81.

109. Ullrich CK, Lehmann L, London WB, et al. End-of-life care patterns associated with pediatric palliative care among children who underwent hematopoietic stem cell transplant. Biol Blood Marrow Transplant 2016;22:1049–55.

110. Harden KL. Early intervention with transplantation recipients to improve access to and knowledge of palliative care. Clin J Oncol Nurs 2016;20:E88–92.

111. Loggers ET, Maciejewski PK, Paulk E, et al. Racial differences in predictors of intensive end-of-life care in patients with advanced cancer. J Clin Oncol 2009;27:5559–64.

112. Johnson KS. Racial and ethnic disparities in palliative care. J Palliat Med 2013;16:1329–34.

113. Smith AK, Earle CC, McCarthy EP. Racial and ethnic differences in end-of-life care in fee-for-service Medicare beneficiaries with advanced cancer. J Am Geriatr Soc 2009;57:153–8.

114. Barnato AE, Anthony DL, Skinner J, et al. Racial and ethnic differences in preferences for end-of-life treatment. J Gen Intern Med 2009;24:695–701.

115. Jaramillo S, Hui D. End-of-Life care for undocumented immigrants with advanced cancer: documenting the undocumented. J Pain Symptom Manage 2016;51:784–8.

116. Smith AK, Sudore RL, Perez-Stable EJ. Palliative care for Latino patients and their families: whenever we prayed, she wept. JAMA 2009;301:1047–57. E1.

117. Sharma RK, Prigerson HG, Penedo FJ, et al. Male-female patient differences in the association between end-of-life discussions and receipt of intensive care near death. Cancer 2015;121:2814–20.

118. Nevadunsky NS, Spoozak L, Gordon S, et al. End-of-life care of women with gynecologic malignancies: a pilot study. Int J Gynecol Cancer 2013;23:546–52.

119. Lefkowits C, W Rabow M, E Sherman A, et al. Predictors of high symptom burden in gynecologic oncology outpatients: who should be referred to outpatient palliative care? Gynecol Oncol 2014;132:698–702.

120. Lefkowits C, Teuteberg W, Courtney-Brooks M, et al. Improvement in symptom burden within one day after palliative care consultation in a cohort of gynecologic oncology inpatients. Gynecol Oncol 2015;136:424–8.

Index

Note: Page numbers of article titles are in **boldface** type.

Clin Chest Med 38 (2017) 377–383
http://dx.doi.org/10.1016/S0272-5231(17)30017-5
0272-5231/17

chestmed.theclinics.com